Intensive Care in the Newborn, III

LEO STERN, M.D.
Professor and Chairman of Pediatrics
Brown University, Providence, Rhode Island

BERNARD SALLE, M.D.
Professor of Pediatrics
Claude Bernard University, Lyon, France

BENT FRIIS-HANSEN, M.D.
Professor of Pediatrics and Neonatology
University of Copenhagen, Denmark

MASSON Publishing USA, Inc.
*New York • Paris • Barcelona • Milan •
Mexico City • Rio de Janeiro*

ISBN 0-89352-114-0

ISSN 0270-1855

Printed in the United States of America

Preface

Since the early 1970s a group of colleagues from different countries have met approximately every two years to exchange views and discuss new developments in the physiologic and biochemical problems that pertain to newborn infants in intensive care units. These gatherings have provided a forum for in-depth exchanges of views and mutual appreciation of each other's work.

The present volume records the proceedings of the most recent meeting of our group, which was held from August 26 to 30, 1979, at the Museé Claude Bernard in St. Julien en Beaujolais, France. As with the previous volumes no attempt is made to cover the entire area of neonatal intensive care, but the contributions once again represent the current interest of the members of the group.

We continue to believe that the rational basis for intensive care can only be expressed in an in-depth understanding of the underlying causes of the conditions being treated. The primary role of the scientific method in both the basic aspects and abnormal processes, as well as in the application of direct therapeutic approaches, remains a hallmark of appropriate care and management of the sick newborn infant. It is for these reasons that our group meets and for the same reasons that these volumes are subsequently published.

Those of us who have acted as editors do so with gratitude and understanding that we represent only the contributors and participants whose work and efforts have made the meetings and the subsequent volumes a realistic possibility.

We hope the reader will enjoy the material and profit by it, as well. As in the past we can only express the wish that the true beneficiaries will be the children in our care, who can only benefit from a better understanding of the nature and causes of the problems that may beset them.

Leo Stern
Providence, R.I., U.S.A.

Bernard Salle
Lyon, France

Bent Friis-Hansen
Copenhagen, Denmark

Introduction

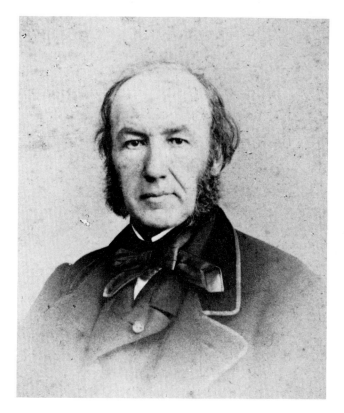

CLAUDE BERNARD (1813–1878)

In 1878 Claude Bernard died in Paris; 1978, therefore, was the centenary of his death. Many commemorations were held in different countries throughout the world, particularly in the United States at Stanford University, and of course, in Lyon.

Claude Bernard was born in 1813 in Saint Julien en Beaujolais in the tiny house behind the Museum. His father was a wine merchant, and Claude Bernard's childhood was that of a simple country boy. He went to primary school in Thoissey and then went to Lyon where he worked as a Chemist's Assistant.

However, Bernard preferred the theatre and literature to chemistry and so, at the age of 21, he went to Paris to become a writer. On the advice of the literary critic Saint Marc Girardin, however, he was persuaded to abandon literature in favor of medicine. He passed his high school exam in Paris and studied medicine, at which he seemed to be a very mediocre student.

As an intern of the hospitals of Paris, he attracted the attention of Magendie, the famous professor of physiology and medicine. Magendie sent Claude Bernard to the College de France. He immediately started his personal research and his experiments led to new discoveries. In 1855, he succeeded Magendie and a chair of general physiology was created.

He was to make the principal discoveries now known throughout the world and wrote "Introduction to Experimental Medicine." His studies remain a model of analysis and experimentation.

First, Bernard insisted on the unity of science. The line of reasoning must be the same for those who study human beings as for those who study inanimate objects, i.e., basic science, he said. He insisted on biochemical research in medicine and was careful to make this research profitable both clinically and experimentally.

Men who see new truths are rare, and in every field of science most practitioners follow and expound the ideas of others. Those who discover, however, promote new and fertile ideas. Claude Bernard solved the problem in a very realistic way, establishing that the evolution of science could be divided in twain: That part which is known and that part which is unknown. In the former all men have the same value and "great" men are not different from any others. It is in the unknown and obscure part that the great man can be distinguished. He is characterized by his genius, which illuminates obscure phenomena and carries science forward. Each time a new and reliable discovery is made in experimental analysis, science progresses in the field wherever this discovery can be applied.

We would like to think that Claude Bernard's principles should occupy our thoughts and make us humble.

Bernard Salle
Lyon

Contributors

ABU ZENT, Y., Research Fellow, Pediatric Children Hospital, Cairo

AMIEL-TISON, C., Port-Royal Maternity Hospital, Paris, France

ANDRE, M., Service de Medecine Neonatale, Maternite Universitaire, Nancy, France

APERIA, A., Department of Pediatrics, Karolinska Institute, St. Goran's Children's Hospital, Stockholm, Sweden

AVERY, G. B., Department of Neonatology, Children's Hospital National Medical Center, Department of Child Health and Development, School of Medicine and Health Sciences, George Washington University, Washington, D.C.

BALLOWITZ, L., Children's Hospital, Free University, Berlin, West Germany

BARD, H., Hopital Sainte-Justine, Montreal, Quebec, Canada,

BARRETT, C. T., Departments of Medicine, Pharmacology, and Pediatrics, UCLA School of Medicine, Los Angeles, California

BAUM, J. D., Department of Paediatrics, University of Oxford, John Radcliffe Hospital Headington, Oxford, England

BERTRAND, J., Unite de Recherches Endocriniennes et Metaboliques chez l'Enfant, Lyon, France

BIEHL, D. R., Assistant Professor of Anesthesia and Perinatology, St. Boniface Hospital, Winnipeg, Canada

BISTOLETTI, P., Research Trainee, Department of Obstetrics and Gynaecology, Karolinska Institute, Huddinge Hospital, Huddinge, Sweden

BRASH, A. R., Departments of Pediatrics and Clinical Pharmacology, Vanderbilt University School of Medicine, Nashville, Tennessee

BROBERGER, O., Department of Pediatrics, Karolinska Institute, St. Goran's Children's Hospital, Stockholm, Sweden

BRODERSEN, R., Professor of Medical Biochemistry, Institute of Medical Biochemistry, University of Aarhus, Denmark

BRYAN, A. C., The Hospital for Sick Children, Toronto, Ontario, Canada,

BRYAN, M. H., The Hospital for Sick Children Toronto, Ontario, Canada

BUCCI, G., Institute of Pediatrics, University of Rome

BURNARD, E. D., Senior Research Fellow, Children's Medical Research Foundation, Royal Alexandra Hospital for Children, Director of Neonatal Intensive Care, The Women's Hospital, Crown Street, Sydney, Australia

CATLIN, D. H., Departments of Medicine, Pharmacology and Pediatrics, UCLA School of Medicine, Los Angeles, California

CHANEZ-BEL, C., Hôpital Port Royal, Paris, France

CHRISTENSEN, K. K., Neonatal Unit Department of Paediatrics, University Hospital, Lund, Sweden

CHRISTENSEN, P., Medical Microbiology, University Hospital, Lund, Sweden

COTTON, R. B., Department of Pediatrics, Vanderbilt University School of Medicine, Nashville, Tennessee

DALISSON, C., Port-Royal Maternity Hospital, Paris, France

DAVID, L., Associate Professor, Department of Pediatrics, Hôpital Edouard Herriot, Lyon, France

DELVIN, E. E., McGill University, Genetics Unit, Shriners Hospital, Montreal, Quebec, Canada

DE ROEVER-BONNET, H., Wilhelmina Gasthuis, University of Amsterdam, The Netherlands

DEMPSTER, W. S., Chief Technologist, Institute of Child Health Laboratories, Red Cross War Memorial Children's Hospital, Cape Town, Republic of South Africa

DESPRATS, R., Hopital La Grave, Toulouse C, France

DUC, G., Department of Pediatrics and Obstetrics, University of Zurich

FERRO, R., Institute of Pediatrics, University of Rome, Rome, Italy

FOREST, M. G., Hôpital Debrousse, Lyon, France

FRIIS-HANSEN, B., Rigshospitalet, Department of Neonatology, Copenhagen, Denmark

FROESE, A. B., The Hospital for Sick Children, Toronto, Ontario, Canada

GAITER, J. L., Departments of Neonatology and Pediatric Psychology, Children's Hospital National Medical Center, Department of Child Health Sciences, George Washington University, Washington, D.C.

GLORIEUX, F. H., McGill University, Shriners Hospital, Genetics Unit, Montreal, Quebec, Canada

GRANDJEAN, H., Hôpital La Grave, Toulouse, France

GRAY, M. E., Departments of Pediatrics and Pathology, Newborn Lung Center, Vanderbilt University School of Medicine, Nashville, Tennessee

GREEN, R. S., Department of Pediatrics, Vanderbilt University School of Medicine, Nashville, Tennessee

HAMON, A., Hôpital Port Royal, Paris, France

HANSON, N., Department of Pediatrics, Division of Neonatology, University Hospital, Groningen, The Netherlands

HEESE, H. DE V., Departments of Paediatrics and Child Health, Obstetrics and Gynaecology, and Chemical Pathology, University of Cape Town, Republic of South Africa

HERIN, P., Department of Pediatrics, Karolinska Institute, St. Goran's Children's Hospital, Stockholm, Sweden

HICKEY, D., Departments of Pediatrics and Clinical Pharmacology, Vanderbilt University School of Medicine, Nashville, Tennessee

HORNYCH, H., Port-Royal Maternity Hospital, Paris, France

HYTE, M., The Neonatology Service and Laboratory, Department of Pediatrics, Tufts-New England Medical Center Hospital, Boston, Massachusetts

ISACCHI, G., Department of Hematology, University of Rome

JOHNSON, A. A. S., Department of Neonatology, Children's Hospital National Medical Center, Department of Psychology George Washington University, Washington, D.C.

JOLLER, P., Department of Pediatrics and Obstetrics, University of Zurich, Switzerland

JORI, G., Department of Pediatrics and C. N. R. Center for the Physiology and Biochemistry of Hemocyanins and Other Metallo-Proteins, Institute of Animal Biology, University of Padova, Padova, Italy

KILDEBERG, P., Professor of Pediatrics, Odense University Hospital, Odense, Denmark

KNIGHT, G. J., Head, Department of Computer Services, Red Cross War Memorial Children's Hospital, Cape Town, Republic of South Africa

KOPPE, J. G., Department of Neonatology, Wilhelmina Gathuis, University of Amsterdam, The Netherlands

KORDON, C., Hôpital Port Royal, Paris, France

KOROBKIN, R., Port-Royal Maternity Hospital, Paris Cedex, France

LAGERCRANTZ, H., Department of Physiology, Karolinska Institute, and Department of Paediatrics, Karolinska, Hospital, Stockholm, Sweden

LASSEN, N. A., Bispebjerg Hospital, Department of Clinical Physiology, Copenhagen, Denmark

LAURENTI, F., Institute of Pediatrics, University of Rome, Rome, Italy

LeCOQ, A., Hôpital Debrousse, Lyon, France

LINDSTROM, D. P., Department of Applied Medical Electronics, Chalmers University of Technology, Gothenburg, Sweden

LOEWER-SIEGER, D. H., Wilhelmina Gasthuis, University of Amsterdam, The Netherlands

LOU, H. C., Roskilde Hospital, Department of Neurology, Roskilde, Denmark

MALAN, A. F., Departments of Paediatrics and Child Health, Obstetrics and Gynaecology, and Chemical Pathology, University of Cape Town, Republic of South Africa

MALAGNINO, F., Department of Hematology, University of Rome, Rome, Italy

MANDELLI, F., Department of Hematology, University of Rome, Rome, Italy

MANDYLA-SFAGOU, E., Registar, Newborn Intensive Care Unit, First Department of Paediatrics, Athens University, Athens, Greece

MARAGHI, S., Departments of Pediatrics and Clinical Pathology, Cairo University, Cairo, Egypt

MARAVELIAS, C., Research Registrar in Physiology, Newborn Instensive Care Unit, 1st Department of Paediatrics, Athens University, Athens, Greece

MARZETTI, G., Institute of Pediatrics, University of Rome, Rome, Italy

MATSANIOTIS, N., Professor and Chairman, First Department of Paediatrics, Athens University, Athens, Greece

MEYER, J., Registered Medical Technologist, Institute of Child Health Laboratories, Red Cross War Memorial Children's Hospital, Cape Town, Republic of South Africa

MILLAR, R. P., Departments of Paediatrics and Child Health, Obstetrics and Gynaecology, and Chemical Pathology, University of Cape Town, Republic of South Africa

MINKOWSKI, A., Hôpital Port Royal, Paris, France

MONIN, P., Service de Medecine Neonatale, Maternite Universitaire Nancy, France

MORSELLI, P. L., Department de Recherche Clinique, LERS, Synthelabo, Paris, France

DE MOUSON, J., Hopital La Grave, Toulouse, France

MULLER, N. L., The Research Institute, The Hospital for Sick Children, Toronto, Ontario, Canada

MURPHY, K., The Neonatology Service and Laboratory, The Department of Pediatrics, New England Medical Center Hospital, Boston, Massachusetts

NIELSON, L., The Neonatology Service and Laboratory, The Department of Pediatrics, Tufts-New England Medical Center Hospital, Boston, Massachusetts

NIERMEYER, S., Department of Pediatrics, Vanderbilt University School of Medicine, Nashville, Tennessee

NYLUND, L., Research Trainee, Department of Obstetrics and Gynaecology, Karolinska Institute, Huddinge Hospital, Huddinge, Sweden

OKKEN, A., Department of Pediatrics, Division of Neonatology, University Hospital, Groningen, The Netherlands

OLSSON, T., Department of Applied Medical Electronics, Chalmers University of Technology, Gothenburg, Sweden

PERKETT, E., Departments of Pediatrics and Pathology, Newborn Lung Center, Vanderbilt University School of Medicine, Nashville, Tennessee

PIERCY, W. N., Departments of Paediatrics and Obstetrics and Gynaecology, Queen's University, Kingston, Ontario, Canada

PONTONNIER, G., Hôpital La Grave, Toulouse, France

PRIAM, M., Hôpital Port Royal, Paris, France

PUTET, G., Neonatal Department, Hôpital Edouard Herriot, Lyon, France

ROBINSON, J. S., Departments of Medicine, Pharmacology, and Pediatrics, UCLA

School of Medicine, Los Angeles, California

ROJAS, J., Department of Pediatrics, Vanderbilt University School of Medicine, Nashville, Tennessee

ROKICKI, W., Clinic of Pathological Pregnancy, Institute of Obstetrics and Gynecology, Silesian Academy of Medicine, Bytom, Poland

ROOS, P. J., Departments of Paediatrics and Child Health, Obstetrics and Gynaecology, and Chemical Pathology, University of Cape Town, Republic of South Africa

ROSSI, E., Department of Pediatrics and C.N.R. Center for the Physiology and Biochemistry of Hemocyanins and Other Metallo-Proteins, Institute of Animal Biology, University of Padova, Padova, Italy

ROSSINI, M., C.N.R. Center for Respiratory Viruses, University of Rome, Rome, Italy

ROVEI, V., Department de Recherche Clinique, Laboratoire LERS, Synthelabo, Paris, France

RUBALTELLI, F. F., Department of Pediatrics and C.N.R. Center for the Physiology and Biochemistry of Hemocyanins and Other Metallo-Proteins, Institute of Animal Biology, University of Padova, Padova, Italy

SALLE, B., Professor of Pediatrics, Chief of Neonatal Department, Hopital Edouard Herriot, Lyon, France

SANJUAN, C., Department de Recherche Clinique, Laboratoire LERS, Synthelabo, Paris, France

SEGER, R., Department of Pediatrics and Obstetrics, University of Zurich, Zurich, Switzerland

SENTERRE, J., Maitre de Recherches of the National Foundation for Scientific Research, Department of Pediatrics, State University of Liege, Hopital de Baviere, Liege, Belgium

SHAMS EL-DIN, A., Professor of Pediatrics, Cairo University, Cairo, Egypt

SHNIDER, S. M., Professor of Anesthesia, Obstetrics, Gynecology and Reproductive Sciences, University of California, San Francisco, California

SMITH, S., Research Fellow, Department of Paediatrics and Child Health, University of Cape Town, Cape Town, Republic of South Africa

SMITH, B. T., Scholar, Medical Research Council of Canada, Department of Pediatrics, Harvard Medical School, Boston, Massachusetts

STAHLMAN, M., M.D., Departments of Pediatrics and Pathology, Newborn Lung Center, Vanderbilt University School of Medicine, Nashville, Tennessee

STEIGERWALD, A., Children's Hospital, Free University, Berlin, Federal Republic of Germany

SVENNINGSEN, N. W., Neonatal Unit Department of Paediatrics, University Hospital, Lund, Sweden

TANSWELL, A. K., Fellow, Canadian Cystic Fibrosis Foundation and the William T. McEachern Foundation, Department of Paediatrics, Queen's University, Kingston, Ontario, Canada

TEMPLE, C. J., Department of Neonatology, Children's Hospital National Medical Center, Washington, D.C.

THOMAS, D. B., Neonatologist, The Women's Hospital, Crown Street, Sydney, Australia

VALAES, T., The Neonatology Service and Laboratory, Department of Pediatrics, Tufts-New England Medical Center Hospital, Boston, Massachusetts

VEILLEUX, A., Neonatal Department, Hôpital Edouard Herriot, Lyon, France

VERT, P., Service de Medecine Neonatale, Maternite Universitaire, Nancy, France

VIBERT M., Service de Medecine Neonatale, Maternite Universitaire, Nancy, France

WATERMEYER, S., Research Assistant, Department of Paediatrics and Child Health, University of Cape Town, Cape Town, Republic of South Africa

WARSHAW, J. B., Division of Perinatal Medicine, Departments of Pediatrics and Obstetrics and Gynecology, Yale University School of Medicine, New Haven, Connecticut

WENDER, D. F., Division of Perinatal Medicine, Departments of Pediatrics and Obstetrics and Gynecology, Yale University School of Medicine, New Haven, Connecticut

WHITE, N. B., Epidemiology and Biometry Research Program, National Institute of Child Health and Human Development, Bethesda, Maryland

WIESE, G., Childrens Hospital, Free University, Berlin, Federal Republic of Germany

WIMBERLEY, P. D. Bispebjerg Hospital, Department of Clinical Physiology, Copenhagen, Denmark

WOODS, D. L., Departments of Paediatrics and Child Health, Obstetrics and Gynaecology, and Chemical Pathology, University of Cape Town, Republic of South Africa

WORTHINGTON, D., Departments of Paediatrics and Obstetrics and Gynaecology, Queen's University, Kingston, Ontario, Canada

XANTHOU, M., Associate Professor Paediatrics, Director of the Newborn Intensive Care Unit, First Department of Paediatrics, Athens University, Athens, Greece

ZETTERSTROM, R., Department of Pediatrics, Karolinska Institute, St. Goran's Children's Hospital, Stockholm, Sweden

Contents

1

Sympathoadrenal Activity in the Foetus during Delivery and at Birth

H. LAGERCRANTZ, M.D.,[1] P. BISTOLETTI, M.D.,[2] and L. NYLUND, M.D.[2]

The function of the sympathoadrenal system is to sustain homeostasis during stress. Increased sympathoadrenal activity has been demonstrated in conditions such as physical exercise,[9] asphyxia,[9] mental stress,[10] haemorrhage,[9] surgery,[9] aeroplane transport,[9] and parachute jumping.[10] Less attention has been paid to the role of the sympathoadrenal system during birth, which probably constitutes one of the most severe challenges to the homeostatic mechanisms during life. However, during the last decade, several reports on the catecholamine concentrations at birth have appeared.[1, 8, 14, 20, 21]

We have studied sympathoadrenal activity during delivery and at birth by analysing catecholamines in foetal scalp and umbilical cord blood samples. This approach gives only a reflection of the sympathoadrenal activity, and the data must be interpreted cautiously. By comparison between the levels of catecholamines in the infant and corresponding levels of catecholamines causing physiological effects in the foetal sheep, we can obtain some idea about the function of the sympathoadrenal system during birth in the human.

METHODS

I. The initial part of this investigation is an extension of a previously published study,[20] where the methodological details are given. In brief: umbilical arterial and venous blood were collected at birth after double clamping of the umbilical cord. The plasma was separated, stored in a freezer, passed through small columns with alumina oxide, and analysed fluorimetrically for

[1] Department of Physiology, Karolinska Institute, and Department of Paediatrics, Karolinska Hospital, Stockholm, Sweden
[2] Research trainees, Department of Obstetrics & Gynaecology, Karolinska Institute, Huddinge Hospital, Huddinge, Sweden

its content of noradrenaline and adrenaline. The sensitivity of the method allowed determination of 2 nmol/liter catecholamines. The values were corrected for the average 25% losses of amines in the columns.

II. In the second part of this study, the catecholamines were determined in foetal scalp blood samples by a radioenzymatic method based on catechol-*O*-methylation with radioactive methyl groups.[26] The lowest concentration of adrenaline and noradrenaline which could be determined by us with this method was 0.24 nmol/liter (= the double blank) and less than 100 μl plasma was required.[25] Infant plasma with known amounts of catecholamines was run in parallel and therefore no correction of the values was necessary.

More recently we have analyzed catecholamines in cooperation with Dr. P. Hjemdahl by high performance liquid chromatography (HPLC) with electrochemical detection,[13] and some values obtained by this method are included in Figure 2 and Tables VI and VII.

Altogether 149 umbilical arterial and 101 venous blood samples and 43 scalp blood analyses are included in this report. The catecholamine concentrations were correlated to the blood gases in the umbilical arterial blood and *p*H in the scalp blood, which were determined with a Radiometer BMS (Copenhagen). The Apgar score was routinely evaluated. The gestational age was assessed according to Dubowitz in doubtful cases.

Classification of the Cases

I. Umbilical Cord Samples. The cases have been grouped according to four main obstetrical factors: (A) gestational age; (B) vaginal delivery vs. Caesarean section; (C) mode of vaginal delivery; and (D) asphyxia. The independent subgroups have been compared with each other using the nonparametric statistical analyses according to Mann-Whitney.[30]

The subgroups have been defined in the following way:

A. Noninstrumental vertex deliveries
   i.   Full-term infants appropriate in weight for gestational age (AGA) (n = 82)
   ii. Preterm AGA infants with a gestational age less than 37 weeks (n = 15)
   iii. Full-term small-for-gestational-age infants (SGA) (n = 14)
B. Full-term AGA infants
   i.   Uncomplicated vertex deliveries with no clinical signs of foetal asphyxia and umbilical arterial pH $\geqslant$ 7.25 (n = 19)
   ii. Elective Caesarean section indicated by contracted pelvis or for psychological reasons (n = 14)
   iii. Emergency Caesarean section, usually caused by the appearance of abnormal foetal heart rate patterns (n = 24)
C. Full-term AGA infants
   i.   Noninstrumental vertex deliveries (n = 59)
   ii. Vaginal deliveries by vacuum extraction (n = 26)
   iii. Breech deliveries (n = 9)
D. Asphyxiated infants. Asphyxia defined as pH < 7.25 in the umbilical arterial blood

i. Full-term AGA infants ($n = 24$)

ii. Preterm AGA infants ($n = 7$)

iii. Full-term SGA infants ($n = 9$)

II. Scalp Blood Samples. In the second part of this study scalp blood plasma catecholamines were assayed in foetuses from which scalp pH was determined during routine clinical management.[29] The indication for this sampling was usually the occurrence of abnormal foetal heart rate patterns or long-lasting delivery. Only one scalp blood sample with pH $\geq$ 7.25 was included in Table III from each patient. In a few cases, who developed asphyxia, two scalp and the umbilical arterial blood samples *were* included (Fig. 2) as examples.

For comparison some preliminary data are included of the catecholamine concentrations in mothers during vaginal delivery and Caesarean section. We have also determined catecholamines in normoglycaemic infants of diabetic mothers and infants with respiratory distress at the age of 12 hr. The blood was collected from the umbilical artery.

The project has been approved by the local ethics committee.

RESULTS

I. Table I shows the noradrenaline and adrenaline concentrations in the umbilical artery and vein directly after noninstrumental vertex delivery. The noradrenaline and adrenaline concentration was higher in the full-term SGA and AGA infants than in the preterm AGA infants.

The mean foetal catecholamine concentration was significantly lower at elective Caesarean section than after vaginal vertex delivery, even when this was uncomplicated with no clinical signs of asphyxia (Table II). Emergency Caesarean section (Table II), instrumental delivery and particularly breech delivery were associated with considerably increased noradrenaline levels (Table III).

In Figure 1 the catecholamine concentrations in all the asphyxiated cases (pH $<$ 7.25) are plotted and grouped according to gestational age and size. The asphyxiated preterm infants had lower levels of amines at birth than the asphyxiated full-term AGA and SGA infants.

TABLE I

Catecholamine Concentrations at Birth; Noninstrumental Vertex Deliveries

Birth Weight (kg)	Apgar Score (1 min)	[H$^+$] (nmol/ liter)	pH	Venous			Arterial		
				Noradrena-line (nmol/ liter)	Adrena-line (nmol/ liter)	n	Noradrena-line (nmol/ liter)	Adrena-line (nmol/li-ter)	n
Full-term AGA	3.5 ± 0.5	8.0 ± 1.6	55.7 ± 10.0	(7.25)	38.2 ± 48.8	7.4 ± 9.7	82	62.4 ± 58.7	8.7 ± 11.7 59
Preterm AGA	1.9 ± 0.6^a	6.3 ± 3.0^a	61.0 ± 25.1^b	(7.21)	26.7 ± 35.6^b	4.9 ± 6.7	15	38.5 ± 21.6^b	2.5 ± 4.4^b 8
Full-term SGA	2.7 ± 0.3^b	8.2 ± 1.3	53.9 ± 11.4	(7.27)	32.4 ± 48.0	6.3 ± 9.3	14	44.8 ± 28.4	4.7 ± 4.7 8

^{a} ±SD: $p < 0.01$.
^{b} ±SD: $p < 0.05$.

TABLE II

Catecholamine Concentrations in the Umbilical Artery at Birth; Vaginal Delivery vs. Caesarean Section

	Birth Weight (kg)	Apgar Score (1 min)	[H$^+$] (nmol/ liter)	pH	Noradrena-line (nmol/ liter)	Adrena-line (nmol/ liter)	n
Uncomplicated vertex delivery	3.3 ± 0.6	7.9 ± 0.9	47.7 ± 4.8	(7.33)	30.0 ± 27.0	5.6 ± 6.1	19
Elective Caesarean section	3.3 ± 0.4	7.7 ± 1.11	50.3 ± 4.1	(7.30)	14.6 ± 8.6^a	3.0 ± 8.6^b	14
Emergency Caesarean section	3.2 ± 0.5	6.3 ± 2.4^a	58.6 ± 0.8^b	(7.23)	64.9 ± 51.9^c	6.8 ± 7.3	24

^{a} ±SD: $p < 0.01$.
^{b} ±SD: $p < 0.05$.
^{c} ±SD: $p < 0.001$.

TABLE III

Catecholamine Concentrations in the Umbilical Artery at Birth due to Mode of Delivery

	Birth Weight (kg)	Apgar Score (1 min)	[H$^+$] (nmol/ liter)	pH	Noradrena-line (nmol/ liter)	Adrenaline (nmol/ liter)	n
Vertex delivery noninstrumental	3.5 ± 0.5	8.0 ± 1.6	55.7 ± 10.0	(7.25)	62.4 ± 58.1	8.7 ± 11.7	59
Vacuum extraction	3.5 ± 0.6	7.3 ± 1.6^a	60.5 ± 8.4^b	(7.22)	93.3 ± 53.3^a	12.7 ± 14.8	26
Breech delivery	3.3 ± 0.7	6.5 ± 2.3^a	62.3 ± 15.4^b	(7.20)	141.8 ± 102.6^a	14.1 ± 28.8	9

^{a} ±SD: $p < 0.001$.
^{b} SD: $p < 0.01$.

The inverse correlation coefficient between catecholamine concentration and Apgar score was very weak (Table IV). The noradrenaline concentration seemed to correlate somewhat better with the blood gases, particularly with the hydrogen concentration (Table IV).

II. Analyses of catecholamines in foetal scalp blood samples obtained at three levels of cervix dilatation showed a successive increase of the amine levels towards birth (Table V). All these samples had a pH above 7.25. In Figure 2 four examples of complicated deliveries are shown (from Ref. 25), in comparison with the "normal" values. Case 1 was a breech delivery who had an abnormal foetal heart rate pattern and was delivered by emergency Caesarean section. Case 2 had an entangled cord and was meconium stained and acidotic, but had a normal Apgar score. The amine level was extremely high. Cases 3 and 4 were delivered by vacuum extraction which seemed to be associated with increased amine concentrations.

There was a significant correlation between the total catecholamine concentration and pH in the scalp blood samples (Fig. 3).

The catecholamine levels at birth were in general considerably higher than

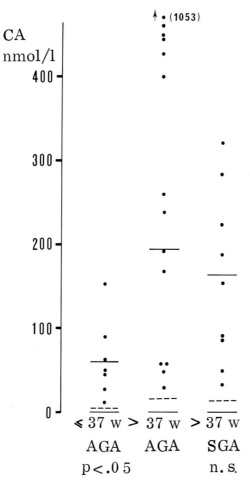

Fig. 1. Catecholamine (CA) concentrations in the umbilical artery with asphyxia ($pH < 7.25$) in preterm and fullterm AGA and SGA infants. The mean total catecholamine levels are indicated by the continuous bars and the mean adrenaline levels by the hatched bars.

TABLE IV

Correlation Matrix ($n = 149$)

Umbilical Arterial	Apgar Score (1 min)	p	PO_2	p	PCO_2	p	$[H^+]$	p	Base Deficiency	p
Nor-adrenaline	−0.20	<0.01	−0.16	<0.05	0.33	<0.001	0.42	<0.001	0.15	n.s.
Adrenaline	0.10	n.s.	0.04	n.s.	0.04	n.s.	0.21	<0.01	0.23	<0.01

in the mother during pregnancy and delivery (Table VI). They were also higher than in infants in the nursery with moderate problems of neonatal adaptation (Table VII).

TABLE V

Catecholamine Concentrations in Foetal Scalp Blood Samples ($pH \geq 7.25$)

Cervix Dilatation (cm)	Noradrenaline (nmol/liter)	Adrenaline (nmol/liter)	n
3–5	7.15 ± 4.14	2.03 ± 3.20	11
6–8	10.43 ± 8.07	2.66 ± 3.10	12
9–10	17.20 ± 11.16[a]	5.63 ± 4.07[a]	11

[a] ±SD: $p < 0.05$.

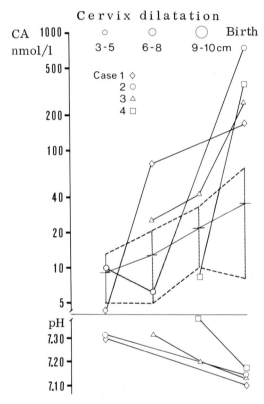

Fig. 2. Catecholamine (CA) concentrations in scalp blood samples obtained at different degrees of cervix dilatation and in the umbilical artery at birth. The mean values of the non-asphyxiated infants are from Tables V and II. For comparison the catecholamine concentrations in four full-term infants who sustained complicated deliveries are demonstrated. Case 1: breech delivery, which was terminated by Caesarean section. Apgar score 2.6. Case 2: entangled cord, Apgar score 8.10. Case 3: vacuum extraction, Apgar score 4.7. Case 4: vacuum extraction, Apgar score 9.10. The pH in the scalp blood and umbilical artery is shown below.

DISCUSSION

The Catecholamine Assay. Until recently the commonly used catecholamine assay has been the fluorimetric method. Large plasma volumes (about 10 ml) were required for accurate measurements.[33] However, the catecholamine con-centration at birth is considerably higher than in the resting adult,[14, 20] and

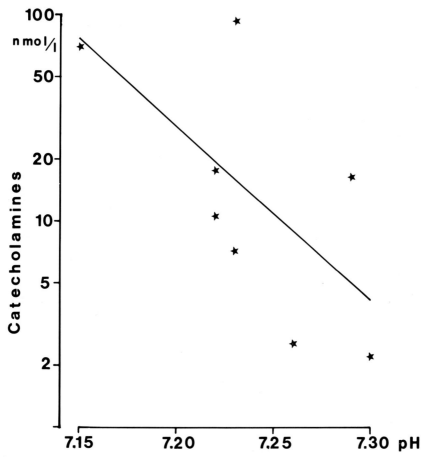

Fig. 3. $\log_{10}$ catecholamine concentrations vs. pH in foetal scalp blood samples obtained during the first stage of labour. The correlation coefficient was -0.67, which was significant ($p < 0.05$).

TABLE VI

Catecholamine Concentrations in the Mothers (Peripheral vein)

	Noradrenaline (nmol/liter)	Adrenaline (nmol/liter)	n
During vaginal delivery	4.0 ± 2.2	1.0 ± 1.1	8
During Caesarean section	3.3 ± 2.4	0.9 ± 1.7	16

(Irestedt and Lagercrantz, to be published).

TABLE VII

Catecholamine Concentrations in Infants 12 Hr after Birth (Abdominal aorta)

	Noradrenaline (nmol/liter)	Adrenaline (nmol/liter)	n
Normoglucaemic infants of diabetic mothers	4.67 ± 2.30	2.25 ± 0.96	8
Preterm infants with respiratory distress	7.09 ± 3.58	3.34 ± 2.00	6

therefore it has been possible to assay the catecholamines in smaller volumes of umbilical cord blood.

The radioenzymatic method allows determination of catecholamines in volumes down to 100 μl plasma.[25, 26] The differentiation between noradrenaline and adrenaline is better than with the fluorimetric method. However, the method is tedious and expensive.

The high performance liquid chromatography with electrochemical detection (HPLC) is not as sensitive as the radioenzymatic method. It has, however, a number of advantages: an internal standard can be added to each sample and losses during chromatography can be corrected; any disturbance or poor sensitivity can be detected and corrected before proceeding with the analyses.[13]

A satisfactory agreement between the fluorimetric and radioenzymatic methods was found, except in samples with very low amounts of catecholamines, when the values obtained by the fluorimetric assay tended to be too high, probably due to blank problems. Thus, the amine levels at elective Caesarean section have been found to be lower in our most recent studies. HPLC has been found to show excellent agreement with the radioenzymatic method in our institute.[13]

Bioassays have been used to determine catecholamines in umbilical cord blood.[14] Even if the bioassay is very sensitive, its specificity can be questioned, particularly since many kinds of vasoactive substance are released at birth.

Catecholamine Concentrations at Birth

The noradrenaline and adrenaline concentrations in both the umbilical artery and vein are remarkably high at birth after "normal" vertex delivery, about tenfold higher than in the resting adult (=1–3 nmol/liter).[26] At asphyxia extremely high amine concentrations have often been found that are only seen in adults with phaeochromocytoma.[33]

The catecholamines in the umbilical artery originate mainly from the foetus since: (i) the arteriovenous difference is about 1.5–2:1; (ii) the maternal amine levels are considerably lower than the foetal during the delivery; (iii) radioactive noradrenaline injected into women during abortion was found in very low concentrations in the foetus (10–12% of the maternal level)[28]; (iv) the placenta has a high amine metabolizing capacity.[28]

Lower catecholamine concentrations were seen after elective Caesarean section than after uncomplicated vaginal delivery, indicating that vaginal parturition is associated with increased sympathoadrenal activity.

The high catecholamine concentrations with asphyxia suggest that the hypoxia or acidosis triggers the amine release as in the foetal sheep.[5, 16] For pH values below 7.25, the correlation coefficient between pH and $\log_{10}$ catecholamines was found to be −0.71.[20] However, in the entire material the correlation between catecholamines and blood gases was less apparent, suggesting that the squashing and squeezing through the birth canal could also be important factors. This is indicated by the very high amine levels seen in vacuum extracted infants, even in those without asphyxia. The correlation between catecholamines and hydrogen concentration, particularly below pH 7.25, might also be due to lactate formation secondary to the amine release.[18]

Preterm infants had generally lower amine levels than full-term infants sustaining comparable degree of asphyxia, possibly because their sympathoadrenal system is not completely developed.[11, 22] SGA infants have previously been reported to have a deficient adrenaline response to hypoglycaemia,[31] but their amine concentrations at asphyxia were in the same range as for the fullterm AGA infants.

The duration of the asphyxia is probably of importance. Long-term asphyxia seemed to be associated with lower catecholamine concentrations at birth, possibly due to partial depletion.[20]

Catecholamines in Foetal Scalp Blood Samples

The plasma catecholamine concentration during the first stage of labour was about double that of the resting adult and more than twofold higher than in the undisturbed chronically catheterized foetal sheep (Rosén and Lagercrantz, to be published). Uterine contractions and the pain caused by the scalp blood sampling procedure probably elevated the amine levels. Furthermore, these deliveries were not strictly uncomplicated, since there was always some clinical indication for the scalp blood sampling (see Methods). Thus the values in Figure 2 might represent the upper limit of the nonasphyxiated foetuses. There seemed to be a successive increase in catecholamine release towards the completion of the delivery. In the four asphyxiated foetuses the amine release was considerably increased.

The catecholamine concentrations correlated fairly well with the hydrogen ion concentration in the scalp blood (Fig. 3).

The Origin of the Foetal Catecholamines

The catecholamines in adult plasma originate mainly from sympathetic overflow and to a lesser extent from the adrenal medulla.[9] In the foetus, the sympathetic nervous system may not be completely developed,[11] while the adrenal medulla constitutes a relatively larger mass.[5] Furthermore, the foetuses are provided with paraganglia containing nearly as much catecholamines as the adrenal glands.[12]

After adrenalectomy by infusion of formalin to chronic foetal sheep preparations, there was only a minor decrease of the noradrenaline levels while the adrenaline concentration became very low (Jones and Lagercrantz, to be published). Studies of aborted human foetuses have shown that hypoxia causes a depletion of the paraganglia, prior to that of the adrenal medulla.[12] Thus, the paraganglia might contribute substantially to the plasma catecholamines, a fact also indicated by the dominance of noradrenaline.

The Physiological Significance of Catecholamine Release

We need to critically evaluate to what extent these occasional samples reflect the sympathoadrenal activity during delivery. The half-life of the catecholamines is about 3 min in the human adult.[19] In the foetus, conditions which stimulate the secretion of catecholamines, such as hypoxia or labour, do not produce transient changes but maintain an elevated plasma concentration.[16, 17]

Eliot *et al.*[8] have recently shown that the catecholamine concentration remained fairly high during the first 3 hr after birth in peripheral venous blood (about 6 nmol/liter). At 12 and 24 hr the level had decreased to about 2 nmol/liter—the normal value of the resting adult.

What is the functional role of this high catecholamine release during birth? Some idea can be obtained by comparing the amine concentrations we have measured with those causing physiological effects in animals. However, usually considerably higher circulating catecholamine concentrations are required than what is released from the nerve terminals.[4] On the other hand, the foetus seems to be more sensitive to circulating catecholamines than the adult, possibly due to the fact that the sympathetic nerve plexa and thus the termination of action are not completely developed at birth.[11]

The following effects of the catecholamines might be of particular value for the foetus during the delivery, especially with asphyxia:

   i.   Vasoconstriction of blood vessels to the gastrointestinal organs, the kidneys, the skin, and the muscles and distribution of the blood towards the most vital organs, the placenta, the heart, and the brain[6]

   ii.   Increasing cardiac performance particularly with asphyxia[7]

   iii.   Mobilization of glucose. Inhibition of insulin release[18]

   iv.   Stimulation of lung liquid absorption[23, 24]

   v.   Enhancement of surfactant release[23]

   vi.   Stimulation of central nervous system—arousal[10]

   vii.   Increasing muscular tone[10]

   viii.   Stimulation of peripheral chemoreceptors[27]

   ix.   Activation of nonshivering thermogenesis[24]

All these actions of the catecholamines might be of fundamental importance for neonatal adaptation. In fact the catecholamines seem to increase four of the five parameters in the Apgar score: heart rate (ii), respiration (vi and viii), muscular tone (vii), irritability (vi).

The effect particularly of adrenaline on lung liquid absorption and surfactant release might possibly explain why infants delivered by Caesarean section who have low catecholamines often develop tachypnea and respiratory distress syndrome.[32] It is interesting, that β-stimulating drugs like terbutaline prevent respiratory distress to some extent.[2] We cannot exclude the possibility that the extremely high catecholamine levels might have some negative effects, particularly a vasoconstrictive action on the pulmonary and intestinal blood vessels.[6]

Future Directions

With the new sensitive catecholamine assays it is possible to assess the sympathoadrenal activity during birth. This might be of interest in the evaluation of cardiotocography. The appearance of abnormal foetal heart rate patterns is both poorly correlated to catecholamine levels and with clinical outcome.[3] However, ST–T changes in the foetal electrocardiogram, which seems to be a more reliable indicator of foetal asphyxia than cardiotocography, were found to be highly correlated with the catecholamine concentrations during asphyxia in chronic foetal sheep preparations (see Ref. 15; Rosén and Lagercrantz, unpublished observations). Studies of the role of the sympathoadrenal system in metabolic adaptation might also be of considerable interest.

CONCLUSIONS

During delivery the foetal sympathoadrenal system is activated, particularly with asphyxia as indicated by the high scalp and umbilical arterial plasma levels. We believe that this is of importance to sustain homeostasis and facilitate neonatal adaptation.

ACKNOWLEDGMENTS

Supported by the Swedish Medical Research Council (Project No. 5234), Expressen's and Odd Fellow's Prenatal Research Foundations, Majblommans Stiftelse, and Stiftelsen Allmänna BB.

REFERENCES

1. Artal, R., Lam, R. W., Eliot, J., Hobel, C. J., and Fisher, D. A., Circulating Catecholamines Prior to and after Delivery, in *Catecholamines: Basic and Clinical Frontiers*, E. Usdin, I. J. Kopin, and J. Barchas, Eds. Pergamon Press, New York, 1979, p. 951.
2. Bergman, B., and Hedner, T., Antepartum administration of terbutaline and the incidence of hyaline membrane disease in preterm infants. *Acta Obstet. Gynecol. Scand.* **57,** 217 (1978).
3. Bistoletti, P., Lagercrantz, H., and Lunell, N. O., Evaluation of fetal heart rate deceleration and baseline variability during last hour of labour. *Acta Obstet. Gynecol. Scand.*, in press.
4. Celander, O., The range of control exercised by the sympatico-adrenal system. *Acta Physiol. Scand.* **32, Suppl.** 116 (1954).
5. Comline, R. S., and Silver, M., Development of activity in the adrenal medulla of the foetus and newborn animal. *Br. Med. Bull.* **22,** 16 (1966).
6. Dawes, G. S., *Foetal and Neonatal Physiology.* Yearbook Publishers, Chicago, 1968.
7. Downing, S. E., Gardner, T. H., and Rocamora, J. M., Adrenergic support of cardiac function during hypoxia in the newborn lamb. *Am. J. Physiol.* **217,** 728 (1969).
8. Eliot, R. J., Lam, R., Leake, R., Hobel, C. J., and Fisher, D. A., Plasma catecholamine concentrations in infants at birth and during the first 48 hours of life. *J. Pediatr.* **96,** 311 (1980).
9. Euler, U. S. v., *Noradrenaline.* C. Thomas, Springfield, 1956.
10. Frankenhaeuser, M., Behavior and circulating catecholamines. *Brain Res.* **31,** 241 (1971).
11. Friedman, W. F., The Intrinsic Physiological Properties of the Developing heart, in *Neonatal Heart Disease*, W. F. Friedman, M. Lesch, and E. H. Sonnenblick, Eds. Grune and Stratton, New York, 1973, p. 21.
12. Hervonen, A., and Korkola, O., The effects of hypoxia on the catecholamine content of human fetal abdominal paraganglia and adrenal medulla. *Acta Obstet. Gynecol. Scand.* **51,** 17 (1972).
13. Hjemdahl, P., Daleskog, M., and Kahan, T., Determination of plasma catecholamines by high performance liquid chromatography with electrochemical detection: Comparison with a radioenzymatic method. *Life Sci.* **25,** 131 (1979).
14. Holden, K. R., Young, R. B., Piland, J. H., and Hurt, W. G., Plasma pressors in the normal and stressed newborn infant. *Pediatrics* **49,** 495 (1972).

15. Hökegård, K. H., Karlsson, K., Kjellmer, I., and Rosén, K. G., ECG-changes in the fetal lamb during asphyxia in relation to beta-adrenoceptor stimulation and blockade. *Acta Physiol. Scand.* **105**, 195 (1979).

16. Jones, C. T., and Robinson, R. O., Plasma catecholamines in foetal and adult sheep. *J. Physiol. (Lond.)* **248**, 15 (1975).

17. Jones, C. T., and Ritchie, J. W. K., The cardiovascular effects of circulating catecholamines in fetal sheep. *J. Physiol. (Lond.)* **285**, 381 (1978).

18. Jones, C. T., and Ritchie, J. W. K., The metabolic and endocrine effects of circulating catecholamines in fetal sheep. *J. Physiol. (Lond.)* **285**, 395 (1978).

19. Kopin, I. J., Plasma Catecholamines: A Brief Overview, in *Catecholamines: Basic and Clinical Frontiers*, E. Usdin, I. J. Kopin, and J. Barchas, Eds. Pergamon Press, New York, 1979, p. 897.

20. Lagercrantz, H., and Bistoletti, P., Catecholamine release in the newborn infant at birth. *Pediatr. Res.* **11**, 889 (1977).

21. Lagercrantz, H., Bistoletti, P., and Lunell, N.-O., Catecholamine Release in the Human Fetus and Newborn Infant, in *Catecholamines: Basic and Clinical Frontiers*, E. Usdin, I. J. Kopin, and J. Barchas, Eds. Pergamon Press, New York, 1979, p. 912.

22. Lagercrantz, H., Sjöquist, B., Bremme, K., Lunell, N.-O., and Somell, C., Catecholamine metabolites in amniotic fluid as indicators of intrauterine stress. *Am. J. Obstet. Gynecol.* **136**, 1067 (1980).

23. Lawson, E. E., Brown, E. R., Torday, J. S., Madansky, D. L., and Taeusch, H. W., The effect of epinephrine on tracheal fluid flow and surfactant efflux in fetal sheep. *Am. Rev. Respir. Dis.* **118**, 1023 (1978).

24. Moore, R. E., Control of heat production in newborn mammals: Role of noradrenaline and mode of action. *Fed. Proc.* **22**, 920 (1963).

25. Nylund, L., Bistoletti, P., and Lagercrantz, H., Catecholamines in foetal blood during birth. *J. Dev. Physiol.* **1**, 427 (1980).

26. Peuler, J. D., and Johnson, G. A., Simultaneous single isotope-radioenzymatic assay of plasma norepinephrine, epinephrine and dopamine. *Life Sci.* **21**, 625 (1977).

27. Purves, M. J., and Biscoe, T. J., Development of chemoreceptor activity. *Br. Med. Bull.* **22**, 56 (1966).

28. Saarikoski, S., Fate of noradrenaline in the human foetoplacental unit. *Acta Physiol. Scand. Suppl.* 421, 93 (1975).

29. Saling, E., Neues Vorgehen zur Untersuchung des Kindes unter der Geburt. *Arch. Gynaekol.* **197**, 108 (1962).

30. Siegel, S. *Non-parametric Statistics.* McGraw-Hill, New York, 1956.

31. Stern, L., Sourkes, T. L., and Raihä, N., The role of the adrenal medulla in the hypoglycemia of foetal malnutrition. *Biol. Neonate* **11**, 129 (1967).

32. Usher, R., Allen, A. C., and McLean, F. M., Risk of respiratory distress syndrome related to gestational age, route of delivery, and maternal diabetes. *Am. J. Obstet. Gynecol.* **111**, 826 (1971).

33. Vendsalu, A., Studies on adrenaline and noradrenaline in human plasma. *Acta Physiol. Scand.* **49**, *Suppl.* 173 (1960).

34. Walters, D. V., and Olver, R. E., The role of catecholamines in lung liquid absorption at birth. *Pediatr. Res.* **12**, 239 (1978).

2

Neurotransmitters in Early Life and in Intrauterine Growth Retardation

C. CHANEZ-BEL, M. PRIAM, A. HAMON, C. KORDON, and
A. MINKOWSKI

INTRODUCTION

Early restriction of nutrients influences to a considerable extent the somatic development of experimental animals.[1-139] Malnutrition can have significant repercussions on the ontogeny of the central nervous system. Dobbing and co-workers[1, 32-36] refer to the brain "growth spurt" as a vulnerable period of development, during which animals or specific organs are most sensitive to the state of nutrition and injury can have important and permanent consequences.

The purpose of this study was to assess the influence of *in utero* restricted blood supply on the developing nervous system. The experimental intrauterine growth retardation (IUGR) in the fetus is induced in the latter part of fetal life at the end of the period of neuronal proliferation.

Recent studies have proven that alterations in electrophysiological properties, behavior, and neurotransmitter metabolism are induced in the fetus or newborn rat by protein deprivation during pregnancy and the lactation period.[146] As the development of brain serotonin (5HT) neurons provoked by changes in free tryptophan occurring during the early neonatal period shows that underfeeding or malnutrition affects free tryptophan, dopamine, and norepinephrine levels, it was thought interesting to obtain information on the influence of restricted blood supply on 5HT and catecholamine metabolism in IUGR rats.

BIOLOGICAL BASIS

Figure 1 illustrates how tryptophan,[149] the precursor of serotonin (5HT), passes from the blood stream to the neuron and is then transformed to 5HTP

Centre de Recherches de Biologie du Développement Foetal et Néonatal, Hôpital Port-Royal, Université René Descartes, Paris, France

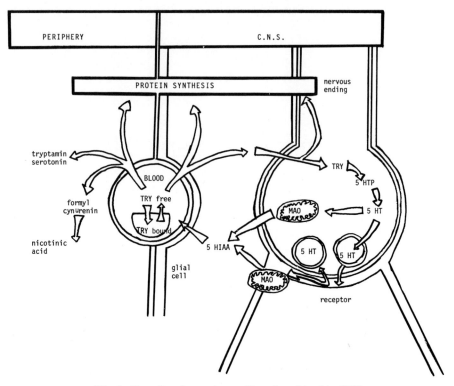

Fig. 1. Transfer of neurotransmitters from blood to CNS.

and 5HT and finally to the metabolite 5HIAA (5 hydroxyindolacetic acid) (Fig. 1b).

According to Hamon and co-workers,[142, 143] the free tryptophan level in neonatal rat serum is 10 times higher than in the adult animal (probably due to a low rate of binding with albumin[141] and to the high level of NEFA, which is a potent inhibitor of amino acid binding, in newborn rat serum). The high level of tryptophan immediately points to the relationship of neurotransmitters to nutrition.

Finally it should be emphasized that the majority of the serotonin is located in the gastrointestinal tract (90%), with the rest in platelets and only 2% in the central nervous system. The main site of neurotransmitters is in the forebrain: median raphe for serotonin, locus coerulaeus for catecholamines.[140] This explains why it is so difficult to study them in the human as their presence in the blood stream is meaningless. Studies estimating serotonin in human cerebrospinal fluid have been proven to be of a very little value.[148]

MATERIAL AND METHODS

Female rats of the Sherman strain were used. Intrauterine growth retardation of the fetus was obtained by clamping the uterine vessels of one horn on

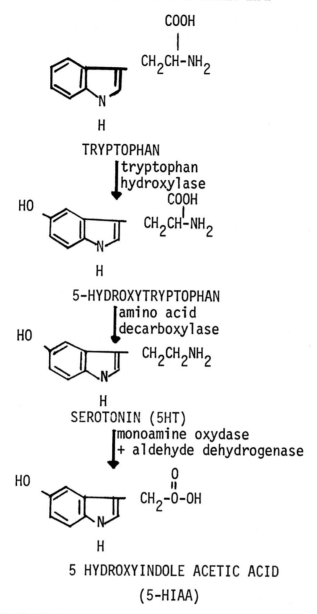

Fig. 1b. Metabolic pathway for serotonin synthesis and degradation.

the 17th day of gestation according to Wigglesworth's procedure.[147] The opposite horn was left as a control (Fig. 2). The animal was considered hypotrophic (intrauterine growth retardation) when body weight reduction was at least 30% compared to controls of the same age. At birth, the difference in weight between IUGR and control rats reaches 40%. This difference in body

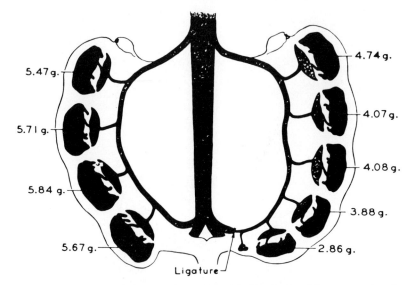

Fig. 2. Schematic diagram of the experimental model. The fetal weights were taken from one experiment. Modified from Wigglesworth's procedure.[61]

weight persists up to adulthood and IUGR rats never reach the weight of control rats whatever the rearing conditions (Fig. 3).

All organs undergo a significant reduction,[145] particularly in the liver and in brown adipose tissue. The brain weight is reduced by only about 10% (Fig. 4). At weaning, the average reduction of the organs levels off at about 30%, with the brain relatively unchanged. This organ benefits from a privileged distribution of blood flow during intrauterine life (six times more than in fetal lamb's liver). During the experiments, mothers are fed *ad libitum* with a standard diet and are maintained in individual cages with six to eight newborns.

Both males and females were used at random and sacrificed at 1, 8, 15, and 22 days (between 10 and 12 AM). Blood was collected from trunk vessels. Serum was obtained by centrifugation in the cold at 3,000 *g* for 30 min. The brain was removed quickly and the forebrain and brain stem were dissected, weighed, and homogenized in 3 ml of an ethanol–water solution. After storage at −30°C, the homogenate was centrifuged; serotonin, dopamine, and norepinephrine (5HT, DA, NE) were isolated from the supernatant by ion exchange chromatography on Amberlite CG 50. They were estimated in eluates according to the spectrofluorimetric methods of Bogdanski *et al.*, Laverty and Taylor, and Euler and Lishajko.

Tryptophan was isolated from Amberlite effluent using a Dowex column AG 50 W × 4 200/400 mesh, and after 5HIAA contained in the Dowex effluent was absorbed on Sephadex G 10, the amino acid levels were measured by the spectrofluorimetric method of Denckla and Dewey. For measuring 5HIAA concentrations, the same 5HT method was employed. Total and free tryptophan were measured on samples of serum and ultrafiltrates after centrifugation by the same procedure used for brain tryptophan.

Experimental Material

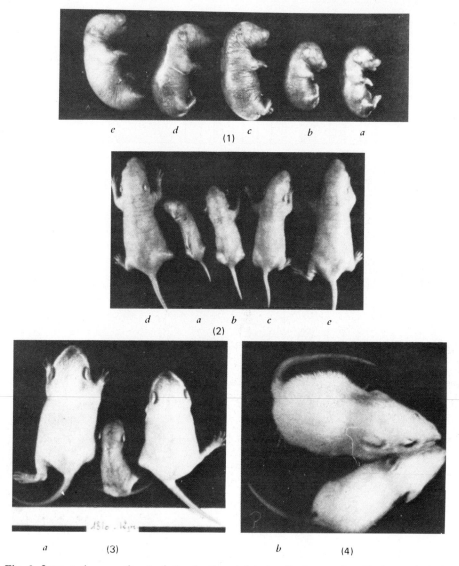

Fig. 3. Intrauterine growth retardation in the rat (uterine ligation on day 17 of gestation). (1) Fetuses at day 21 (1 day before natural delivery): a and b, IUGR; c, d, and e, controls. (2) Six days after birth (a, b, and c, IUGR). (3) Twelve days after birth. (4) Seventeen days after birth.

RESULTS

Changes in Tryptophan Concentration in Plasma and Brain during Development

In Figure 5 it can be noted that in the plasma the estimated percentage of free tryptophan versus total tryptophan is higher in IUGR rats at 8 and 15 days than in control animals. The difference is statistically significant. During

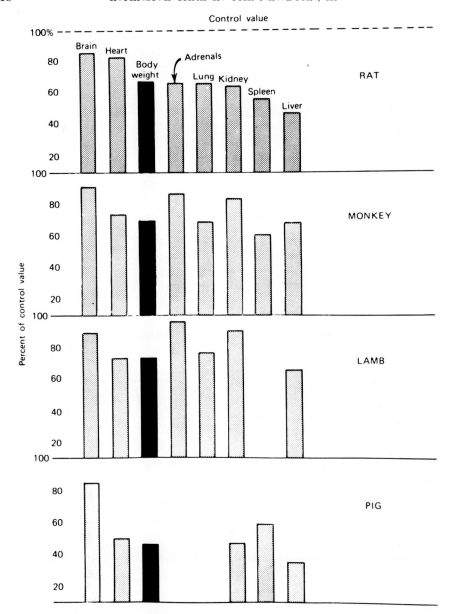

Fig. 4. Mean body and organ weights of IUGR rats (56), monkeys (38), lambs (10), and pigs (59), plotted as percentages of the control values.

that period the percentage of free tryptophan remains stable in IUGR rats, whereas it decreases in control animals.

In Figure 6 one can follow the concentration of tryptophan in the forebrain and the brain stem in control and IUGR animals. From birth on, one can see that its concentrations are higher in the IUGR animals in both central nervous

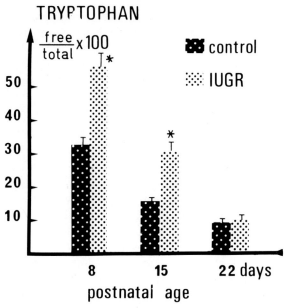

Fig. 5. Percentage of serum free tryptophan in intrauterine growth retardation rats (hatched bars) and control rats (black bars) at various ages after birth.

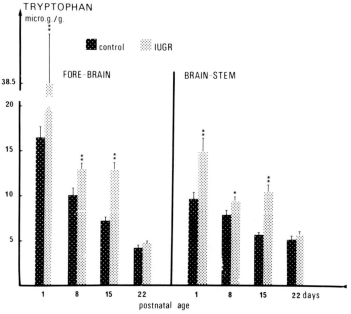

Fig. 6. Tryptophan levels in the forebrain and the brain stem of intrauterine growth retardation (hatched bars) and controls rats (black bars). The results are given at various ages after birth and are expressed in $\mu g/g$ of wet tissue. Each bar represents the mean based on 20 to 30 samples. The asterisks denote statistically significant differences in comparison to the values for control animals. Control by Student's t test (** at least $p < 0.01$; * at least $p < 0.05$).

system structures at all ages studied. As for serum values, central nervous system tryptophan values decrease regularly with age in the control animals until weaning, whereas those values remain constant in IUGR at 8 and 15 days. The tryptophan concentration then remains higher during the lactation period. At 22 days, in both groups of animals, the values in the forebrain and the brain stem are approximately those of adults.

Changes in Serotonin (5HT) and 5-Hydroxyindolacetic acid (5HIAA) in Developing Control and IUGR Rat Brains

The concentration of 5HT (Fig. 7) in the forebrain increases slowly with age. At 22 days, those values hardly represent the ones of adult age. The values of 5HTP in IUGR animals are significantly higher than in controls at age 1 and 15 days. At 8 days, concentrations of 5HT are slightly higher in IUGR. At the time of weaning, the values are identical in both groups. As expected, the values are higher in the brain stem (main site for 5HT) than in forebrain in both groups. At 22 days, the values reach the adult level.

In Figure 8, one can see the course of 5HIAA concentration, the main product of 5HT catabolism in the brain. As for 5HT, values of 5HIAA are lower in the forebrain than in the brain stem. They increase during the first 3 weeks of life. The values in IUGR rats parallel the control ones, but are at a significantly higher level at days 1, 15, and 21.

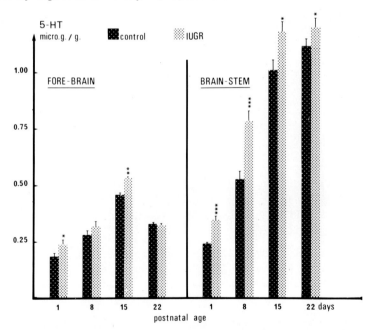

Fig. 7. Serotonin (5HT) levels in the forebrain and the brain stem of intrauterine growth retardation (hatched bars) and control rats (black bars). The results are given at various ages after birth and are expressed in $\mu g/g$ of wet tissue. Each bar represents the mean based on 20 to 30 samples. The asterisks denote statistically significant differences in comparison to the values for control animals. Control by Student's t test (** at least $p < 0.01$; * at least $p < 0.05$).

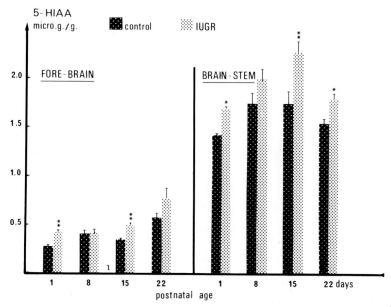

Fig. 8. Hydroxyindolacetic acid (5-HIAA) levels in the forebrain and the brain stem of intrauterine growth retardation (hatched bars) and control rats (black bars). The results are given at various ages after birth and are expressed in μg/g of wet tissue. Each bar represents the mean based on 20 to 30 samples. The asterisks denote statistically significant difference in comparison to the values for control animals. Control by Student's t test (** at least $p < 0.01$; * at least $p < 0.05$).

In the brain stem, however, the pattern differs from the 5HT one. At 24 hr, the concentrations of 5HIAA are nearly as high as in the adult animals. They increase and are at a maximum at day 15. After the third week, they decrease slightly.

At all ages studied, 5HIAA concentrations are higher in IUGR than in controls. The comparison between the amine and its metabolite in both forebrain and brain stem can be visualized by the ratio 5HIAA/5HT during development. In both structures, it is higher in young animals than in adults. In addition to this, it is higher in IUGR brain stem than in controls.

Changes in Dopamine (DA) and Norepinephrine (NE) in Developing Control and IUGR Rat Brains

In this study (Table I), the dopamine values are significantly higher in the forebrain for IUGR rats at 1, 15, and 21 days postnatally. At 8 days, they are still higher, though not significantly so.

In the forebrain and in the brain stem, the values of norepinephrine are higher in the IUGR animals at all ages studied.

COMMENTS AND DISCUSSION

Decreasing blood flow in the gestant rat alters the metabolism of 5HT during the first postnatal 3 weeks of the IUGR rat. At the different ages selected in

TABLE I

Dopamine (DA) and Norepinephrine (NE) Levels in the Forebrain and the Brain Stem of Intrauterine Growth Retardation and Control Rats at 1, 8, 15, and 22 Days Postnatal[a]

Age	1 day		8 days		15 days		22 days	
	Control	IUGR	Control	IUGR	Control	IUGR	Control	IUGR
Norepineph-rine Fore-brain	0.127 0.009 ($n = 18$)	0.158* 0.016 ($n = 19$)	0.131 0.005 ($n = 19$)	0.146[N.S.] 0.008 ($n = 18$)	0.151 0.008 ($n = 12$)	0.154[N.S.] 0.008 ($n = 15$)	0.191 0.008 ($n = 14$)	0.187[N.S.] 0.012 ($n = 14$)
Norepineph-rine brain stem	0.30 0.010 ($n = 13$)	0.326[N.S.] 0.029 ($n = 18$)	0.315 0.021 ($n = 18$)	0.362[N.S.] 0.015 ($n = 18$)	0.420 0.018 ($n = 16$)	0.472[N.S.] 0.025 ($n = 14$)	0.555 0.021 ($n = 14$)	0.559[N.S.] 0.029 ($n = 14$)
Dopamine Forebrain	0.232 0.010 ($n = 18$)	0.282** 0.013 ($n = 18$)	0.339 0.007 ($n = 16$)	0.348[N.S.] 0.007 ($n = 18$)	0.421 0.014 ($n = 14$)	0.470* 0.014 ($n = 14$)	0.419 0.012 ($n = 13$)	0.564* 0.022 ($n = 14$)

[a] Data are expressed in μg/g of wet tissue (n) in parentheses indicate numbers of animal. The asterisks denote significant differences. Control by Student's t test (** at least $p < 0.01$; * at least $p < 0.05$).

the present study (1, 8, 15, and 22 days), the concentration of 5HT is significantly higher in the IUGR rat. The concentration values have a parallel course compared to the concentrations obtained in the control rats.

In our study, the correlation coefficient between the brain weight and the amine has been found to be weak. We preferred then to express our results in micrograms per gram of tissue.

Cerebral catabolism of 5HT is more important in the young than in the adult rat. The very significant increase of 5HIAA observed in the IUGR rat from birth on until weaning, indicates that the speed of renewal of the neurotransmitters is higher in the IUGR rats. The increase of serotonin and its main metabolite in the brain should be seen in relation to the precursor, tryptophan; in newborn rat brains, tryptophan is 5–10 times higher than in the adult. In fact at birth, tryptophan is 90% free, whereas it is bound to albumin in the adult. It is known that only the free tryptophan could cross the hematoencephalic barrier and then contribute to the synthesis of 5HT.

Experimentally varying the concentrations of plasma tryptophan by overloading, one obtains, in general, an increase in endogenous 5HT with a parallel increase in 5HIAA.

In summary, any increase in the brain tryptophan, either directly or via any increase in plasma tryptophan, increases brain tryptophan and then serotonin. That relationship also exists in the IUGR rats, but with significantly higher values.

As for the so-called problem of acceleration of maturation, it should be emphasized that:

all IUGR rats opened their eyes one day before the control rats;

after daily injections of 5 HTP† to control rats, they opened their eyes one day in advance of the untreated animals (13th day instead of 14th in the control).

---

† 5HTP = Hydroxytryptophan, precursor of serotonin

We believe that this is a result of a modification of the neurochemical profile. As for the so-called acceleration of neurological maturation observed after stress during pregnancy, there are some reservations: We have never seen any advance in maturation in EEG tracings. As for the clinical advance, our collaborators find only a modification of passive tone not in the active tone. We think, therefore, that this concept is open to discussion and certainly not a proven one.

Finally it should be pointed out that serotonin may play a role in brain growth, in the differentiation of neurons. Thus, from the third week on in the rat[140] 5HT appears correlated with quiet sleep activity and catecholamines with paradoxical sleep.

At the present time, these investigations are only possible in experimental animals, but they indicate a line of thinking to be followed in developmental neurophysiology.

REFERENCES

1. Adlard, B. P. F., and Dobbing, J., Elevated cholinesterase activity in adult rat brain after undernutrition in early life. *Brain Res.* **30,** 198–199 (1971).
2. Adlard, B. P. F., and Dobbing, J., Vulnerability of developing brain. III. Development of four enzymes in the brains of normal and undernourished rats. *Brain Res.* **28,** 97–107 (1971).
3. Adlard, B. P. F., Dobbing, J., and Smart, J. L. Adult brain nerve-ending content and acetylcholinesterase activity in rats growth retarded for different periods in early life. *Biochem. Soc. Trans.* **2,** 124–127 (1974).
4. Aghajanian, G., and Bloom, F. E., The formation of synaptic junctions in developing rat brain: A quantitative electron microscopic study. *Brain Res.* **6,** 716 (1967).
5. Allen, E., The cessation of mitosis in the central nervous system of the albino rat. *J. Comp. Neurol.* **22,** 547 (1912).
6. Altman, J., Das, G. D., and Sudarshan, K., The influence of nutrition on neural and behavioral development. I. Critical review of some data on the growth of the body and the brain following dietary deprivation during gestation and lactation. *Dev. Psychobiol.* **3,** 281–301 (1970).
7. Anden, N-E., Dahlstrom, A., Fuxe, K., Larsson, K., Olson, L., and Ungerstedt, U., Ascending monoamine neurons to the telencephalon and diencephalon. *Acta Physiol. Scand.* **67,** 313–326 (1966).
8. Badger, T. M., and Tumbleson, M. E. Protein-calorie malnutrition in young miniature swine: Brain free amino acids. *J. Nutr.* **104,** 1329–1338 (1974).
9. Barnes, D., and Altman, J., Effects of different schedules of early undernutrition on the preweaning growth of the rat cerebellum. *Exp. Neurol.* **38,** 406–419 (1973).
10. Barnes, D., and Altman, J., Effect of two levels of gestational-lactational undernutrition on the postweaning growth of the rat cerebellum. *Exp. Neurol.* **38,** 420–428 (1973).
11. Bass, N. H., Netsky, M. G., and Young, E., Effect of neonatal malnutrition on developing cerebrum. I. Microchemical and histologic study of cellular differentiation in the rat. *Arch. Neurol.* **23,** 289–302 (1970).
12. Bass, N. H., Netsky, M. G., and Young, E., Effect of neonatal malnutrition on developing cerebrum. III. Micro-chemical and histologic study of myelin formation in the rat. *Arch. Neurol.* **23,** 303–313 (1970).
13. Benton, J. W., Moser, H. W., Dodge, P. R., and Carr, S., Modification of the schedule of myelination in the rat by early nutritional deprivation. *Pediatrics* **38,** 801–807 (1966).
14. Bloom, F. E., The formation of synaptic junctions in developing brain. In *Structure and Function of Synapses*, G. D. Pappas and D. P. Purpura (eds.), Raven Press, New York, 1972, pp. 101–120.

15. Bloom, F. E., Amino acids and polypeptides in neuronal function. *Neurosci. Res. Prog. Bull.* **10,** No. 2 (1973).

16. Bloom, F. E., and Aghajanian, G. K., Fine structural cytochemical analysis of the staining of synaptic junctions with phosphotungstic acid. *J. Ultrastruct. Res.* **22,** 361–375 (1968).

17. Borgman, R. F., Bursey, R. G., and Caffrey, B. C., Influence of dietary fat upon rats during gestation and lactation. *Am. J. Vet. Res.* **36,** 795–798 (1975).

18. Borgman, R. F., Bursey, R. G., and Caffrey, B. C., Influence of maternal dietary fat upon rat pups. *Am. J. Vet. Res.* **36,** 799–805 (1975).

19. Brown, R. E., Organ weight in malnutrition with special reference to brain weight. *Dev. Med. Child. Neurol.* **8,** 512–522 (1966).

20. Buchanan, A. R., and Roberts, J. E., Relative lack of myelin in optic tracts as result of underfeeding in the young albino rat. *Proc. Soc. Exp. Biol. Med.* **69,** 101–104 (1948).

21. Burns, E. M., Richards, J. G., and Kuhn, H., An ultrastructural investigation of the effect of perinatal malnutrition on E-PTA stained synaptic junctions. *Experientia* **32,** 1451–1453 (1975).

22. Burton, K., A study of the conditions and mechanisms of the diphenylamine reaction for the colorimetric estimation of deoxyribonucleic acid. *Biochem. J.* **62,** 315 (1956).

23. Chase, H. P., Lindsley, W. F. B., and O'Brien, D., Undernutrition and cerebellar development. *Nature (Lond.)* **221,** 554–555 (1968).

24. Cheney, D. L., Racagni, G., Zsilla, G., and Costa, E., Differences in the action of various drugs on striatal acetylcholine and choline content in rats killed by decipation or microwave radiation. *J. Pharm. Pharmacol.* **28,** 75–77 (1976).

25. Clos, J., Rebiere, A., and Legrand, J., Differential effects of hypothyroidism and undernutrition on the development of glia in the rat cerebellum. *Brain Res.* **63,** 445–449 (1973).

26. Cohen, E. L., and Wurtman, R. J., Brain acetylcholine: Control by dietary choline. *Science* **191,** 561–562 (1976).

27. Cragg, B. G., The development of cortical synapses during starvation in the rat. *Brain* **95,** 143–150 (1972).

28. Culley, W. J., and Lineberger, R. O., Effect of undernutrition on the size and composition of the rat brain. *J. Nutr.* **96,** 375–381 (1968).

29. Dalton, M. M., Hommes, O. R., and Leblond, C. P., Correlation of glial proliferation with age in the mouse brain. *J. Comp. Neurol.* **134,** 397 (1968).

30. Daly, M., Early stimulation of rodents: A critical review of present interpretations. *Br. J. Psychol.* **64,** 435–460 (1973).

31. Davidson, J. N., and Leslie, I., Nucleic acids in relation to issue growth: A review. *Cancer Res.* **10,** 587 (1950).

32. Dobbing, J., Effects of experimental undernutrition on development of the nervous system. In *Malnutrition, Learning, and Behavior*, N. S. Scrimshaw and J. Gordon (eds.), M.I.T. Press, Cambridge, 1968.

33. Dobbing, J., and Smart, J. L., Early undernutrition, brain development, and behavior. In *Ethology and Development*, S. A. Barnett (ed.), Lippincott, Philadelphia, 1973, pp. 16–36.

34. Dobbing, J., and Smart, J. L. Vulnerability of developing brain and behavior. *Br. Med. Bull.* **30,** 164–168 (1974).

35. Dobbing, J., and Widdowson, E., The effect of undernutrition and subsequent rehabilitation of myelination of rat brain as measured by its composition. *Brain* **88,** 357–366 (1965).

36. Dobbing, J., Hopewell, J. W., and Lynch, A., Vulnerability of developing brain. VII. Permanent deficit of neurons in cerebral and cerebellar cortex following early mild undernutrition. *Exp. Neurol.* **32,** 439–477 (1971).

37. Eayrs, J. T., and Horn, G., Development of cerebral cortex in hypothyroid and starved rats. *Anat. Rec.* **121,** 53 (1955).

38. Eckhert, C. D., Levitsky, D. A., and Barnes, R. H., Postnatal stimulation: The effects on cholinergic enzyme activity in undernourished rats. *Proc. Soc. Exp. Bio. Med.* **149,** 860–863 (1975).

39. Eidelberg, E., and Stein, D. G., Functional recovery after lesions of the nervous system. *Neurosci. Res. Prog. Bull.* **12,** No. 2 (1974).

40. Enesco, M., and Leblond, C. P., Increase in cell number as a factor in the growth of the organs of the young male rat. *J. Embryol. Exp. Morphol.* **10**, 530 (1962).
41. Engsner, G., Belete, S., Sjogren, I., and Vahlquist, B., Brain growth in children with marasmus. *Ups. J. Med. Sci.* **79**, 116–128 (1974).
42. Engsner, G., Hobte, D., Sjogren, I., and Vahlquist, B., Brain growth in children with kwashiorkor. *Acta Paediatr. Scand.* **63**, 687–694 (1974).
43. Enwonwu, C. O., and Worthington, B. S., Concentrations of histamine in brain of guinea pig and rat during dietary protein malnutrition. *Biochem. J.* **144**, 601–603 (1974).
44. Enwonwu, C. O., and Worthington, D. S., Elevation of brain histamine content in protein-deficient rats. *J. Neurochem.* **24**, 941–945 (1975).
45. Fernstrom, J. D., and Hirsch, M. J., Rapid repletion of brain serotonin in malnourished corn-fed rats following L-tryptophan injection. *Life Sci.* **17**, 455–464 (1975).
46. Fish, I., and Winick, M., Effect of malnutrition on regional growth of the developing rat brain. *Exp. Neurol.* **25**, 534–540 (1969).
47. Fishman, M. A., Prensky, A. L., and Dodge, P. R., Low content of cerebral lipids in infants suffering from malnutrition. *Nature (Lond.)* **221**, 552–553 (1969).
48. Fishman, M. A., Prensky, A. L., Tumbleson, M. E., and Daftari, B., Relative resistance of the later phase of myelination to severe undernutrition in miniature swine. *Am. J. Clin. Nutr.* **25**, 7–10 (1972).
49. Gaetani, S., Mengheri, E., Spadoni, M., Rossi, A., and Toschi, G., Effects of litter size on protein, choline acetyltransferase, and dopamine-β-hydroxylase of a mouse sympathetic ganglion. *Brain Res.* **86**, 75–84 (1975).
50. Gambetti, P., Autilio-Gambetti, L., Gonatas, N., Shafer, B., and Steiber, A., Synapses and malnutrition: Morphological and biochemical study of synaptosomal fractions from rat cerebral cortex. *Brain Res.* **47**, 477–484 (1972).
51. Gambetti, P., Autilio-Gambetti, L., Rizzuto, N., Shafer, B., and Pfaff, L., Synapses and malnutrition: Quantitative ultrastructural study of rat cerebral cortex. *Exp. Neurol.* **43**, 464–473 (1974).
52. Gourdon, J., Clos, J., Coste, C., Dainat, J., and Legrand, J., Comparative effects of hypothyroidism, hyperthyroidism, and undernutrition on the protein and nucleic acid content of the cerebellum in the young rat. *J. Neurochem.* **21**, 861–871 (1973).
53. Griffin, W. S. T., and Woodward, D. J., Neurological manifestations of undernutrition in rat cerebellum: A Golgi-Cox analysis (submitted for publication).
54. Griffin, W. S. T., Woodward, D. J., and Chanda, R., Malnutrition and brain development: Cerebellar weight, DNA, RNA, protein, and histological correlations (submitted for publication).
55. Guthrie, H. A., and Brown, M. L., Effect of severe undernutrition in early life on growth, brain size, and composition in adult rats. *J. Nutr.* **94**, 419–426 (1968).
56. Haltia, M., Postnatal development of spinal anterior horn neurons in normal and undernourished rats. *Acta Physiol. Scad. (suppl.)* 352 (1970).
57. Hatai, S., The effect of partial starvation on the brain of the white rat. *Am. J. Physiol.* **12**, 116 (1904).
58. Hatai, S., Effects of partial starvation followed by a return to normal diet on the growth of the body and central nervous system of albino rats. *Am. J. Physiol.* **18**, 309 (1907).
59. Hatai, S., Preliminary note on the size and condition of the central nervous system in albino rats severely stunted. *J. Comp. Neurol.* **18**, 151 (1908).
60. Heller, I. H., and Elliot, K. A. G., Desoxyribonucleic acid content and cell density in brain and human tumors. *Can. J. Biochem. Physiol.* **32**, 584–592 (1954).
61. Hernandez, R. J., Developmental pattern of the serotonin synthesizing enzyme in the brain of postnatally malnourished rats. *Experienta* **29**, 1487–1488 (1973).
62. Howard, E., and Granoff, D. M., Effect of neonatal food restriction in mice on brain growth, DNA, and cholesterol, and on adult delayed response learning. *J. Nutr.* **95**, 111–121 (1968).
63. Im, H. S., Barnes, R. H., and Levitsky, D. A., Postnatal malnutrition and brain cholinesterase in rats. *Nature (Lond.)* **233**, 269–270 (1971).

64. Im, H. S., Barnes, R. H., Levitsky, D. A., and Pond, W. G., Postnatal malnutrition and regional cholinesterase activities in brains of pigs. *Brain Res.* **63,** 461–465 (1973).
65. Jackson, C. M., and Stewart, C. A., The effects of inanition in the young upon the ultimate size of the body and of the various organs in the albino rat. *J. Exp. Zool.* **30,** 97–128 (1920).
66. Johnson, J. E., Jr., and Yoesle, R. A., The effects of malnutrition on the developing brain stem of the rat: A preliminary experiment using the lateral vestibular nucleus. *Brain Res.* **89,** 170–174 (1975).
67. Kasa, D., Histochemistry of choline acetyltransferase. In *Cholinergic Mechanisms,* P. G. Waser (ed.), Raven Press, New York, 1975, pp. 271–281.
68. Kissane, J. O., and Hawrylewicz, E. J., Development of Na^+-K^+-ATPase in neonatal rat brain synaptosomes after perinatal protein malnutrition. *Pediatr. Res.* **9,** 146–150 (1975).
69. Latham, M. C., Protein-calorie malnutrition in children and its relation to psychological development and behavior. *Physiol. Rev.* **54,** 541–565 (1974).
70. Lee, C-J., Catecholamine-binding brain protein in mice exposed to perinatal malnutrition and neonatal infection. *Pediatr. Res.* **9,** 645–652 (1975).
71. Lee, C-J., and Dubos, R., Lasting biological effects of early environmental influences. VIII. Effects of neonatal infection, perinatal malnutrition, and crowding on catecholamine metabolism of brain. *J. Exp. Med.* **36,** 1031–1042 (1972).
72. Lewis, P. D., Balazs, R., Patel, A. J., and Johnson, A. L., The effect of undernutrition in early life on cell generation in the rat brain. *Brain Res.* **83,** 235–247 (1975).
73. Lichtenteiger, W., Effect of endocrine manipulations on the metabolism of hypothalamic monoamines. In *Neurochemical Aspects of Hypothalamic Function,* L. Martini and J. Meites (eds.), Academic Press, New York, 1970, pp. 101–133.
74. Manocha, S. L., and Olkowski, Z., Cytochemistry of experimental protein malnutrition in primates: Effect on the spinal cord of the squirrel monkey *Siamiri sciureus. Histochem. J.* **4,** 531–544 (1972).
75. Manocha, S. L., and Olkowski, Z., Experimental protein malnutrition in primates: Cytochemical studies on the cerebellum of the squirrel monkey *Siamiri sciureus. Histochem. J.* **5,** 105–118 (1972).
76. Martes, M. P., Bauchy, M., and Schwartz, J. C., Histamine synthesis in the developing rat brain: Evidence for a multiple compartmentation. *Brain Res.* **83,** 261–275 (1975).
77. Munro, H. N., and Fleck, A., Analyis of tissues and body fluids for nitrogenous constituents. In *Mammalian Protein Metabolism.* H. N. Munro (ed.), Academic Press, New York, 1968, Vol. 3, p. 424.
78. Newton, G., and Levine, S. *Early Experience and Behavior.* Charles C Thomas, Springfield, Ill., 1968.
79. Ordy, J. M., Postnatal protein-calorie deficiency effects or learning and neurochemistry of infant monkeys (abstract). *Trans. Am. Soc. Neurochem.* **2,** 99 (1971).
80. Paoletti, R., and Galli, C., Effects of essential fatty acid deficiency on the central nervous system in the growing rat. In *Lipids, Malnutrition and the Developing Brain,* CIBA Foundation Symposium, Elsevier, Amsterdam, 1972, pp. 121–140.
81. Patel, A. J., Balazs, R., and Johnson, A. L., Effect of undernutrition on cell formation in the rat brain. *J. Neurochem.* **20,** 1151–1165 (1973).
82. Persson, L., and Sima, A., The effect of pre- and postnatal undernutrition on the development of the cerebellar cortex in the rat. II. Histochemical observations. *Neurobiology* **5,** 151–166 (1975).
83. Platt, B. S., Pampiglione, G., and Stewart, R. J. C., Experimental protein-calorie deficiency, clinical, EEG and neuropathological changes in pigs. *Dev. Med. Child Neurol.* **7,** 9 (1965).
84. Platt, B. S., and Stewart, R. J. C., Effects of protein-calorie deficiency on dogs. II. Morphological changes in the nervous system. *Dev. Med. Child Neurol.* **11,** 174–192 (1969).
85. Plaut, S. M., Studies on undernutrition in the young rat: Methodological considerations. *Dev. Psychobiol.* **3,** 157–167 (1970).
86. Prewitt, J. M. S., Reece, D. K., Hutchinson, G., and Jackson, C. K., *Decide: An Expandable System for Medical Decision-Making,* Informatique Médicale, Toulouse, 1974, pp. 153–182.

87. Pysh, J. J., and Perkins, R. E., Undernutrition and Purkinje cell development. *Neurosci. Abstr.* **1,** 756 (1975).

88. Rajalakshmi, R., Parameswaran, M., Telang, S. D., and Ramakrishnan, C. V., Effect of undernutrition and protein deficiency on glutamate dehydrogenase and decarboxylase in rat brain. *J. Neurochem.* **23,** 129–133 (1974).

89. Reis, D. J., Weinbren, M., and Corvelli, A., A circadian rhythm of norepinephrine regionally in rat brain: Its relationship to environmental lighting and to regional diurnal variations in brain serotonin. *J. Pharmacol. Exp. Ther.* **164,** 135–145 (1968).

90. Richter, D., and Crossland, J., Variation in acetylcholine content of brain with physiological state. *Am. J. Physiol.* **159,** 247–255 (1949).

91. Roeder, L. M., and Chow, B. P., Pituitary hormone regulated systems of the progeny of underfed dams. In *Endocrinology, Proceedings of IV International Congress of Endocrinology,* R. O. Scow (ed.), Excerpta Medica, Amsterdam, 1973, pp. 1091–1097.

92. Rossier, J., Bauman, A., Rieger, F., and Benda, P., Immunological studies on the enzymes of the cholinergic system. In *Cholinergic Mechanisms,* D. G. Waser (ed.), Raven Press, New York, 1975, pp. 283–293.

93. Rozovski, J., Noroa, F., Arbarzua, J., and Monckeberg, F., Cranial transillumination in early and severe malnutrition. *Br. J. Nutr.* **25,** 107–111 (1971).

94. Schonback, J., Hu, K. H., and Friede, R., Cellular and chemical changes during myelination: Histologic, autoradiographic, histochemical, and biochemical data on myelination in the pyramidal tract and corpus callosum of rat. *J. Comp. Neurol.* **134,** 21 (1968).

95. Schwartz, J. C., Lampart, C., and Rose, C., Histamine formation in rat brain *in vivo*. Effects of histidine loads. *J. Neurochem.* **19,** 801–810 (1972).

96. Segal, D. S., Sullivan, J. L., Kuczenski, R. T., and Mandell, A. J., Effects on long-term reserpine treatment on brain tyrosine hydroxylase and behavioral activity. *Science* **173,** 847–849 (1971).

97. Selivonchick, D. P., and Johnston, P. V., Fat deficiency in rats during development of the central nervous system and susceptibility to experimental allergic encephalomyelitis. *J. Nutr.* **105,** 288–300 (1975).

98. Sereni, F., Principi, N., Perletti, L., and Piceni-Sereni, L., Undernutrition and developing rat brain. I. Influence on acetylcholinesterase and succinic acid dehydrogenase activities and on norepinephrine and 5-OH-tryptamine tissue concentrations. *Biol. Neonate* **10,** 254–265 (1966).

99. Shambaugh, G. E., and Wilber, J. F., The effect of caloric deprivation upon thyroid function in the neonatal rat. *Endocrinology* **94,** 1145–1149 (1974).

100. Shoemaker, W. J., The effect of perinatal undernutrition on the metabolism of catecholamines in the rat brain. Doctoral thesis, M.I. T., Cambridge, Mass., 1971.

101. Shoemaker, W. J., and Bloom, F. E., A quantitative electronmicroscopic study of undernourished rat brain utilizing ethanolic phosphotungstic acid (in preparation).

102. Shoemaker, W. J., and Dallman, M. F., Pituitary-adrenal function in perinatally undernourished rats. *Fed. Proc.* **32,** 909 (1973).

103. Shoemaker, W. J., and Wurtman, R. J., Perinatal undernutrition: Accumulation of catecholamines in rat brain. *Science* **171,** 1017–1019 (1971).

104. Shoemaker, W. J., and Wurtman, R. J., Effect of perinatal undernutrition on the metabolism of catecholamines in the rat brain. *J. Nutr.* **103,** 1537–1547 (1973).

105. Shoemaker, W. J., Coyle, J. T., Jr., and Bloom, F. E., Perinatal undernutrition. Effect of neurotransmitters, transmitter synthetic enzymes, and the number of synaptic connections. *Trans. Am. Soc. Neurochem.* **4,** 100 (1974).

106. Shrader, R. E., and Zeman, F. J., Effect of maternal protein deprivation on morphological and enzymatic development of neonatal rat tissue. *J. Nutr.* **99,** 401–421 (1969).

107. Siassi, F., and Siassi, B., Differential effects of protein-calorie restriction and subsequent repletion on neuronal and nonneuronal components of cerebral cortex in newborn rats. *J. Nutr.* **103,** 1625–1633 (1973).

108. Sima, A., Relation between the number of myelin lamellae and axon circumference in fibers of ventral and dorsal roots and optic nerve in normal undernourished and rehabilitated rats. *Acta Physiol. Scand.* (Suppl.) 410 (1974).

109. Sima, A., and Persson, L., The effect of pre- and postnatal undernutrition on the development of the rat cerebellar cortex. I. Morphological observations. *Neurobiology* **5,** 23–24 (1975).

110. Sobotka, T. J., Cook, M. P., and Brodie, R. E., Neonatal malnutrition: Neurochemical, hormonal, and behavioral manifestations. *Brain Res.* **65,** 443–457 (1974).

111. Sourander, P., Sima, A., and Haltia, M., Malnutrition and morphological development of the nervous system. In *Early Malnutrition and Mental Development Symposia of the Swedish Nutrition Foundation XII,* J. Cravioto, I. Hambraeus, and B. Vahlquist (eds.), Almquist and Wiksell, Stockholm, 1974, pp. 39–64.

112. Stern, W. C., Forbes, W. B., Resnick, O., and Morgane, P. J., Seizure susceptibility and brain amine levels following protein malnutrition during the development in the rat. *Brain Res.* **79,** 375–384 (1974).

113. Stern, W. C., Miller, M., Forbes, W. B., Morgane, P. J., and Resnick, O., Ontogeny of the levels of biogenic amines in various parts of the brain and in peripheral tissues in normal and protein malnourished rats. *Exp. Neurol.* **49,** 314–326 (1975).

114. Stewart, C. A., Weights of various parts of the brain in normal and underfed albino rats at different ages. *J. Comp. Neurol.* **29,** 511 (1918).

115. Stewart, C. A., Changes in the relative weights of the various parts, systems and organs of young albino rats underfed for various periods. *J. Exp. Zool.* **25,** 301 (1918).

116. Stewart, R. J. C., Merat, A., and Dickerson, J. W. T., Effect of a low protein diet in mother rats on the structure of the brains of the offspring. *Biol. Neonate* **25,** 425–434 (1974).

117. Sugita, N., Comparative studies on the growth of the cerebral cortex. VII. On the influence of starvation at an early age upon the development of the cerebral cortex: albino rat. *J. Comp. Neurol.* **29,** 177–242 (1918).

118. Tigner, J. C., and Barnes, R. H., Effect of postnatal malnutrition on plasma corticosteroid levels in male albino rats. *Proc. Soc. Exp. Biol. Med.* **149,** 80–82 (1975).

119. Treherne, J. E., The nutrition of the central nervous system in the cockroach, *Periplanta americana* L: The exchange and metabolism of sugars. *J. Exp. Biol.* **37,** 513–533 (1960).

120. Tricklebank, M. D., and Adlard, B. P. F., Regional brain 5-hydroxytryptamine turnover in adult rats growth retarded in early life. *Biochem. Soc. Trans.* **2,** 127–129 (1974).

121. Weiner, N., Regulation of norepinephrine biosynthesis. *Annu. Rev. Pharmacol.* **10,** 273 (1970).

122. Weiner, S. G., Post-weaning rehabilitation of catecholamine levels in the rat brain and heart after perinatal undernutrition. Master's thesis, M.I.T., Cambridge, Mass., 1972.

123. Wiggins, R. C., Benjamins, J. A., Krigman, M. R., and Morell, P., Synthesis of myelin proteins during starvation. *Brain Res.* **80,** 345–349 (1974).

124. Wigglesworth, V. B., The nutrition of the central nervous system in the cockroach, *Periplanta americana* L: The role of perineurium and glial cells in the mobilization of reserves. *J. Exp. Biol.* **37,** 500–512 (1960).

125. Winick, M., Fetal malnutrition and growth process. *Hosp. Pract.* **5,** 33 (1970).

126. Winick, M., and Noble, A., Quantitative changes in DNA, RNA, and protein during prenatal and postnatal growth in the rat. *Dev. Biol.* **12,** 451 (1965).

127. Winick, M., and Noble, A., Cellular response in rats during malnutrition at various ages. *J. Nutr.* **89,** 300–306 (1966).

128. Winick, M., and Rosso, P., The effect of severe early malnutrition on cellular growth of human brain. *Pediatr. Res.* **3,** 181 (1969).

129. Winick, M., Fish, I., and Rosso, P., Cellular recovery in rat tissues after a brief period of neonatal malnutrition. *J. Nutr.* **95,** 623 (1968).

130. Winick, M., Rosso, P., and Waterlow, J., Cellular growth of cerebrum, cerebellum, and brain stem in normal and marasmic children. *Exp. Neurol.* **26,** 393–400 (1970).

131. Wood, J. G., Positive identification of intracellular biogenic amine reaction product with electron microscopic x-ray analysis. *J. Histochem. Cytochem.* **22,** 1060–1063 (1974).

132. Wood, J. G., Use of the analytical electron microscope (AFM) in cytochemical studies of the central nervous system. *Histochemistry* **41,** 233–240 (1975).

133. Wurtman, R. J., and Fernstrom, J. D., L-Tryptophan, L-tyrosine, and the control of brain monoamine biosynthesis. In *Perspectives in Neuropharmacology,* S. J. Synder (ed.), Oxford University Press, New York, 1972, pp. 143–193.

134. Yu, M. C., Lee, J. C., and Bakay, L., The ultrastructure of the rat central nervous system in chronic undernutrition. *Acta Neuropathol.* **30**, 197–210 (1974).
135. Zamenhof, S., Van Marthens, E., and Margolis, F., DNA (cell number) and protein in neonatal brain: Alteration by maternal dietary protein restriction. *Science* **160**, 322–323 (1968).
136. Salas, M., Diaz, S., and Nieto, A., Effects of neonatal food deprivation on cortical spines and dendritic development of the rat. *Brain Res.* **73**, 139–144 (1974).
137. Cordero, M. E., Diaz, G., and Araya, J., Neocortex development during severe malnutrition in the rat. *Am. J. Clin. Nutrition* **29**, 358–365 (1976).
138. Greenough, W. T., and Volkmar, F. R., Pattern of dendritic branching in occipital cortex of rats reared in complex environments. *Exp. Neurol.* **40**, 491–504 (1973).
139. Greenough, W. T., Volkmar, F. R., and Juraska, J. M., Effects of rearing complexity on dendritic branching in frontolateral and temporal cortex of the rat. *Exp. Neurol.* **41**, 371–378 (1973).
140. Adrien, J., Bourgoin, S., and Hamon, M., Midbrain raphe lesion in the newborn rat. *J. Neurophys. Brain Res.* **127**, 99–110 (1977).
141. Bourgoin, S., Faivre-Bauman, A., Hery, F., Ternaux, J. P., and Hamon, M., Characteristics of Tryptophan binding in the serum of the newborn rat. *Biol. Neonat.* **31**, 141–154 (1977).
142. Hamon, M., Bourgoin, S., Morot-Gaudry, Y., Hery, F., and Glowinski, J., Role of active transport of tryptophan in the control of 5-HT biosynthesis. In *Serotonin—New Vistas*, E. Costa, G. L. Gessa, and M. Sandler (eds.), Raven Press, New York, 1974, Vol. 11, pp. 153–162.
143. Hamon, M., and Glowinski, J., Regulation of serotonin synthesis. *Life Sci.* **15**, 1533–1548 (1974).
144. Lauder, J. M., and Krebs, H., Serotonin as a differentiation signal in early neurogenesis. *Devel. Neurosc.* **1**, 15–30 (1978).
145. Minkowski, A., Roux, J. M., Tordet-Caridroit, C., Pathophysiologic changes in Intra Uterine Malnutrition. In *Nutrition and Fetal Development*, M. Winick (ed.), Wiley, New York, 1974.
146. Morgane, P. J., Miller, M., Kemper, T., Stern, W., Forbes, W., Hall, R., Bronzino, J., Kissane, J., Hawrylewicz, E., and Resnick, O., The effects of protein malnutrition or the developing central nervous system in the rat. *Neurosci. Biobehav. Rev.* **2**, 137–221 (1978).
147. Roux, J. M., Chanez-Bel, C., Degremont, C., Gaben-Cogneville, A. M., Fulchignoni-Lataud, M.C., Swierczewski, E., Tordet-Caridroit, C., Minkowski, A., Effect of Intrauterine growth retardation on cellular proliferation and differentiation in developing rat. *Ann. Biol. Anim. Bioch. Biophys.* **19**, 135–150 (1979).
148. Shaywitz, S. E., Cohen, D. J., and Shaywitz, B. A., The biochemical basis of minimal brain dysfunction. *J. Pediatr.* **92**, 179–187 (1978).
149. Yuwiler, A., Conversion of D and L trytophan to brain serotonin and 5-hydroxy-indoacetic acid and to blood serotonin. *J. Neurochem.* **20**, 1099–1109 (1973).

3

The Effect of Maternal Stress and General Anesthesia on Plasma Catecholamines and Uterine Blood Flow in the Pregnant Ewe

SOL M. SHNIDER, M.D.[1] and DIANE R. BIEHL, M.D.[2]

INTRODUCTION

Adrenergic stimulation can constrict uterine vessels and reduce uterine blood flow.[1-8] High blood epinephrine levels achieved by inadvertent intravascular injection produce alpha effects with consequent uterine vasoconstriction, increase in uterine activity, and decrease in uterine blood flow. In ewes given 0.10–1.00 μg/kg/min epinephrine, maternal blood pressure rose to 50–65% above control values, and uterine blood flow was reduced 55–75%.[6]

Exogenous norepinephrine infusion[9] or electrical stimulation of the major sympathetic branch of the hypogastric plexus[4] also significantly reduces uterine blood flow in the pregnant ewe.

In pregnant monkeys anesthetized with pentobarbitol, fetuses regularly develop hypoxia, acidosis, and bradycardia as the monkeys are awakening.[10] These changes are reversed by reestablishing anesthesia.

It now appears that maternal stress, anxiety, and pain may adversely affect the fetus. The result of such stress may be an increase in the rate of spontaneous abortion,[11-14] premature delivery or fetal growth retardation,[15-18] or perinatal death.[19-21] The cause of the fetal compromise induced by maternal anxiety probably involves a number of factors, including abnormal metabolism of

[1] Professor of Anesthesia, Obstetrics, Gynecology and Reproductive Sciences, University of California—San Francisco, California 94143
[2] Assistant Professor of Anesthesia and Perinatology, St. Boniface Hospital, Winnipeg, Canada

corticoids and other steroid hormones, or of protein hormones from the central nervous system. Increased maternal secretion of catecholamines with a consequent decrease in uteroplacental blood flow may also be a factor. We have recently reported the relationship between stress, endogenous catecholamines, and uterine blood flow.[22]

Eight awake, unmedicated pregnant ewes near term (mean gestational age 133 days, range 124–138 days, term 147–150 days) were studied. At least 24 hr before each study a preparatory surgical procedure was performed. During halothane-oxygen anesthesia, the gravid uterus was exposed and a fetal hind limb extracted through a small hysterotomy. A polyvinyl catheter (#4 French, 0.048″ OD) was inserted into a hind-limb artery, and the limb returned to the uterus. The fetal catheter was used for monitoring arterial blood presure, heart rate, and acid-base status. A polyvinyl catheter (#8 French, 0.105″ OD) was inserted into the uterine cavity to allow amniotic fluid pressure measurement, and the uterine incision was closed. Through the abdominal incision, a Statham precalibrated, electromagnetic flow probe was secured on a main branch of the uterine artery supplying the pregnant horn. Polyvinyl #8-French catheters were placed in the maternal aorta via a femoral artery and the inferior vena cava via a femoral vein. The maternal-artery catheter allowed measurement of blood-gas and norepinephrine values, blood pressure, and heart rate. Fluids were infused via the femoral-vein catheter.

Fetal and maternal blood pressure and heart rate values and amniotic fluid pressure were measured continuously using Statham P23DC strain gauges connected to a Grass polygraph recorder. Fetal blood pressure was corrected by subtracting intra-amniotic fluid pressure from the recorded fetal-artery pressure. Uterine blood flow was measured continuously with a Statham SP2022 blood-flowmeter with a nonocclusive zero. Arterial blood-gas values were measured immediately after sampling* and were corrected for body temperature, measured by a Yellow Springs rectal probe. Base excess values were calculated using the Severinghaus slide rule. Hemoglobin concentration was determined using a cyanmethemoglobin method and spectrophotometer (Bausch and Lomb Spectronic 20).

Prior to all studies, maternal and fetal acid-base status, heart rate, blood pressure, maternal temperature, feeding habits, and general physical status appeared normal. At the beginning of each study the animal was placed in the left lateral position and oxygen was administered by face mask to prevent hypoxia from atelectasis. Following a 30-min control period of stable maternal and fetal cardiovascular and acid-base values, we examined the effects of maternal stress. We induced maternal stress by applying a uniform electrical stimulus of 30 V at a frequency of 167 Hz to the ewe's skin for 30–60 sec (Model PS-50X, Winston Electronics Co., Box 16156, San Francisco, California). All sheep were thus stressed on two occasions separated by an interval of at least 15 min to allow all values to return to control levels. We obtained maternal plasma from the electrically stimulated ewes during and 1, 3, and 10 min

---

* Instrumentation Laboratory 313 Blood Gas Analyzer

following this stress for measurement of norepinephrine levels using a radio-isotopic enzymatic assay.[23]

Control values for maternal and fetal blood pressure, heart rate, and uterine blood flow were means of six determinations made at 5-min intervals. Control values for maternal and fetal arterial blood acid-base status and maternal norepinephrine levels were the means of two determinations taken at 15-min intervals. During and following maternal stress, cardiovascular values reported were those found at the time of the maximum maternal blood pressure response during stress and 1, 3, 5, and 10 min later. Acid-base data reported following stress were obtained 10 min after each stress episode. Results from each animal were averaged, and cardiovascular and norepinephrine values were presented as percentage changes from control.

Analysis of variance, one-way classification, was used to examine the cardiovascular and norepinephrine data for statistical analysis. The Student t test was used for the acid-base data, and regression analysis was used where indicated. $P < 0.05$ was considered significant.

Control values for cardiovascular, acid-base and plasma norepinephrine data are given in Table I. The maximum maternal cardiovascular response occurred 30–45 sec after initiation of an electrical stimulus. At this time plasma norepinephrine levels were increased 25%, with an associated increase in maternal blood pressure of 50% and a decrease in uterine blood flow of 52% (Fig. 1). In every animal, stimulation produced a simultaneous increase in plasma norepinephrine and decrease in uterine blood flow. At 3 min uterine blood flow and blood pressure had returned to control values, while norepinephrine levels were still increased. Ten minutes after electrical stimulation plasma norepinephrine had returned to control values. Regression analysis indicated a significant correlation between increase in plasma norepinephrine ($r = 0.76$) (Fig. 2) and the simultaneous decrease in uterine flow during and after acute maternal stress. Maternal and fetal acid-base status and fetal heart rate were

TABLE I

Control Data

Maternal			
Blood pressure (torr)	107	±	7
Uterine blood flow (ml/min)	548	±	37
Heart rate (beats/min)	92	±	4
Arterial blood norepinephrine (pg/ml)	1886	±	601
pH	7.47 ±		0.01
PCO_2 (torr)	36	±	1
Base excess (mEq/liter)	−2.2	±	1.2
PO_2 (torr)	265	±	22
Fetal			
Blood pressure (torr)	59	± 5	
Heart rate (beats/min)	153	± 8	
pH	7.34 ± 0.01		
PCO_2 (torr)	45	± 2	
Base excess (mEq/liter)	−1.1	± 1.0	
PO_2 (torr)	25	± 1	

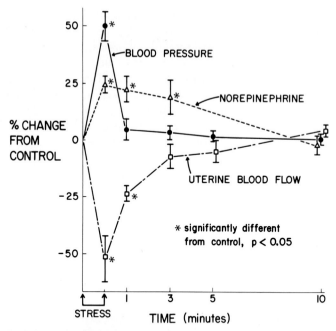

Fig. 1. Effects of electrically induced stress (30–60 sec) on maternal mean arterial blood pressure, plasma norepinephrine levels, and uterine blood flow. All values subsequent to control are given as mean percentage changes ±SE. Reprinted by permission from Shnider, *et al*, Uterine blood flow and plasma norepinephrine changes during maternal stress in the pregnant ewe. *Anesthesiology* **50**, 524–527 (1979).

unchanged following stress. Fetal blood pressure increased 9% during stress and returned to the control level 1 min later.

EFFECTS OF GENERAL ANESTHESIA

In a subsequent series of experiments we studied the effects of general anesthesia on uterine blood flow and plasma norepinephrine. Anesthetic agents modify sympathetic activity. Halothane reduces plasma norepinephrine in rats[23] and nitrous oxide increases serum norepinephrine in human volunteers.[24] We postulated that nitrous oxide anesthesia may decrease uterine blood flow through elevation of endogenous norepinephrine and that this potentially deleterious effect might be avoided by the addition of low concentrations of halothane or enflurane. Using our chronic maternal fetal sheep preparation described above, we performed the following experiments in 12 pregnant sheep near term.

Following a 30-min control period with the animal lying quietly on her side breathing 100% oxygen, anesthesia was induced with thiopental 4 mg/kg. Intubation was facilitated with 0.25 mg/kg of succinylcholine. On separate days anesthesia was maintained by positive pressure ventilation with one of three anesthetic mixtures, N_2O 50% or N_2O 50% and halothane 0.5% or N_2O

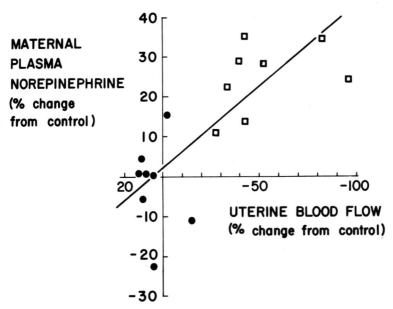

Fig. 2. Least-square regression of maternal norepinephrine on uterine blood flow. Simultaneous changes in each of eight animals in maternal norepinephrine levels and uterine blood flow during the period of electrically induced maternal stress, indicated by open box □, and 10 min later during recovery, indicated by closed circles ●. Regression line slope = 0.370. Regression line Y intercept = 2.563. $r = 0.76$; $P < 0.05$. Reprinted by permission from Shnider, *et al.*, Uterine blood flow and plasma norepinephrine changes during maternal stress in the pregnant ewe. *Anesthesiology* **50**, 524–527 (1979).

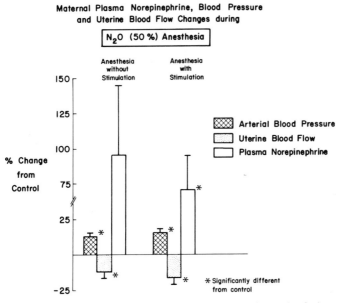

Fig. 3. Effects of nitrous oxide anesthesia, with and without noxious stimulation, on maternal plasma norepinephrine, blood pressure, and uterine blood flow in the pregnant ewe. Reprinted by permission from Shnider, S. M., and Levinson, G., Inhalation Analgesia and Anesthesia for Vaginal Delivery, in *Anesthesia for Obstetrics*, Shnider, S. M., and Levinson, G., Eds. The Williams and Wilkins Co., Baltimore, 1979.

50% and enflurane 1.0%. Each study consisted of two sequential periods of 30 min each: a period of anesthesia with noxious stimulation superimposed (electrical stimulation, see above) and a period of anesthesia without noxious stimulation. Selection of anesthesia and sequence of the two periods were randomly assigned.

RESULTS

Intravenous induction with thiopental followed by direct laryngoscopy and endotracheal intubation resulted in an increase in plasma norepinephrine of 89% from control. Blood pressure rose 65%, uterine blood flow fell 24%, and uterine vascular resistance rose 42%. These acute cardiovascular changes quickly diminished with termination of airway manipulation. Noxious stimulation during $N_2O:O_2$ anesthesia was associated with an increase in maternal blood pressure of 15%, a decrease in uterine blood flow of 16%, and an increase in plasma norepinephrine of 71% from the awake control state (Fig. 3). By contrast noxious stimulation during $N_2O:O_2$ anesthesia that was supplemented with either 0.5% halothane or 1% enflurane did not increase plasma catecholamines. Blood pressure remained unchanged in both groups and uterine blood flow increased 22% with halothane but did not change with enflurane.

DISCUSSION

If maternal stress causes catecholamine release and thereby decreases uterine blood flow, then maternal stress may represent a preventable cause of fetal distress. We found that the discomfort produced by a uniform electric stimulus resulted in maternal hypertension and decreased uterine blood flow. Norepinephrine levels were consistently increased. We did not, however, find that maternal stress compromised fetal well-being. This is not surprising, since healthy lamb fetuses do not undergo hypoxemia or acidosis with *transient* profound depressions of uterine blood flow.[25] However, an already compromised fetus will not tolerate even a minimal decrease in uterine blood flow. Myers reported that hypoxic and acidotic fetuses became more hypoxic and acidotic during acute maternal psychological stress. Morishima, et al.[26] studied the effects of maternal agitation, induced by exposure to bright light, upon fetal well-being in pregnant rhesus monkeys. Fetuses were classified as "healthy" or "asphyxiated" according to their initial acid-base status. While both groups showed decreases in arterial oxygenation, more profound hypoxia was seen in the "asphyxiated" group, and recovery was slower.

Based on our studies and those of others we postulate that prevention of maternal stress during labor may contribute to the normal maintenance of uteroplacental blood flow. In a recent study, Lederman, et al.[27] suggested that patients given regional anesthesia during labor tended to have lower levels of plasma epinephrine following the block. These investigators, however, studied only two patients given epidural anesthesia during labor and six given spinal anesthesia for delivery. With this small population, statistically significant differences could not be demonstrated, nor did these investigators relate catecholamine levels to the clinical and biochemical conditions of the newborn. The relationship of obstetric anesthesia to maternal plasma catecholamines and fetal and neonatal health deserves further investigation.

In the pregnant ewe it is apparent that the addition of halothane or enflurane to nitrous oxide prevents the elevation of plasma norepinephrine associated with the use of nitrous oxide alone.

REFERENCES

1. Ahlquist, R. P., and Woodbury, R. A., Influence of drugs and uterine activity upon uterine blood flow. *Fed. Proc.* **6**, 305 (1947).
2. Berry, F. A. Jr., Vasopressors in pregnancy. *Va. Med. Mon.* **94**, 697–701 (1967).
3. Greiss, F. C., Jr., A clinical concept of uterine blood flow during pregnancy. *Obstet. Gynecol.* **30**, 595–603 (1967).
4. Greiss, F. C., Jr., and Gobble, F. L., Jr., Effect of sympathetic nerve stimulation on the uterine vascular bed. *Am. J. Obstet. Gynecol.* **97**, 962–967 (1967).
5. Greiss, F. C., Jr., and Pick, J. R., Jr., The uterine vascular bed: Adrenergic receptors. *Obstet. Gynecol.* **23**, 209–213 (1964).
6. Greiss, F. C., Jr., The uterine vascular bed: Effect of adrenergic stimulation. *Obstet. Gynecol.* **21**, 295–301 (1963).
7. Martin, C. B., Jr., and Gingerick, B., Uteroplacental physiology. *J. Obstet. Gynecol. Nurs. (suppl.)* **5**, 16–25 (1976).
8. Nimwegan, D. V., and Dyer, D. C., The action of vasopressors on isolated uterine arteries. *Am. J. Obstet. Gynecol.* **118**, 1099–1103 (1974).
9. Barton, M. D., Killam, A. P., and Meschia, G., Response of ovine uterine blood flow to epinephrine and norepinephrine. *Proc. Soc. Exp. Biol. Med.* **145**, 996–1003 (1974).
10. Myers, R. E., Maternal psychological stress and fetal asphyxia: A study in the monkey. *Am. J. Obstet. Gynecol.* **122**, 47–59 (1975).
11. Janert, C. T., Repeated abortion. *Obstet. Gynecol.* **3**, 420–433 (1954).
12. Berle, B. B., and Janert, C. T., Stress and habitual abortion: Their relationship and the effect of therapy. *Obstet. Gynecol.* **3**, 298–306 (1954).
13. James, W. H., The problem of spontaneous abortion. X. The efficacy of psychotherapy. *Am. J. Obstet. Gynecol.* **85**, 38–40 (1963).
14. Tupper, C., and Weil, R. J., The problem of spontaneous abortion. IX. The treatment of habitual aborters by psychotherapy. *Am. J. Obstet. Gynecol.* **83**, 421–424 (1962).
15. Shaw, J. A., Wheeler, P., and Morgan, D. W., Mother-infant relationship and weight gain in the first months of life. *J. Am. Acad. Child. Psychiatr.* **9**, 428–444 (1970).
16. Sontag, L. W., Effect of fetal activity on the nutritional state of the infant at birth. *Am. J. Dis. Child.* **60**, 621–630 (1940).
17. Smith, D. J., Jaffe, J. M., and Heseltine, G. F. D., Modification of prenatal stress effects in rats by adrenalectomy, dexamethasone and chlorpromazine. *Fed. Proc.* **33**, 223 (1974).
18. Myers, R. E., The pathology of the rhesus monkey placenta. *Acta Endocrinol. (Suppl.)* **166**, 221–257 (1972).
19. Hockman, C. H., Prenatal maternal stress in the rat: Its effects on emotional behavior in the offspring. *J. Comp. Physiol. Psychol.* **54**, 679–684 (1961).
20. Caldwell, D. F., Stillbirths from adrenal demedullated mice subjected to chronic stress throughout gestation. *J. Embryol. Exp. Morphol.* **10**, 471–475 (1962).
21. James, W. H., The effect of maternal psychological stress on the fetus. *Br. J. Psychiatr.* **115**, 811–825 (1969).
22. Shnider, S. M., Wright, R. G., Levinson, G., *et al.*, Uterine blood flow and plasma norepinephrine changes during maternal stress in the pregnant ewe. *Anesthesiology* **50**, 524–527 (1979).
23. Roizen, M. F., Moss, J., Henry, D. P., *et al.*, Effects of halothane on plasma catecholamines. *Anesthesiology* **41**, 432–439 (1974).

24. Smith, N. T., Eger, E. I., II, Stoelting, R. K., *et al.*, The cardiovascular and sympathomimetic response to the addition of nitrous oxide to halothane in man. *Anesthesiology* **32,** 410–421 (1970).
25. Ralston, D. H., Shnider, S. M., and deLorimier, A. A., Effects of equipotent ephedrine, metaraminol, mephentermine and methoxamine on uterine blood flow in the pregnant ewe. *Anesthesiology* **40,** 354–370 (1974).
26. Morishima, H. O., Pedersen, H., and Finster, M., The influence of maternal psychological stress on the fetus. *Am. J. Obstet. Gynecol.* **131,** 286–290, 1978.
27. Lederman, R. P., McCann, D. S., Work, B., *et al.*, Endogenous plasma epinephrine and norepinephrine in last-trimester pregnancy and labor. *Am. J. Obstet. Gynecol.* **129,** 5–8 (1977).

4

Perinatal Effects of Analgesia

G. PONTONNIER, H. GRANDJEAN, J. de MOUZON, and
R. DESPRATS

Obstetrical analgesic techniques are generally used to resolve various types of pathological labours. The main indications are maternal agitation, with or without functional dystocia, and optimal conditions for trial labour in cases of borderline pelvis. These techniques are now increasingly offered to improve maternal comfort, even in the case of normal labour. It is therefore important to objectively measure their consequences on the fetus. These are the reasons why we performed two successive studies using phenoperidine and peridural analgesia.

Initially we studied the perinatal effects of both analgesic techniques as they are used daily for varied indications, with nonselected patients. Then a randomised trial on preselected normal cases was performed to compare both techniques and evaluate their perinatal effects.

The methodology used to evaluate the perinatal effects of analgesics were the same in both groups. It is based on the records of fetal and neonatal parameters which can be modified in the case of fetal anoxia: fetal heart rate, pH and PCO_2. These parameters were measured within 30 min before analgesia, then during the analgesia. The interpretation of the fetal heart rate curve is done with reference to the intra-amniotic pressure which is simultaneously recorded, studying fetal heart rate between contractions and possible bradycardia induced by contractions. These bradycardias are of two types: early deceleration of Hon or DIP I of Caldeyro Barcia, and late deceleration or DIP II. pH and PCO_2 are simultaneously measured on the mother's finger tip and on the fetal scalp, at birth on the umbilical vessels, then on the heel during the first 2 hr of life. The Apgar score is performed at the first and fifth minutes, and the clinical behaviour of the newborn child is evaluated during the first 6 days.

Inserm U. 168, Hôpital La Grave, 31 052 Toulouse Cédex, France

I. PERINATAL EFFECT OF ANALGESIA IN NONSELECTED CASES

Material and Methods

Sixty-five women received neuroleptanalgesia with intravenous injection of 0.5 mg of atropine and of 10 mg of droperidol and, after 10 min, successive injections of 0.5 mg of phenoperidine approximately every 10 min until disappearance of pain.[3] Analgesia was then maintained by intravenous injection of 0.5 mg of phenoperidine every 20 min. All the women breathed an oxygen enriched mixture through a nasal catheter, at a flow of 3–5 liters of humidified oxygen per minute.

Forty-three women had peridural analgesia achieved by the injection of 12 ml of local anesthesic into the epidural space. Three different drugs were used: lidocaine at 1.5%, with epinephrine at 1/200,000 (nine cases), bupivacaine at 0.5% (18 cases), bupivacaine at 0.5% with epinephrine at 1/200,000 (16 cases). Reinjections of 6 ml of the same product were given when pain reappeared.[8]

Analgesic indications decided by the supervising obstetrical team are summarised in Table I.

The results were interpreted by comparison to a group of normal labours previously studied by the same team.[5]

Results

Spontaneous delivery was obtained in 51% of peridural analgesia cases and in only 12% of the neuroleptanalgesia cases (Table I). In this last series the number of Cesarean sections is high (26%), due to the high proportion of pathological labours.

Evolution of the perinatal parameters is shown in Table II. For the series of peridural analgesia, results concerning the three drugs have been compiled together since the differences between them were very slight and not significant.

Mean basal fetal heart rate was identical in both types of analgesia and

TABLE I

Clinical Data of the First Study

	Neuroleptanalgesia 65 Cases		Peridural Analgesia 43 Cases	
	(*n*)	(%)	(*n*)	(%)
Indication				
Functional dystocia	23	35		
Borderline pelvis	17	26	6	14
Agitation	12	19	11	26
Maternal comfort	13	20	26	60
Method of delivery				
Spontaneous delivery	8	12	22	51
Instrumental extraction	40	62	19	44
Cesarean section	17	26	2	5

TABLE II

Fetal Parameters of the First Study (Mean ± Standard Deviation)

	Neuroleptanalgesia	Peridural Analgesia	Normal Labour Dilatation	
FHR				
Before	142 ± 13	144 ± 13	4–6 cm	138 ± 12
During	146 ± 12	143 ± 12	8–10 cm	136 ± 12
DIP I				
Before	3%	11%	4–6 cm	3%
During	3%	6%	8–10 cm	7%
DIP II				
Before	2%	1%	4–6 cm	4%
During	2%	1%	4–10 cm	4%
pH				
Before	7.36 ± 0.05	7.37 ± 0.05	4–6 cm	7.37 ± 0.05
UA	7.22 + 0.07	7.28 ± 0.05	UA	7.27 ± 0.06
Pco_2				
Before	32 ± 8	37 ± 9	4–6 cm	32 ± 9
UA	44 ± 12	47 ± 14	UA	40 ± 7
Po_2				
Before	19 ± 5	19 ± 4	4–6 cm	18 ± 7
UA	21 ± 4	18 ± 5	UA	15 ± 5
Apgar score ≥7				
1st min	88%	83%		100%
5th min	98%	98%		100%

remains close to normal labour. No variation was observed in the number of bradycardias induced by contractions (DIP I or DIP II).

Before analgesia, the fetal pH, PCO_2, and PCO_2 are identical to those of normal labour. At birth, in the umbilical artery, the PCO_2 is slightly higher in the two series of analgesia and the pH of the neuroleptanalgesia series is significantly lower than in normal labour ($p < 0.01$). However, these values remain within physiological limits. On the other hand, the fetal PCO_2 is higher under neuroleptanalgesia than in normal labour, due to the breathing of the oxygen-enriched mixture.

A few infants had an Apgar score less than 7 in the first minute in the studied series. Under peridural analgesia only one was still depressed at the fifth minute with a score at 5, but recovered fast. Under neuroleptanalgesia one infant remained depressed, he died at 30 min, and we could not find any reason for this death. Apart from this case, all the infants in the two series showed normal clinical behaviour during the first 6 days.

The two treated series involved many pathological labours, but with either of the studied methods, the newborn infants remained in a good state. The main differences between the treated series and the control series concern the pH value in the umbilical arteries and the number of Cesarean sections and instrumental extractions. When analysing the results, it is impossible to tell what was due to pathological labour or due to the specific influence of analgesic techniques. To measure this influence, a randomised trial was performed only on normal cases where analgesia was administered to improve maternal comfort.

II. RANDOMISED TRIAL ON PERINATAL EFFECTS OF ANALGESIA DURING NORMAL LABOUR

Material and Methods

The chosen test to measure any noxious effect on the fetus of the given drugs is the pH of the umbilical artery. Previous studies on normal labour allowed us to fix the average value of the pH at 7.27 with a standard deviation of ±0.06.[6] We considered as pathological a fall of pH of 0.07 and accepted a risk at the most equal to 1% to ignore such a difference, in a test where significance level is 5%. Thus we decided on a group of 30 women to run this test.[7]

The selection was as follows: women with no known previous pathology, having a normal pregnancy, and a normal pelvis, spontaneously starting labour between the 38th and 42nd week of pregnancy and reaching 4 cm of dilatation without any clinical and paraclinical problems. At this stage of dilatation, the women were separated at random, with their consent, into three groups:

A control group receiving no drug at all

A group receiving phenoperidine analgesia, obtained by a direct 1-mg intravenous injection, then a 34-μg/min infusion

A group having peridural analgesia by a 12-ml injection of lidocaine at 1.5% with epinephrine at 1/200,000, and 6-ml reinjected when pain reappeared.

Women of the second group breathed an oxygen enriched mixture identical to the one in the first study.

Results

The results can be found on Table III. The frequency of instrumental extractions is statistically higher in the two series of analgesia. These have been performed because of nonspontaneous expulsion. Only one Cesarean section was necessary due to a narrow pelvis, unknown at selection.

The basal fetal heart rate remained normal in the three series; no important variation was observed in the type I or II DIP contraction percentage.

The average values of pH, PCO_2 and PO_2 measured on the fetal scalp at the beginning of labour were identical in all three series. At birth, in the umbilical artery, there was still no difference as far as pH and PCO_2 were concerned. The only modified parameter was a higher PO_2 in the two treated series compared to the control series.

At the first minute of life, there was no significant difference in the number of infants showing an Apgar score below 7. At the fifth minute, all infants had a score greater than 7.

The pH evolution, measured on the newborn infant's heel during the first 2 hr of life is shown in Table IV. No significant difference was observed among the three series.

The pediatric examination on the sixth day showed no abnormality.

TABLE III

Method of Delivery and Fetal Parameters in the Randomised Trial

	Controls		Phenoperidine		Peridural Analgesia		Statistical Comparison
	(n)	(%)	(n)	(%)	(n)	(%)	
Method of delivery							
Spontaneous	28	93	19	63	20	67	
Instrumental extraction	2	7	10	33	10	33	p < 0.01
Cesarean section	0	0	1	4	0	0	
FHR (beat/min)	3–4 cm	137 ± 10	Before	141 ± 11	Before	141 ± 10	NS
	5–10 cm	136 ± 9	During	138 ± 11	During	141 ± 15	NS
DIP I	3–4 cm	1%	Before	2%	Before	2%	NS
	5–10 cm	4%	During	7%	During	5%	NS
DIP II	3–4 cm	0%	Before	1%	Before	0%	NS
	5–10 cm	1%	During	1%	During	1%	NS
Apgar score ⩾7							
1st min		93%		87%		100%	NS
5th min		100%		100%		100%	NS
pH At 4 cm		7.36 ± 0.04		7.36 ± 0.05		7.38 ± 0.05	NS
UA		7.23 ± 0.07		7.22 ± 0.05		7.24 ± 0.06	NS
PCO_2 At 4 cm		34 ± 9		34 ± 9		36 ± 9	NS
mmHg UA		45 ± 7		49 ± 12		47 ± 9	NS
PO_2 At 4 cm		20 ± 5		20 ± 6		21 ± 5	NS
mmHg UA		13 ± 6		17 ± 7		19 ± 6	p < 0.05

TABLE IV

pH of the Newborn Infants during the First 2 hr of Life (Mean Standard Deviation)

	Controls	Phenoperidine	Peridural Analgesia
1st hr	7.31 ± 0.07	7.32 ± 0.09	7.29 ± 0.07
2nd hr	7.34 ± 0.07	7.36 ± 0.04	7.32 ± 0.07

III. DISCUSSION

The aim of this study was to evaluate the perinatal effects of analgesia during labour. From the study of the first series including many pathological labours, we established that these treatments did not jeopardize the newborn infants. Still there were differences between the infants of the treated groups and the control series. Specifically the pH in the umbilical artery of the infants born under neuroleptanalgesia, even though within physiological limits, was significantly lower than during normal labour.

This is why it seemed essential, at a time when analgesia is used more and more for maternal comfort, to evaluate the real effects on the fetus.

The results of the randomised trial can be given in two main points:

1. The number of instrumental extractions is higher in the two analgesia series, and similar in both of them, due to the decrease of the expulsion

reflexes, caused by the drugs. Still none of these extractions had a traumatic effect on the infants.

2. The comparison of the fetal parameters do not show any noxious influence of the analgesics; specifically, the pH in the umbilical artery, chosen as the main factor of judgment in the trial, is identical in the three series. The only difference comes from the PO_2 which is higher in the two treated series than in the control group. This shows the good quality of fetoplacental exchanges and, for the phenoperidine series, is also due to the breathing of enriched oxygen by the mother.

These results demonstrate that phenoperidine or peridural analgesia used in normal conditions does not jeopardize the infants. Usually accepted for peridural analgesia,[4, 10, 12] it has been more controversial where the morphinics are concerned.[1] Our trial seems to confirm the experience of the authors who attest to the inocuity of these drugs.[2, 9, 11]

REFERENCES

1. Bonica, J. J., Respiratory Insufficiency after Analgesia and Anesthesia, in *Obstetrical Anesthesia*, Shnider P.S.M., Ed. Williams and Wilkins Co., Baltimore, 1970.
2. Corsen, G., Neuroleptanalgesia and anesthesia in Obstetrics. *Clin. Obstet. Gynecol.* **17**, 241 (1974).
3. Grandjean, H., Bertrand, J. C., Grandjean, B., Reme, J. M., Degoy, J., and Pontonnier, G. La neuroleptanalgesie dans la direction du travail. *J. Gynecol. Obstet. Rep.* **6**, 563 (1977).
4. McDonald, J. S., Bjorkman, L. L., and Reed, E. C., Epidural analgesia for obstetrics. A maternal, fetal and neonatal study. *Am. J. Obstet. Gynecol.* **120**, 1055 (1974).
5. Pontonnier, G., Puech, F., Grandjean, H., and Rolland M., Some physical and biochemical parameters during maternal labour. Fetal and maternal study. *Biol. Neonat.* **26**, 159 (1975).
6. Pontonnier, G., Grandjean, H., Derache, P., Reme, J. M., Boulogne, M., and De Mouzon, J., Intérêt de la mesure du pH sanguin dans la surveillance foetale pendant l'accouchement. *J. Gynecol. Obstet. Biol. Rep.* **7**, 1065 (1978).
7. Schwartz, D., Flamant, R., and Lellouch, J., *L'essai thérapeutique chez l'homme*. Flammarion, Paris, 1970.
8. Secherre, V., and Secherre, G., L'accouchement sous anesthésie péridurale. thèse de médecine, Bordeaux, 1977.
9. Stockhammer, H., Stockhammer, J., and Frangenhein, H., Das neuroleptanalgetikum Thalamonal zur medikamentösen geburtserleichterung (Erste Klinische Erfährungen). *Geburtshilfe Frauenheilkd.* **29**, 735 (1960).
10. Thalme, B., Belfrage, P., and Raabe N., Lumbar epidural analgesia in labour. I. Acidbase balance and clinical condition of mothers, fetus and newborn child. *Acta Obstet. Gynecol. Scand.* **53**, 27 (1974).
11. Weiss, V., Thalamonaltropfinfusion für Geburtshilfliche Analgesie. *Anesthesist.* **20**, 56 (1971).
12. Wingate, M. B., Wingate, L., Iffy, L., Freundlich, J., and Gottsegen, D., The effect of epidural analgesia upon fetal and neonatal status. *Am. J. Obstet. Gynecol.* **119**, 1101 (1974).

5

Local Control of Glucocorticoid Levels by Individual Tissues in the Fetus: Commonality among Foregut Derivatives[1]

BARRY T. SMITH,[2, 3] A. KEITH TANSWELL,[4] DENNIS WORTHINGTON, and W. NEIL PIERCY

INTRODUCTION

Glucocorticoids are generally considered to be antianabolic, and thus it would seem logical that the rapidly growing fetus should be provided with a relatively low glucocorticoid environment.[11] Indeed, fetal circulating glucocorticoid levels are lower than adult levels.[5, 8, 12] This likely results from three major influences: (a) a relatively lower "set point" for the fetal pituitary-adrenal axis[5]; (b) inactivation of maternal glucocorticoids on crossing the placenta by oxidation of the 11β-hydroxy group to a ketone[9]; and (c) similar 11-oxidation of active glucocorticoids by many fetal tissues.[10]

The extensive 11-oxidation of glucocorticoids in the fetus is in contrast to adult tissues, where the reverse reaction (11-reduction) predominates, such that inherently inactive 11-oxo steroids (e.g., cortisone) possess biologic activity after conversion to their active counterparts (e.g., cortisol). Certain exceptions to the general 11-oxidizing pattern of fetal tissues have been noted, however. For example, the fetal lung, which depends upon glucocorticoid for normal

Departments of Paediatrics and Obstetrics, and Gynaecology, Queen's University, Kingston, Ontario, Canada
[1] Supported by Grants (MT 5757 and MA 6375) from the Medical Research Council of Canada
[2] Scholar, Medical Research Council of Canada
[3] Present address: Department of Pediatrics, Harvard Medical School, Boston, MA 02115
[4] Fellow, Canadian Cystic Fibrosis Foundation and the William T. McEachern Foundation

development of the surfactant system,[13] possesses the ability to reduce ("activate") the abundant fetal supplies of cortisone to cortisol and this activity increases with gestational age.[4, 14, 15, 20, 21] Indeed, if 11-reduction of cortisone is pharmacologically inhibited, lung maturation is delayed.[12] Similar activity has also been noted in amniotic membranes.[7, 18, 19]

The present study was designed to systematically determine the ability of various tissues to interconvert cortisol and cortisone in late gestation, and to compare this activity to circulating and tissue levels of cortisol.

METHODS

Four accurately timed sheep of mixed breed were used in this study.[16, 22] At 135 days gestation (term = 145 days), the ewes were sacrificed with a lethal intravenous dose of pentobarbital. Duplicate samples of maternal serum, amniotic fluid, and fetal serum were obtained for determination of corticosteroid levels. The fetus was removed by hysterotomy and aliquots of various tissues (Table I) were obtained for determination of cortisol levels and interconversion of cortisol and cortisone.

Measurement of Cortisol Levels. Serum and amniotic fluid steroids were

TABLE I

Cortisol Levels and Cortisol (F) and Cortisone (E) Interconversion by Various Fetal Sheep Tissues. Means ± SD, $n = 4$

Tissue	Cortisol Level (ng/ml or g)	E → F (11-reduction)	F → E (11-oxidation)	C11 Activation
(a) Fluids				
Maternal serum	302 ± 42	—	—	—
Fetal serum	44.5 ± 18.8	—	—	—
Amniotic fluid	33.0 ± 7.3	—	—	—
(b) Foregut derivatives				
Lung:				
Upper lobe	63.4 ± 5.9	38.2 ± 2.9	12.5 ± 3.7	25.7 ± 1.3
Middle lobe	54.0 ± 10.1	29.7 ± 4.5	12.1 ± 6.1	17.6 ± 1.8
Lower lobe	50.4 ± 8.3	18.6 ± 5.1	14.8 ± 3.6	3.8 ± 1.6
Parotid	43.6 ± 11.7	22.6 ± 4.2	11.3 ± 2.7	11.3 ± 1.9
Thyroid	56.0 ± 4.9	26.4 ± 4.4	9.6 ± 2.3	16.8 ± 2.6
Stomach	61.7 ± 11.9	17.3 ± 5.8	6.2 ± 2.1	11.1 ± 3.7
Small intestine	54.7 ± 17.5	31.3 ± 3.9	5.0 ± 3.6	26.3 ± 5.3
Liver	44.2 ± 19.9	30.7 ± 6.6	13.8 ± 3.7	16.9 ± 3.8
Pancreas	50.4 ± 11.9	10.1 ± 2.0	5.4 ± 3.0	4.7 ± 2.9
Pituitary	—	19.8 ± 7.4	5.8 ± 3.8	14.0 ± 4.7
(c) Other tissues				
Skeletal muscle	42.0 ± 12.0	6.1 ± 2.5	7.8 ± 2.7	−1.8 ± 0.7
Large intestine	51.3 ± 14.1	11.0 ± 2.4	14.7 ± 1.5	−3.7 ± 2.6
Kidney	25.7 ± 7.8	16.8 ± 6.1	83.1 ± 5.4	−66.3 ± 10.6
Cerebrum	30.2 ± 4.6	7.3 ± 2.6	29.9 ± 9.6	−22.7 ± 7.6
Cerebellum	39.0 ± 10.5	9.0 ± 3.1	24.4 ± 6.6	−15.3 ± 3.6
Skin	39.9 ± 7.1	4.9 ± 1.4	6.8 ± 1.8	−2.1 ± 0.5
Thymus	35.6 ± 5.9	15.8 ± 6.3	22.3 ± 6.5	−6.6 ± 2.5
Heart	48.8 ± 13.9	8.2 ± 2.6	8.3 ± 2.7	−0.1 ± 0.5

extracted with four volumes of ethyl acetate as previously described.[12, 16] One gram aliquots of fetal tissues were homogenized in 1 N saline to give a 10% (wt: vol) suspension. This was then extracted with 4-vol ethyl acetate, as above.[12] In all cases, tracer amounts of 4-^{14}C-cortisol (New England Nuclear, specific activity 55 Ci/mmole) were added to correct for experimental losses. Cortisol was isolated by thin layer chromatography[16] and assayed by the radiotransinassay of Murphy[6] as previously described.[12, 16, 17]

Interconversion of Cortisol and Cortisone. Duplicate aliquots of 100 mg of each fetal tissue studied were homogenized in 2 ml of bicarbonate-buffered Earle's balanced salt solution, pH 7.4, and incubated at 37°C under an atmosphere of 5% CO_2/95% air for 2 hr. The incubation solution contained equimolar concentrations (10^{-7} M) of ^{14}C-cortisone (New England Nuclear, specific activity 59.8 mCi/mmole, 1.2×10^5 dpm) and 1,2-^{3}H-cortisol (New England Nuclear, specific activity 40 mCi/mmole, 1.0×10^6 dpm). At the completion of the incubation, steroids were extracted with 4-vol ethyl acetate, isolated by thin layer chromatography,[16] eluted, and counted in a Searle Isocap 300 liquid scintillation spectrophotometer. From the recovery of ^{14}C and ^{3}H in both cortisone and cortisol, the following data were calculated: (a) conversion (11-reduction) of cortisone to cortisol (biological activation); (b) conversion (11-oxidation) of cortisol to cortisone (biological inactivation); and (c) by arithmetically subtracting (b) from (a), the C11 activation index[14] reflecting the net gain or loss of glucocorticoid activity.

Statistical. Each observation was made in duplicate, and duplicate values all agreed within 10%. The means of these duplicate values were then combined among the four experimental animals studied and expressed as means ± standard deviations, $n = 4$. The means of different groups were compared using Student's t test.[2] The relationship of tissue cortisol levels and the C11 activation index was compared using the least-squares linear regression technique.[3]

RESULTS

As shown in Table I, part a, cortisol levels in the fetal compartment (fetal serum and amniotic fluid) were considerably lower than in maternal serum. Cortisol levels in individual fetal tissues varied widely, within the range of 25.7 ± 7.8 ng/g tissue and 63.4 ± 5.9 ng/g. When tissue cortisol levels of foregut derivatives (Table I, part b) were compared to other fetal tissues (Table I, part c), the levels of the former were noted to be significantly higher (53.2 ± 6.9 ng/g vs. 39.1 ± 8.6 ng/g, $t = 3.7467$, $p < .01$).

The interconversion of cortisol (F) and cortisone (E), as expressed by the C11 activation index and shown in Table I, also differed between foregut derivatives and other fetal tissues in that the former all showed net activation of cortisone to cortisol, while the latter showed net inactivation. As shown in Figure 1, the relationship of tissue cortisol levels and C11 activation index shows a highly significant correlation, indicating this to be an important regulator of tissue glucocorticoid concentration.

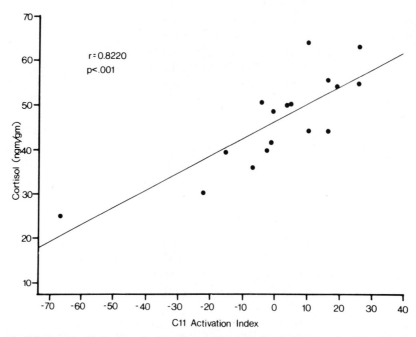

Fig. 1. Relationship of tissue cortisol levels and C11 activation index in various tissues collected from fetal sheep at 135 days gestation. The solid line represents the linear regression line calculated by the method of least squares.[3]

DISCUSSION

These studies indicate that, as with the lung, other foregut derivatives convert inactive 11-oxo steroids to their active 11β-hydroxy counterparts in the fetus near term. This results in higher tissue glucocorticoid concentrations. As has been noted,[12, 13] such activity has physiologic relevance with respect to lung development. A similar conclusion may be drawn about the other foregut derivatives, many of which are also developmentally regulated by glucocorticoid hormones.

Of the non-foregut-derived fetal tissues studied, it is of interest that those with the greatest capacity to inactivate glucocorticoids, and the lowest tissue cortisol concentrations, are those in which toxic effects of pharmacological doses of corticosteroids in the fetus have been noted (cerebrum, cerebellum, and kidney). Thus, inactivation of circulating glucocorticoids by nontarget tissues may have a protective effect. In this regard, concern should be expressed that synthetic glucocorticoids used for prenatal administration[13] in part derive their enhanced activity from structural alterations which allow them to resist 11-oxidation. Thus, unlike endogenous glucocorticoids, their administration would result in delivery of equipotent concentrations to all fetal tissues.

The ability of the pituitary (derived as an outpouch of the foregut: Rathke's pouch) to convert cortisone to cortisol may be of particular interest. While the amount of tissue was too small to allow determination of the pituitary cortisol concentration, this activity would imply that the fetal pituitary may "see" higher cortisol levels than are actually circulating, and may be one mechanism by which the fetal pituitary-adrenal "set point" is down-regulated.

It is of note that the C11 activation index and cortisol levels were highest in the upper lobe of the lung and decreased in the middle and lower lobes, respectively. This appears to be in keeping with the known sequence of lung maturation in this species.

Commonality among foregut derivatives is not a new concept. Indeed, the possibility of glucocorticoid regulation of fetal lung development was first proposed by Buckingham, *et al.* in 1968,[1] by analogy to the known effect of glucocorticoids on the developing foregut. Exploration of other developmental events which may be shared by foregut derivatives should be pursued.

REFERENCES

1. Buckingham, S., McNary, W. F., Sommers, S. C., and Rothschild, J., Is lung an analog of Moog's developing intestine? I. Phosphatases and pulmonary alveolar differentiation in fetal rabbits. *Fed. Proc.* **27,** 328 (1968) (Abstract).
2. Colton, T., *Statistics in Medicine*. Little and Brown, Boston, 1974, p. 127.
3. Colton, T., *Statistics in Medicine*. Little and Brown, Boston, 1974, p. 207.
4. Giannopoulos, G., Uptake and metabolism of cortisone and cortisol by the rabbit fetal lung. *Steroids* **22,** 845–853 (1974).
5. Henning, S. J., Plasma concentrations of total and free corticosterone during development in the rat. *Am. J. Physiol.* **235,** 451–456 (1978).
6. Murphy, B. E. P., Some studies of the protein-binding of steroids and their application to the routine micro and ultramicro measurement of various steroids in body fluids by competitive protein-binding radioassay. *J. Clin. Endocrinol. Metab.* **27,** 973–980 (1967).
7. Murphy, B. E. P., Chorionic membrane as an extra-adrenal source of fetal cortisol in human amniotic fluid. *Nature* **266,** 179–180 (1977).
8. Murphy, B. E. P., and Diez d'Aux, R. C.: Steroid levels in the human fetus: Cortisol and cortisone. *J. Clin. Endocrinol. Metab.* **35,** 678–683 (1972).
9. Murphy, B. E. P., Clark, S. J., Donald, I. R., Pinsky, M., and Vedady, D., Conversion of maternal cortisol to cortisone during placental transfer to the human fetus. *Am. J. Obstet. Gynecol.* **118,** 538–540 (1974).
10. Pasqualini, J. R., Nguyen, B. L., Uhrich, F., Wiqvist, N., and Diczfalusy, E., Cortisol and cortisone metabolism in the human foeto-placental unit at midgestation. *J. Steroid Biochem.* **1,** 209–219 (1970).
11. Reinisch, J. M., Simon, N. G., Karow, W. G., and Gandelman, R., Prenatal exposure to prednisone in humans and animals retards intrauterine growth. *Science* **202,** 436–438 (1978).
12. Smith, B. T., The role of pulmonary corticosteroid 11-reductase activity in lung maturation in the fetal rat. *Pediatr. Res.* **12,** 12–14 (1978).
13. Smith, B. T., Prevention of Hyaline Membrane Disease: An Attempt to Mimic a Physiologic Process, in *Pediatrics Update*, Moss, A. J., Ed. Elsevier-North-Holland, New York, 1979, pp. 151–167.
14. Smith, B. T., and Giroud, C. J. P., Effect of cortisol on serially propogated fibroblast cell cultures derived from the rabbit fetal lung and skin. *Can. J. Physiol. Pharmacol.* **53,** 1037–1041 (1975).
15. Smith, B. T., Torday, J. S., and Giroud, C. J. P., The growth promoting effect of cortisol on human fetal lung cells. *Steroids* **22,** 515–524 (1974).
16. Smith, B. T., Worthington, D., and Piercy, W. N., The relationship of cortisol and cortisone to saturated lecithin concentration in ovine amniotic fluid and fetal lung liquid. *Endocrinology* **101,** 104–109 (1977).
17. Smith, B. T., Worthington, D., and Maloney, A. H. A., Fetal lung maturation. III. The amniotic

fluid cortisol/cortisone ratio and the risk of respiratory distress syndrome. *Obstet. Gynecol.* **49,** 527–531 (1977).

18. Tanswell, A. K., and Smith, B. T., The relationship of amniotic membrane 11-oxidoreductase activity to lung maturation in the human fetus. *Pediatr. Res.* **12,** 957–960 (1978).

19. Tanswell, A. K., Worthington, D., and Smith, B. T., Human amniotic membrane corticosteroid 11-oxidoreductase activity. *J. Clin. Endocrinol. Metab.* **45,** 721–725 (1977).

20. Torday, J. S., Smith, B. T., and Giroud, C. J. P., The rabbit fetal lung as a glucocorticoid target tissue. *Endocrinology* **96,** 1462–1467 (1975).

21. Torday, J. S., Olson, E. B., and First, N. L.: Production of cortisol from cortisone by isolated perfused fetal rabbit lung. *Steroids* **27,** 869–880 (1976).

22. Worthington, D., Piercy, W. N., and Smith, B. T., Modification of ovine fetal respiratory-like activity by chronic diazepam administration. *Am. J. Obstet. Gynecol.* **131,** 749–754 (1978).

6

Fetal Red Cell Oxygen Affinity, Hemoglobin Type, 2,3-Diphosphoglycerate, and pH as a Function of Gestational Age*

HARRY BARD, M.D.

INTRODUCTION

The oxygen affinity of fetal blood is higher than that of adult blood in all mammals that have been investigated. After birth the oxygen affinity decreases to the adult levels. The time course of this decrease in oxygen affinity varies with species and is mainly due to the intrinsic structure of the hemoglobin molecule and the specific action of 2,3-diphosphoglycerate (DPG) on the hemoglobin molecule[8, 26] and the nonspecific effects of changes of the red cell pH.[1, 10]

Studies have previously been carried out during fetal life in sheep to determine the relationship of 2,3-diphosphoglycerate (DPG), the intracellular red cell and extracellular pH, and the switchover to adult hemoglobin synthesis in regulating the position of the fetal red cell oxygen-affinity curve *in utero*.[4] These studies have shown that adult hemoglobin first appears near 120 days of gestation. The decrease in the red cell oxygen affinity after 120 days of gestation correlated with the amount of adult hemoglobin present in the fetus. This decrease could only be attributed to the amount of the adult-type hemoglobin present, and not to DPG, or to changes in the ΔpH between plasma and red blood cells, because both remained unchanged during the last trimester.

Perinatal Service and Research Center of Hopital Sainte-Justine, Department of Pediatrics, University of Montreal, Montreal, Canada.

* This paper was supported by Grant MA-5120 from Medical Research Council of Canada

The interrelationship of 2,3-diphosphoglycerate (2,3-DPG) and P_{50} levels during fetal and postnatal life have also been determined in two mammalian species which do not have a switchover of hemoglobin type at the end of their fetal development.[6] In the guinea pig and rabbit, the 2,3-DPG levels remain low and stable during fetal life and increase only after birth, remaining elevated throughout adult life. The adult levels are reached at 2 days of age in the guinea pig and the 20th day in rabbit. Fetal P_{50} values increase only after birth, paralleling the rise in the 2,3-DPG. The rapidity of the postnatal rise in 2,3-DPG and decrease in P_{50} can be related to the maturity of the newborn animal at birth in these species.

In the human fetus, adult hemoglobin appears around 8 weeks of gestation,[29] but it is after 30 weeks when there is an acceleration in the switchover from the fetal type hemoglobin (HbF) synthesis to the adult type (HbA).[2] At 5 months after birth HbA synthesis has almost completely replaced HbF, and only a small residual synthesis of HbF persists for the rest of life.[3]

Several studies[13, 23, 27] have been reported on changes of oxygen affinity in newborn infants. They agree on one hand that fetal oxygen affinity decreases as gestation progresses, but on the other hand the interrelationship of adult and fetal hemoglobin, 2,3-DPG, and intracellular pH on red cell oxygen affinity during *in utero* life remains unclear.

Since the regulation of fetal oxygenation is of utmost importance in perinatal medicine, a study was planned using placental cord blood obtained immediately at birth from viable nonstressed fetuses of varying gestational ages to determine *in utero* changes in human fetal oxygen affinity 2,3-DPG, ΔpH between plasma and red blood cells as well as the proportions of adult and fetal hemoglobin.

MATERIALS AND METHODS

In an attempt to reflect fetal conditions as closely as possible, heparinized blood was obtained from the placental end of the umbilical vein immediately after delivery of preterm and term infants of no known risk, except premature labor. The gestational age according to maternal history was always confirmed by physical examination of the newborn infant.[16] The cord samples used for the study were obtained from uncomplicated pregnancies that ranged from 24 to 42 weeks of gestation, which resulted in a newborn who was normal, nonasphyxiated, and appropriate in weight for gestational age.[20] All blood analysis was carried out immediately upon obtaining the sample.

Erythrocyte DPG concentration was determined on fresh heparinized blood according to the method of Keitt[18] and expressed as μmol/gHb and μmol/ml RBC. The reagents were obtained from Sigma Chemical Company.* Also, to compare the relationship between the intracellular concentration of DPG and pH, the intracellular and extracellular pH was determined by a freeze-thaw technique.[7]

The P_{50} was determined by gas mixing tonometry using an IL Blood gas

---

* *Sigma Chemical Company, St. Louis, Mo. 63118*

Laboratory† (213 blood gas analyzer tonometer, 208 gas mixing system, and 182 coximeter). The P_{50} was expressed in mmHg at a temperature of 37°C a pH 7.40 and PCO_2 of 40 mmHg. In brief, samples for fresh blood were equilibrated in a tonometer for 30 min at 37° C with a gas mixture containing 40 mmHg (±0.05 mmHg) CO_2, varying proportions of O_2 and N_2. The tonometer permitted an equilibration and sampling of successive aliquots of blood at different O_2 tensions. Measurement of O_2 saturation, pH, and PO_2 provided the information for plotting the O_2 dissociation curve, and P_{50}. The PO_2 was always converted to a pH 7.4 using a Bohr effect of 0.485,[17] the pH values ranged from 7.20 to 7.44, and the mean was 7.32 ± 0.07. There were at least four experimental points for each oxygen dissociation curve. The standard deviation of the mean P_{50} obtained on the same blood sample was 0.84 mmHg, $N = 10$. The oxygen saturation obtained by use of the co-oximeter was frequently checked by determining the oxygen contents of blood samples equilibrated in the tonometer by use of the Lex-O$_2$-Con.‡

The percentage of adult and fetal hemoglobin at birth was obtained by eluting fetal and adult hemoglobin from DEAE Sephadex A50 using a decreasing pH gradient (7.8–7.1) of Tris-HCl buffer by methods previously described.[15] The absorbance of the protein fractions was determined at 280 nm.

Thirty-seven different samples were analyzed for this study. 2,3-DPG levels, intracellular and extracellular pH were done on all samples. Because of the variation in cord blood volume obtained, P_{50} was determined on 35 and hemoglobin chromatographic separations on 31 of the samples, respectively.

DPG levels were expressed in µmol/gHb for correlation purposes and as µmol/ml RBC for comparison with other studies. When pH values were used for statistical correlation they were converted to hydrogen ion concentration (nEq/liter). Thirteen nonpregnant laboratory technicians had their red cell DPG and P_{50} determined as laboratory controls. The mean values and SD obtained was 13.53 ± 1.07 and 26.4 ± 0.8, respectively. These values correspond well within the norms that exist in the literature.[11, 24]

RESULTS

The change in P_{50} as gestational age advances is shown on Figure 1. There was a significant positive correlation between P_{50} and gestational age ($r = 0.6$, $P < 0.001$). The regression line increased from 17.8 mmHg at 24 weeks to 22.5 mmHg at 42 weeks of gestation. However, during fetal development there is no evidence of a relationship between P_{50} and DPG nor between the level of DPG and the concentration of HbA (Figs. 2 and 3).

The mean percentage of HbA increased with gestational age (GA) similarly to that previously reported[5]; the mean value rose from 3% at 24 weeks to 25% at 42 weeks of gestation (the linear regression was %HbA = 1.49 × GA + 37.68; $r = 0.75$, $P < 0.001$). When P_{50} and the percentage of HbA is correlated, there

† Instrumentation Laboratory Inc., Lexington, Mass. 02173
‡ Lexington Instruments Corporation, Waltham, Mass. 02154

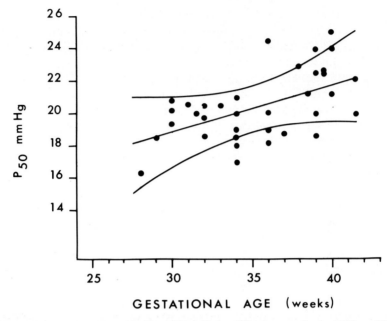

Fig. 1. Blood P_{50} in relation to fetal age. The calculated linear regression and 95% confidence limits are shown by solid lines. $r = 0.67$, $P < 0.001$.

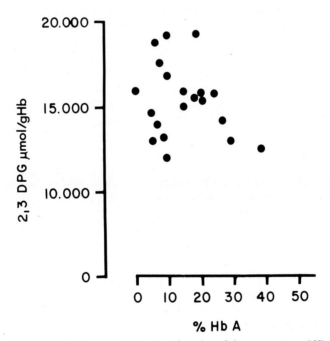

Fig. 2. The 2,3-DPG concentration as a function of the percentage of HbA.

is also a significant positive correlation ($r = 0.7$, $P < 0.001$; $P_{50} = 0.18 \times$ HbA + 17.9).

The relationship of 2,3-DPG and gestational age is demonstrated in Table I. There was no effect of gestational age on 2,3-DPG levels. The mean and SD was 14.86 ± 2.04 μmol/gHb. The mean and SD of the DPG levels when calculated for three different intervals of fetal development either as μmol/gHb or μmol/ml RBC were not significantly different. Similarly the *p*H differences between the fetal red cells and plasma during the different intervals of gestation remained stable (Table II). The mean *in vivo* *p*H was 7.317 ± 0.066, and within the *p*H range of this study the difference between intracellular and extracellular *p*H was constant (ΔpH $= 0.186 \pm$ SD 0.032). However, there was a significant inverse correlation between red cell hydrogen ion concentration and DPG levels ($r = 0.5$, $P < 0.025$; DPG $= -0.31 \times \{\text{H}^+\} + 38.80$).

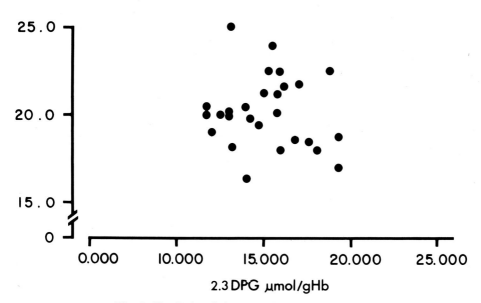

Fig. 3. The P_{50} in relation to 2,3-DPG concentration.

TABLE I
DPG in Relation to Fetal Age (FA)

FA (weeks)	μmol/gHb	μmol/ml RBC	N
<32	14.27 ± 1.31	4.617 ± 0.555	8
32–37	15.35 ± 2.94	5.004 ± 1.005	15
38–42	14.47 ± 1.48	4.704 ± 0.469	14

TABLE II

Extracellular vs. Intracellular pH Differences in Relation to Fetal Age

FA (weeks)	pH			N
	ECF	ICF	ICF − ECF	
<32	7.296 ± 0.089	7.121 ± 0.115	0.175 ± 0.040	8
32–37	7.340 ± 0.055	7.152 ± 0.076	0.188 ± 0.034	15
38–42	7.305 ± 0.065	7.114 ± 0.055	0.191 ± 0.028	14

DISCUSSION

The multiple molecular forms of hemoglobin in normal man and other animals that have developed in the course of evolution appear to confer a physiological advantage within the period of ontogeny during which that particular hemoglobin is present in high concentration. In humans, it is the switch from fetal to adult hemoglobin synthesis that has evolved as the main method for the change in red cell oxygen affinity from the fetal to the air environment. The oxygen dissociation curve of normal fetal blood represents the reaction of the intracellular hemoglobin type (HbA and HbF) with oxygen as modified by the ligands present in the intracellular environment. The ligands of physiological importance are hydrogen ions and DPG.

The DPG levels obtained in this study are similar to those reported on in cord blood at delivery by others[28]; also the mean P_{50} of the term infants of this report (22.1 mmHg) is similar to the average value (22.4 mmHg) of 15 authors listed in a review article by Novy.[22] A possible explanation of the low levels of DPG obtained in preterm infants by others[13, 23] is that the authors did not consider the possible effects of adverse clinical conditions which may occur in preterm deliveries that can induce extracellular changes in pH which in turn have a direct effect on the intraerythrocytic environment[14] and alter DPG synthesis.[25] The acid-base instability of the preterm infants has been observed by several authors.[19, 21] The greater incidence of complicated deliveries and asphyxia associated with preterm birth compared to term delivery could result in more preterm infants being acidotic as compared with term infants.

To date, all mammalian fetuses where fetal red cell organic phosphates were determined at different gestational ages showed no changes in 2,3-DPG levels during fetal life.[4, 5, 9, 12] This report suggests that in the human fetus the decrease in oxygen affinity of fetal red cells during last trimester of gestation is mainly due to the increase in the amount of adult type hemoglobin.

There are no changes in 2,3-DPG or ΔpH as gestation advances, but there is a change in the percentage of adult hemoglobin and a causative relationship is proposed between the increase in adult hemoglobin and P_{50}. Also DPG levels are inversely related to intracellular hydrogen ion concentration which parallels that of whole blood. These data can be useful to investigators in evaluating pathological as well as therapeutic effects on the concentration of DPG in the fetal red blood cell.

REFERENCES

1. Astrup, P., Rorth, M., and Thorshauge, L., Dependency on acid-base status of oxyhemoglobin dissociation and 2,3 diphosphoglycerate levels in human erythrocytes. *Scand. J. Lab. Clin. Invest.* **26,** 47–52 (1970).
2. Bard, H., Postnatal fetal and adult hemoglobins synthesis in early preterm newborn infants. *J. Clin. Invest.* **52,** 1789–1795 (1975).
3. Bard, H., The postnatal decline of hemoglobin F synthesis in normal full-term infants. *J. Clin. Invest.* **55**(2), 395–398 (1975).
4. Bard, H., Fouron, J. C., Robillard, J. E., Cornet, A., and Soukini, M. A., Red cell oxygen affinity in fetal sheep: The role of 2,3 DPG and adult hemoglobin. *J. Appl. Physiol.: Respir. Environ. Exercise Physiol.* **45**(1), 7–10 (1978).
5. Bard, H., Makowski, E. L., Meschia, G., and Battaglia, F. C., The relative rates of synthesis of hemoglobins A and F in immature red cells of newborn infants. *Pediatrics* **45,** 766–772 (1970).
6. Bard, H., and Shapiro, M., Perinatal changes of 2,3 diphosphoglycerate and oxygen affinity in mammals not having fetal type hemoglobins. *Pediatr. Res.* **13,** 167–169 (1979).
7. Battaglia, F. C., Behrman, R. E., Hellegers, A. E., and Battaglia, J. D., Intracellular hydrogen ion concentration changes during acute respiratory acidosis and alcalosis. *J. Pediatr.* **66,** 737–742 (1965).
8. Bauer, C. H., Ludwig, I., and Ludwig, M., Different effects of 2,3 phosphoglycerate and adenosine triphosphate on the oxygen affinity of adult and foetal human hemoglobin. *Life Sci.* **7**(1), 1339–1343 (1968).
9. Baumann, R., Teischel, F., Zoch, R., and Bartels, H., Changes in red cell, 2,3-diphosphoglycerate concentration as cause of the postnatal decrease of pig blood oxygen affinity. *Respir. Physiol.* **19,** 153–161 (1973).
10. Bellingham, A. J., Detter, J. C., and Lenfant, C., Regulatory mechanisms of hemoglobin oxygen affinity in acidosis and alkalosis. *J. Clin. Invest.* **50,** 700–706 (1971).
11. Bellingham, A. J., and Lenfant, C., Hb affinity for O$_2$ determined by O$_2$-Hb dissociation analyze and mixing technique. *J. Appl. Physiol.* **30,** 903–904 (1971).
12. Bunn, H. F., and Kitchen, H., Hemoglobin function in the horse: The role of 2,3 diphosphoglycerate in modifying the oxygen affinity of maternal and fetal blood. *Blood* **42,** 471–479 (1973).
13. Delivoria-Papadopoulos, M., Roncevic, N. P., and Oski, F. A., Postnatal changes in oxygen transport of term premature, and sick infants: The role of red cell 2,3 diphosphoglycerate and adult hemoglobin. *Pediatr. Res.* **5,** 235–245 (1971).
14. Desforges, J. F., and Slawsky, P., Red cell 2,3-diphosphoglycerate and intracellular arterial pH in acidosis and alkalosis. *Blood* **40,** 740–746 (1972).
15. Dozy, A. M., Kleihauer, E. F., and Huisman, H. J., Studies on the heterogeneity of hemoglobin XIII: Chromatography of various human and animal hemoglobin types of DEAE-Sephadex. *J. Chromatog.* **32,** 723–727 (1968).
16. Dubowitz, L. M. S., Dubowitz, V., and Goldberg, C., Clinical assessment of gestational age in the newborn infant. *J. Pediatr.* **77,** 1–10 (1970).
17. Hilpert, P., Fleischmann, R. G., Kempe, D., and Bartels, H., The Bohr effect related to blood and erythrocyte pH. *Am. J. Physiol.* **205,** 337–340 (1963).
18. Keitt, A. S., Reduced nicotinamide adenine dinucleotide-linked analysis of 2,3 diphosphoglyceric acid: Spectrophotometric and fluorometric procedures. *J. Lab. Clin. Med.* **77,** 470–475 (1971).
19. Kildeberg, P., Disturbances of hydrogen ion balance occurring in premature infants. I. Early types of acidosis. *Acta Paediatr.* **53,** 505–516 (1964).
20. Lubchenco, L. O., Hansman, C., and Boyd, E., Intrauterine growth in length and head circumference as estimated from live births at gestational ages from 26 to 42 weeks. *Pediatrics* **37,** 403–408 (1966).
21. Malan, A. F., Evans, A., De V. Heese, H., Serial acid-base determinations in normal premature and full-term infants during the first 72 hours of life. *Arch. Dis. Child.* **40,** 645–650 (1965).
22. Novy, M. J., Fetal Oxygenation and Its Relation to Maternal and Fetal Blood Oxygen Affinity,

in *Preservation of Red Blood Cells.* National Academy of Sciences, Washington, D.C., 1973, pp. 101–117.

23. Orzalesi, M. M., and Hay, W. W., The regulation of oxygen affinity of fetal blood. I. In vitro experiments and results in normal infants. *Pediatrics* **48**(6), 857–864 (1971).

24. Rand, P. W., Norton, J. M., Barker, N., and Lovel, M., Influence of athletic training on hemoglobin-oxygen affinity. *Am. J. Physiol.* **224,** 1334–1337 (1973).

25. Rapoport, S., The regulation of glycolysis in mammalian erythrocytes. *Essays Biochem.* **4,** 69–103 (1968).

26. Tyuma, I., and Shimizu, K., Different response to organic phosphates of human fetal and adult hemoglobins. *Arch. Biochem. Biophys.* **129,** 404–405 (1969).

27. Versmold, H., Seifert, G., Riegel, K. P., Blood oxygen affinity in infancy: The interaction of fetal and adult hemoglobin, oxygen capacity, and red cell hydrogen ion and 2,3 diphospho-glycerate concentration. *Respir. Physiol.* **18,** 14–25 (1973).

28. Weiss, R. R., Roginsky, M. S., Mann, L. I., Melber, A., Bachorik, J., Tejani, N., Bhakthavath-salan, A., Evans, M. I., Erythrocyte 2,3-diphosphoglycerate in normal and hypertensive gravid women and their newborn infants. *Am. J. Obstet. Gynecol.* **124,** 692–696 (1976).

29. Wood, W. G., and Weatherall, D. J., Haemoglobin synthesis during human foetal development. *Nature (Lond.)* **244,** 162–165 (1973).

7

The Management of Jaundiced Ill Preterm Infants Using the Sephadex Column Chromatography Bilirubin Binding Test

TIMOS VALAES, M.D., MARILYN HYTE, B.S., KEVIN MURPHY, B.S., and LARS NIELSON, B.S.

INTRODUCTION

The problems with our current criteria for the management of severe neonatal hyperbilirubinemia stem from the fact that prevention of Kernicterus preceded understanding of its pathogenesis.[1] Actually, it was the successful prevention that served as the basis for elucidating the mechanism of bilirubin (BR) toxicity. Because it is difficult to argue with success, more than 25 years worth of advances in our understanding of Kernicterus had little effect on clinical practice. Moreover, the almost complete elimination of Kernicterus made it impossible to design the kind of clinical studies that could evaluate the merits of methods measuring more appropriate parameters than the BR levels used in the original criteria. Yet neither theory nor *in vitro* or animal experiments could substitute for this essential clinical evaluation. This gap between current knowledge and actual practice became critical with the resurgence of Kernicterus in intensive care units among the severely sick preterm infants.[2-4] Moreover, the possibility that BR toxicity included a much wider spectrum of sequelae than previously recognized created a sense of uneasiness regarding the effectiveness of the old criteria in preventing BR encephalopathy.[5-7]

Central to our understanding of the pathogenesis of Kernicterus is BR binding to albumin.[8] Assessing BR binding with a method that is both reliable

The Neonatology Service and Laboratory, The Department of Pediatrics, Tufts-New England Medical Center Hospital, Boston, Massachusetts 02111

and technically feasible for clinical application is the essential first step in improving the criteria for treatment.

Extensive experience with the sephadex column chromatography method in appropriate clinical material demonstrated a close relationship between a 2+ positive result and Kernicterus and more importantly the absence of classical Kernicterus in infants with a negative or 1+ positive result even when BR values were far above 20 mg/dl.[9-11]

In the present work our experience in managing hyperbilirubinemia in sick preterm infants on the basis of the sephadex test will be described.

MATERIALS AND METHODS

Preterm infants transferred in the first 24 hr of life to Boston Floating Hospital (BFH) for the management of a variety of medical or surgical conditions constitute the clinical material of this work. Excluded from the analysis were 22 infants who died before 72 hr of life and three infants with hemolytic disease due to maternal isoimmunization.

For the monitoring of hyperbilirubinemia, total plasma BR (Americal Optical Bilirubinometer), total plasma proteins (TPR) (American Optical TS meter), and the hematocrit were measured, and Sephadex Column Chromatography (Kernlute, Ames) was performed.[10] These determinations were performed as often as every 4–8 hr during the period of rising BR values and less frequently thereafter. Four capillary tubes (total 0.3 ml of blood) were sufficient for the above determinations. In the routine clinical use of the sephadex test no addition of BR to the plasma to estimate the "reserve BR binding capacity" was carried out. A negative test was interpreted as indicating clinically insignificant levels of "loosely bound BR" and moreover absence of significant levels of conjugated-"direct"-BR.[11] When a positive test was obtained, before accepting it as indicating imminent risk of Kernicterus, the presence of "high direct BR" had to be excluded. If the urine tested negative for BR (Ictotest, Ames), this was considered, on the basis of extensive previous experience, as sufficient evidence of absence of "high direct BR." A positive sephadex and urine test was further investigated by measuring the level of "direct BR" by the diazo reaction.[12] Levels of direct reacting pigment of ≥ 2.0 mg/dl were considered as rendering the sephadex test unreliable for assessing the risk of Kernicterus, and in this situation other criteria, based mainly on the level of unconjugated BR, were used to manage the patient.

On obtaining a positive sephadex test and after excluding "high direct BR" the following steps were taken immediately:

a. The patient, provided there were no cardiovascular contraindications, was given 1 gm/kg salt poor human albumin
b. Blood was ordered for exchange transfusion (ET)
c. The sephadex test was repeated 30 min after the infusion of albumin
d. The ET was performed if the repeat sephadex continued to be positive but no ET was done and the patient was closely monitored if the test was negative.

The rest of the management of our patients followed generally recommended practices. Phototherapy was initiated according to widely used recommendations[13] and delivered by units of eight fluorescent tubes (20 W, daylight). For the infants nursed in warmers, two phototherapy units placed obliquely on the one side and the foot of the warmer were used.

RESULTS

In the present material a 2+ result was obtained only in infants with high "direct reacting" BR. Of the total 304 preterm infants, 31 had one or more 1+ positive sephadex tests. Of these infants, only 11 had to be exchanged while in 20 the sephadex became negative after albumin administration (Table I). The incidence of a positive sephadex test and the need for ET were closely related to gestational age. None of the 136 infants over 33 weeks gestational age (GA) had positive sephadex tests (Table I). This difference could not be explained on the basis of the distribution of maximum BR values in the three gestational groups (Fig. 1). When the maximum values of the ratio plasma total BR (mg/dl)/total plasma proteins (gm/dl) (TBR/TPR) were similarly plotted (Fig. 1), none of the infants over 33 weeks had values over 3.5, reflecting the higher total protein levels in the more mature infants. Theoretically the molar ratio of BR to albumin is the appropriate parameter in relation to BR binding to albumin. In our experience the clinical use of such a ratio was limited by the poor reproducibility, lack of acceptable standard, and relative technical difficulties of the available methods for measuring albumin. The ease of performance, need of only one drop of plasma, and high reproducibility of the estimation of plasma proteins by refractometry coupled with the relative narrow range of albumin/total protein ratio in the newborn make the ratio TBR/TPR an attractive alternative for clinical use. The percentage of sephadex positive samples according to the values of either the plasma TBR or the TBR/TPR ratio (samples with "high direct BR" were excluded as well as those drawn after the infusion of albumin) were calculated for 1636 samples from 168 infants of less than 34 weeks of gestation. From Figure 2, it becomes apparent that the expected increase in the percentage of positive tests with

TABLE I

BFH Material—1975 to 1978[a]

	Gestational Age Groups			Total
	≤30	31–33	34–36	
Total in group	81	87	136	304
Sephadex positive	21 (25.9%)	10 (11.5%)	—	31 (10.2%)
Exchange transfused	9 (11.1%)	2 (2.3%)	—	11 (3.6%)

[a] Admitted in the first 24 hr of life, surviving >72 hr, and direct Coombs negative.

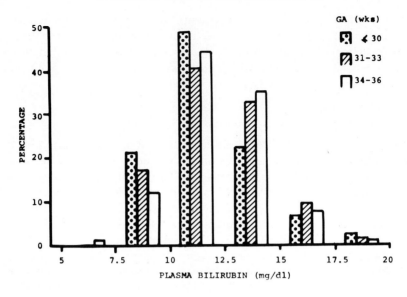

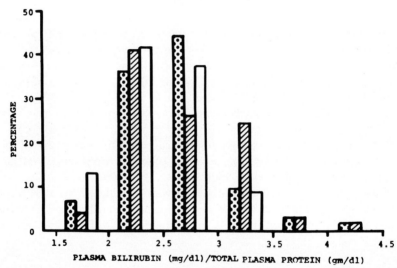

Fig. 1. Distribution of maximum total plasma bilirubin values and of maximum values of the ratio: total plasma bilirubin (mg/dl)/total plasma protein (gm/dl) in three gestational age groups of preterm infants.

increasing values was more clearly seen with the ratio than with the BR values. The value of this ratio closely determined the incidence of positive sephadex tests in the more mature infants but not in those of ≤30 weeks GA in which a higher and at the same time uniform risk was found with values of the ratio between 2.0 and 3.5 (Fig. 3). In none of the infants were symptoms attributed to BR encephalopathy recognized during their hospitalization. Six of the infants died between the 3rd and 10th day of life (Table II). Autopsy was performed in four of them, and none had Kernicterus. Three were positive by sephadex and were treated by either albumin infusion or ET. One of those without autopsy had minimal jaundice, was negative by sephadex, and died after massive intraventricular hemorrhage (IVH). The other infant was the second and much smaller of twins with disseminated intravascular coagulation (DIC), renal failure, metabolic acidosis (pH down to 7.10), and two episodes of massive pulmonary hemorrhage, one at 24 hr of age and the other as a terminal event. Two ETs with heparinized blood, performed also as part of the treatment

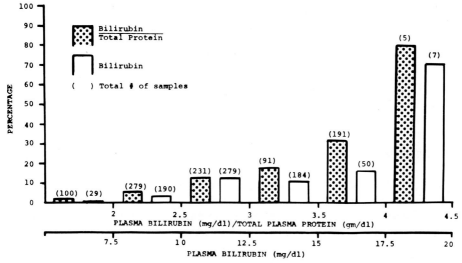

Fig. 2. Percentage of sephadex positive (1+) samples in relation to the values of either total plasma bilirubin or the ratio: total plasma bilirubin (mg/dl)/total plasma protein (gm/dl) in infants ≤33 weeks GA. (Samples with conjugated BR ≥2.0 mg/dl and those drawn immediately after albumin infusion were excluded.)

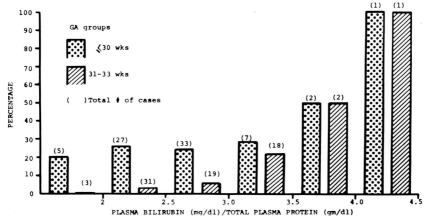

Fig. 3. Percentage of sephadex positive (1+) infants in relation to maximum—before treatment—value of the ratio: total plasma bilirubin (mg/dl)/total plasma protein (gm/dl) and the gestational age group.

TABLE II

Deaths 3rd–10th Day[a]

Sex	BW/GA	Maximum		Sepha-dex	Treat-ment	Age at Death	Diagnosis
		BR	BR/TPR				
M	630/25	10.9	2.42	pos. X2	Alb, none	7 days	No kernicterus IVH
M	680/26	11.8	2.95	pos. X4	ET X2 Alb X2	7 days	No kernicterus IVH
M	1020/28	10.0	1.95	pos.	Alb	7 days	No kernicterus NEC
F	970/32	12.5	2.77	pos. X3	ET X2	85 hr	No autopsy DIC, Pulm. Hem.
M	595/26	6.1	1.35	neg.	—	99 hr	No autopsy IVH
F*	1400/31	10.4	2.38	neg.	—	5 days	No kernicterus IVH, Pulm. Hem.

[a] Among the 304 infants, there were 15 deaths after the 10th day.

of DIC, had only a short-lasting effect on the sephadex test, which was positive for the best part of his life.

At the time the present method of management of jaundice in preterm infants was introduced alternative recommendations were based on the TBR level in relation to birth weight and the clinical status. These recommendations were the result of theoretical considerations and rationalizations rather than of a clinical evaluation. Since then, a retrospective validation of such a set of recommendations was published. By adhering to these preset "exchange levels" no Kernicterus was found among 34 infants that died between the 3rd and 7th day of life.[14] It will be of interest to examine the difference in the management that would have resulted if the TBR criteria were applied to our population. In Table III our material is subdivided into birth weight groups, and the number of infants with positive sephadex test and those actually exchange transfused were compared with the number of infants that fulfilled the criteria for ET based on TBR and the clinical status. Sixty-one infants instead of 11 would have been exchanged according to these criteria. The difference is particularly striking in the smaller weight groups. The group of infants ≤ 1250 g which included the majority of infants with positive sephadex tests was analyzed in more detail. There were 63 infants with birth weight (BW) ≤ 1250 g (Table IV). Twenty infants (group I) had one or more positive sephadex tests and were also positive by the TBR criteria. Twenty-three infants (group II) were negative by the sephadex test but fulfilled the TBR criteria. In this weight group there were no sephadex positive infants that did not fulfill the TBR criteria. Two such infants were found in the >1500 g group. The three groups were similar in birth weight and gestational age. The infants with positive sephadex tests (group I) had TBR and TBR/TPR values (at the time the first positive test was obtained) significantly ($p < 0.05$) higher than the maximum values in the sephadex negative infants (groups II and III). Also group I as judged by the number of early (3rd–10th day) and late (after the 10th day) deaths included the sicker infants.

The 20 infants in group I had a total of 35 separate episodes of being positive by the sephadex test (a new episode was counted if the sephadex became positive again after it was reversed to negative with either albumin or ET treatment). Of the 26 episodes treated initially with albumin the sephadex became negative in 17 while in nine (35%) it remained positive and an ET was performed (Table V). Seven episodes were treated directly by ET either

TABLE III

	Birth Weight Groups (g)				Total
	≤1250	1251–1500	1501–2000	>2000	
Total in group	63	42	67	132	304
Sephadex positive	20	4	5	2	31
	(31.7%)	(9.5%)	(7.5%)	(1.5%)	(10.2%)
Treated with ET	10	—	1	—	11
	(15.9%)		(1.4%)		(3.6%)
Fulfilling TBR criteria[a]	43	13	4	1	61
	(68.2%)	(28.6%)	(6%)	(0.75%)	(20.0%)

[a] As per Ref. 14.

TABLE IV

Infants of Birth Weight ≤1250 g

	I ($N = 20$) Seph. (+) TBR cr. (+)	II ($N = 23$) Seph. (−) TBR cr. (+)	III ($N = 20$) Seph. (−) TBR cr. (−)	p (Ivs II/Ivs II + III)
B.Wt. (g)	927 ± 180	1046 ± 166	1032 ± 170	NS/NS
GA (weeks)	27.8 ± 1.7	28.3 ± 2.9	28.8 ± 2.3	NS/NS
TBR (mg/dl)[a]	12.1 ± 2.4	11.9 ± 1.9	9.6 ± 1.5	NS/<0.05
TBR/TPR[a]	2.73 ± 0.5	2.64 ± 0.3	2.15 ± 0.4	NS/<0.05
Day of life[a]	3.5 ± 1.9	4.0 ± 1.6	2.7 ± 1.5	NS/NS
Deaths:early/late	4/5	−/4	1/2	0.01/0.01[b]

[a] Values are maximum for groups II, III and first sephadex positive for group I.
[b] Chi square, early and late deaths together.

TABLE V

Management of Sephadex Positive Episodes (Infants of ≤1250 g Birth Weight)

	Episode				Total
	First	Second	Third	Fourth	
No. of episodes	20	9	4	2	35
Responded to albumin	12	3	2	—	17[a]
ET after failure of albumin	5	2	1	1	9[a]
ET directly	3	3	1	—	7
Efforts abandoned	—	1	—	1	2

[a] Failure rate of albumin to reverse positive sephadex to negative: 35%.

because in addition to hyperbilirubinemia DIC was present or because congestive heart failure from patent ductus arteriosus was considered a contraindi-
cation to the use of albumin. A total of 16 ETs were performed in 10 babies.
Four received two ETs each and one infant had three ETs. In two infants a
final sephadex positive episode was not treated as the severity of IVH precluded
any effort to salvage them (first and second case in Table II).

In Figures 4 and 5 the values of TBR (Fig. 4) or TBR/TPR (Fig. 5) for each
sephadex positive episode are plotted in relation to the course of corresponding
values in the 43 sephadex negative infants. There is a considerable overlap of
values the extent of which was less after the 4th–5th day of life, i.e., the TBR
or TBR/TPR levels were more important determinants of whether the sephadex was likely to be positive or not after the 4th or 5th day of life than in the
first 4–5 days of life. Or expressed in another way: for a given TBR or TBR/
TPR value the likelihood of a positive sephadex test is higher in the first 4–5
days of life than later.

The group of infants $\leq$ 1250 g were further analyzed to identify other factors
that determine the development of a positive sephadex test. We analyzed both
the total group of infants $\leq$ 1250 g as well as different subgroups (i.e., those

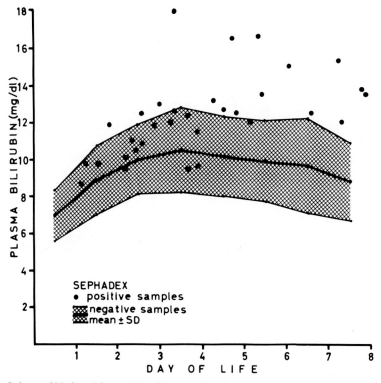

Fig. 4. Infants of birth weight ≤1250 g. Plasma bilirubin values of sephadex positive samples in
relation to the values in the sephadex negative infants. For the calculation of the mean and SD in
the sephadex negative infants, the maximum bilirubin value for each day for each infant was
included.

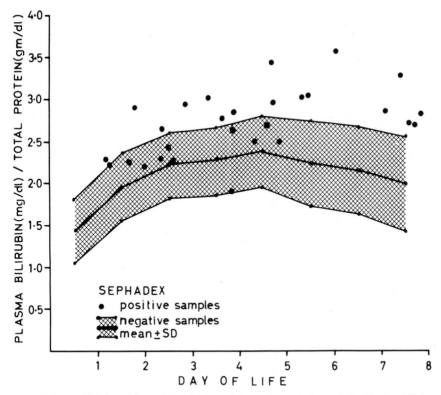

Fig. 5. Infants of birth weight ≤1250 g. Values of the ratio total plasma bilirubin (mg/dl)/total plasma protein (gm/dl) of sephadex positive samples in relation to the values of the ratio in the sephadex negative infants. Mean and SD calculated as in Figure 4.

≤1000 g, the birth asphyxia group, the ventilation group) comparing the sephadex positive with the sephadex negative infants (Table VI).

In all the comparisons TBR and TBR/TPR levels emerged as important factors (Table IV). Individual abnormalities such as hypoxia or acidosis measured by either the degree and total number of episodes up to the time the sephadex positive test was obtained or in only the previous 24 hr did not seem to significantly influence the incidence of positive tests. Similarly, there was no correlation with the caloric intake. On the other hand, such a general index of severity as the need for mechanical ventilation was significantly associated with the development of a positive test. When adverse factors such as low birth weight, low Apgar, need for mechanical ventilation, major complications (occurring before the positive test or the maximum values in those negative by sephadex), and early rise in BR were combined to give a score of clinical severity, this was significantly higher in the sephadex positive group (Table VI). Nevertheless, when the values of this score were plotted against the values of the TBR/TPR ratio in the sephadex positive and negative infants, there was considerable overlap (Fig. 6), making inaccurate the prediction of the outcome of the sephadex test on the basis of this score and the TBR/TPR

TABLE VI
Perinatal Characteristics (Infants of ≤1250 g Birth Weight)

	Sephadex (+) (No. 20)	Sephadex (−) (No. 43)	p
Complications of			
Pregnancy	4	8	NS[b]
Labor	8	15	NS[b]
Delivery	14	23	NS[b]
5′ Apgar ≤5	9	14	NS[b]
SGA	2	6	NS[b]
B.Wt. ≤ 1000 g	10	15	NS[b]
Moderate or Severe			
HMD	7	13	NS[b]
Respirator	16	17	<0.01[b]
Score of clinical severity[a]	9.2 ± 2.9	5.3 ± 2.5	<0.02[c]

[a] Includes the following factors: (a) Birth weight 1001–1250 g = 1, 801–1000 g = 2, ≤800 g = 3. (b) Low Apgar (5′ ≤ 5) = 1. (c) Mechanical ventilation = 2. (d) Major clinical complications (documented sepsis, pneumothorax, NEC, PDA with CHF) before peak of bilirubin or positive sephadex = 1–2. (e) Maximum bilirubin before 5th day = 2. (f) Episodes of abnormal arterial blood gases in the 24 hr previous to the maximum bilirubin values or positive sephadex. Acidotic episodes ($pH \le 7.15$) ≤ 2 = 1 ≥ 3 = 2. Hypoxic episodes ($PO_2 \le 40$ torr) ≤2 = 1, ≥3 = 2.
[b] Chi square test.
[c] Student's t test.

ratio. The overlap was even more pronounced when the values of TBR were used.

DISCUSSION

The results of including tests of bilirubin binding in the clinical management of neonatal jaundice cannot be properly evaluated without examining the state of the art regarding BR encephalopathy and its prevention.

The exact mechanism of BR entry in the neurons and the sequence of events at the cellular and subcellular level that lead to neuron death have not been fully elucidated. The concept that bilirubin toxicity is related to the status of bilirubin binding to albumin is based on solid clinical and experimental data recently reviewed.[15] Conditions that are expected to lead to less tight holding of bilirubin by the albumin molecule such as increasing bilirubin and/or decreasing albumin concentration and the presence of competing or interfering substances both in clinical situations[16, 17] and in experimental settings[18–20] have been shown to increase bilirubin toxicity. Other events such as acidosis, hypoxia, hypothermia, hypoglycemia either experimentally[21] or on anecdotal clinical evidence[2–4] have also been associated with increased risk of bilirubin toxicity, but it is not clear whether this is related to their effect on bilirubin binding or to increased vulnerability of the central nervous system or to both.

Bilirubin encephalopathy cannot be treated but can and has been effectively prevented. Therefore, we need laboratory and/or clinical criteria to select for preventive treatment those at risk for manifesting bilirubin toxicity. Because Kernicterus has a high mortality and the survivors exhibit severe sequelae, it

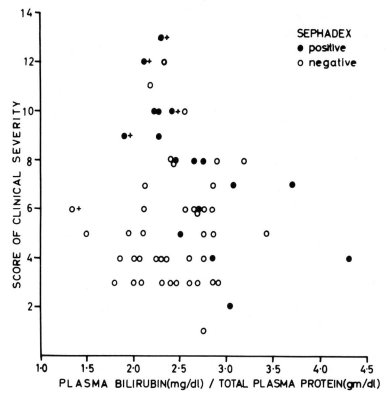

Fig. 6. Individual scores of clinical severity in relation to maximum values of the ratio total plasma bilirubin/total plasma protein of the sephadex negative infants or the values of the first positive sample in the sephadex positive. A cross indicates the infants that died.

becomes mandatory to include in the preventive treatment even infants at low risk. Inevitably this will result in the treatment of a much larger number of infants than the number that would develop bilirubin encephalopathy without intervention. This situation will continue to be acceptable provided the benefit/risk ratio remains favorable. The ratio was definitely favorable when the cutoff point of 18–20 mg/dl of TBR was used for the prevention of Kernicterus in infants with Rh hemolytic disease.[1] This level was recommended on the basis that the incidence of Kernicterus was zero[22] in one series and very low in another[1] if bilirubin remained below this level. Similar success in preventing Kernicterus was achieved in two other common hemolytic conditions in the newborn: ABO incompatibility and G-6-PD deficiency. In the latter condition as well as in infants with marked nonspecific hyperbilirubinemia, both characterized by peak bilirubin levels around the 4th–5th day of life, the cutoff point was raised to 25 mg/dl TBR with equal success in preventing Kernicterus.[23] These criteria for treating hyperbilirubinemia to prevent Kernicterus in term infants were almost universally accepted and have been in practice for over 25 years.

The indications for treatment in preterm infants without hemolytic disease remained controversial decades after clear-cut guidelines were established for term infants. Opinions ranged from using the same (18–20 mg/dl) or lower critical levels of TBR[24–27] to altogether questioning the need for ET in the absence of hemolytic disease.[28, 29] The only randomized controlled study of ET versus no treatment at all showed no conclusive advantage of ET even when the neurological outcome at 12–24 months was taken into consideration.[30] The authors of the study concluded that ET should be reserved for premature infants with levels of TBR over 24 mg/dl with perhaps lower levels used for infants with serious complications. By the late 1960s, early feeding,[31–33] phototherapy,[34, 35] and induction of liver enzymes with phenobarbital[36–38] dramatically reduced the number of preterm infants with bilirubin levels near or above 18 mg/dl, and thus the agonizing question of when to perform an ET was rarely asked. However, the development of intensive care techniques created a new population of jaundiced infants. They are surviving despite extreme immaturity, despite episodes of severe hypoxia and acidosis, despite infections and a variety of near-catastrophic complications. They are nursed in open warmers which up to recently did not provide for effective overhead phototherapy units. Feeding is withheld for prolonged periods and thus an active enterohepatic circulation of BR further reduces the effectiveness of phototherapy. [The above explains why in our series hyperbilirubinemia was both accentuated (Fig. 1) and prolonged (Fig. 4) in relation to preintensive care series of preterm infants treated with phototherapy.[35]] The population of infants that do not survive has also changed. Death is now a slow process and usually comes after a prolonged period of failing vital functions and repeated episodes of cardiopulmonary arrests and resuscitations. It is pertinent to ask how all these affect both the susceptibility to and the manifestations of bilirubin toxicity. Theoretically susceptibility may change in response to factors affecting bilirubin binding and to factors influencing the vulnerability of the central nervous tissue to a given level of the "toxic" species of BR. Obviously in order to resolve this issue, we need to know which is the "toxic" form of BR and be able to measure it in a large enough group of infants so that variability in the incidence and the manifestations of toxicity not accounted for by the level of the "toxic" substance will become apparent.

Regarding the manifestations of bilirubin toxicity in this population, there are questions about the significance of bilirubin staining of the brain in those infants that come to autopsy and the nature of the neurological sequelae in those that survive. In the majority of cases of Kernicterus described in these infants no symptoms attributed to bilirubin toxicity were recognized during life, and from the clinical course and the autopsy findings there was convincing evidence for some other complication being the direct cause of death.[2, 4, 39] The question thus is raised whether these infants died from Kernicterus or died with Kernicterus as a terminal inconsequential event. It is conceivable that under certain circumstances BR staining of the brain represents neuronal damage from a variety of causes with circulating BR entering the already damaged or dead neurons. If this is proven to be the correct explanation for some cases of "Kernicterus" with low BR levels occurring in very sick preterm babies, obviously BR binding is irrelevant in these cases and BR staining of the brain will occur however low the BR level is maintained.[39] The fact that Kernicterus both in newborns and experimental models as a rule occurs from the direct result of BR toxicity and in the absence of any previous neuronal damage does not exclude the possibility of BR staining of the brain occasionally being a secondary event. Another possibility, e.g., previous neuronal damage facilitating the entry of BR in the neuron, thus leading to further damage, has been suggested by the production of Kernicterus in asphyxiated newborn monkeys.[21] Kernicterus was not seen in our series and in the series managed according to quite low "exchange levels."[14] In another recent series[39] the infants with Kernicterus had significantly higher levels of "free" BR than those that died without Kernicterus. These observations indicate that even in the intensive care population most of the cases of BR staining of the brain are the result of preventable BR toxicity.

The classical description of Kernicterus includes characteristic symptomatology during the acute stage of jaundice,[40, 41] BR staining of specific areas of the brain in the infants that die,[42] and in those that survive the development of choreoathetotic cerebral palsy corresponding to damage of the same areas of the brain.[42-44] Within the framework of choreoathetosis, the degree of disability is variable with mental deficiency and even microcephaly seen in a minority of cases and then only in combination with devastating motor dysfunction (personal material). Sensorineural hearing loss centered around 1000 cps is also seen with or without the acute neurological syndrome and subsequent choreoathetosis.[45-47] Bilirubin encephalopathy as described above is seen almost always only with unconjugated BR levels above 18–20 mg/dl with the exception of isolated sensorineural hearing loss that occurred in some infants with maximum BR levels as low as 15–16 mg/dl.[46, 47]

The discussion as to whether BR toxicity includes a much wider spectrum of neurological sequelae was revived by a number of recent reports.[48-53] Two reports from the material of the NINCDS Collaborative Perinatal Project argued that hyperbilirubinemia in excess of 10–14 mg/dl was associated with impaired motor development at 8–12 months.[48, 51] This effect was clinically significant only in the preterm infants with the surprising exception of the under 1500 g group. Although sophisticated statistical analyses were used to exclude confounding factors, the key question of whether both higher BR levels and depressed motor development could be due to a common factor but not causally related was not answered. At the time of the follow-up examination at 8 and 12 months no correction was made for the degree of prematurity. This becomes an important issue since in the analyses wide birth weight/gestational age (BW/GA) groups were used. For instance the group of 1501–2500 g and ≤36 weeks which showed the strongest association between BR levels and outcome at 8–12 months must have included preterm infants between 28 and 36 weeks of gestation. Since the less mature infants were most likely overrepresented in the higher BR groups while by 8–12 months their difference in postconceptional age was still an important determinant of their performance, this factor alone could account for the described association between depressed scores and BR levels. This explanation is strengthened by the results of the follow-up at 4 and 7 years of age which failed to demonstrate a clear-cut association between central nervous system dysfunction and BR levels up to 23 mg/dl.[50, 53] Another report from the Collaborative project stressed the importance of amniotic fluid infections in potentiating the toxicity of BR.[52] This is an example of yet another confounding factor. The complexity of the relationship between perinatal factors and outcome was further demonstrated by the fact that again the association between amniotic fluid infection, hyper-bilirubinemia, and outcome was weakened as the age at assessment increased. Moreover, although, in the tables, from the total material a continuous effect with increasing BR values was apparent, elsewhere it was pointed out that long-term impairment in association with hyperbilirubinemia and amniotic fluid infection was present only in infants of ≤ 34 weeks of gestation. The data presented so far from the Collaborative project cannot be considered conclusive regarding the existence of a continuum of BR toxicity starting at BR levels of 8–10 mg/dl and ranging in manifestations from minimal brain dysfunction to the classical Kernicterus and which is independent of other complicating perinatal factors (prematurity, infections, etc.). The detailed analysis of peri-natal factors, BR levels, and outcome presented by Johnson and Boggs[6] comes close to being persuasive. Although no case of choreoathetosis and sensori-neural hearing loss was found at the 4-year follow-up, abnormal ratings in the psychometric tests and the neurological examination were associated with BR levels ≥15 mg/dl. The association became stronger when the albumin-binding reserve (HBABA method) was taken into consideration. It should be noted that other studies[47, 54] failed to find evidence for an expanded spectrum of brain damage due to BR toxicity.

Information on the effects of hyperbilirubinemia on the neurological outcome of survivors of the intensive care era is scanty. In one report concerning the follow-up to 2 years of age of infants with BW < 1001 g no relationship was found.[55] But these infants should be considered at low risk as BR levels of 10 mg/dl or less were used as indications for ET and only one infant had a BR level in excess of 15 mg/dl.

The difficulties in the clinical evaluation of the management of hyperbili-rubinemia in preterm infants have been illustrated in the preceding review. There is no well-tested and accepted management to compare with any new method. Moreover, the end point is uncertain. BR staining of the brain might not always represent BR toxicity and in the survivors choreoathetosis and hearing loss might not be the only sequelae. For this reason, it is essential to evaluate new tests assessing the risk of BR encephalopathy in a population of newborns in which jaundice is the only significant complication, the risk of BR toxicity is high and clinical and autopsy Kernicterus an easily recognizable end point. In this first step the discriminating power of the test should prove superior to that of TBR level. This evaluation has already been carried out for the sephadex column chromatography test (Kernlute).[9–11] In all 18 cases of definite Kernicterus in term infants a 2+ result was obtained (no false negatives) and approximately one-half of the infants with a 2+ result had Kernic-terus. Conversely no case of Kernicterus was seen among 205 term infants with a negative or 1+ positive result. Several of these infants had BR levels in excess of 30 mg/dl.[11] The frequency with which the BR-binding status changes in individual patients independently from the TBR concentration also became apparent.[10] Thus the results of the test even when additions of BR are used to determine the reserve binding (BR titration point) are valid only for a limited period of time.

The method of management presented in this work was based on this initial evaluation. The key element of the system is the frequent repetition of the test during the critical period of rising BR values and unstable clinical condition in the sick infants. (In the present material an average of 10 tests were performed in the infants < 34 weeks GA.) This policy guarantees that the change from a negative to a positive test will be detected early and no patient will progress to a 2+ result. Prompt action on obtaining a positive result is the second important element of the system. The infusion of albumin was introduced as a way of protecting the patient while preparations for ET were carried out. In ⅔ of the cases this was sufficient to reverse the test from positive to negative, and no further treatment was carried out. Obviously, albumin alone should not be assumed to be effective in protecting every patient without checking the BR-binding status after the infusion. These results of albumin infusion represent *in vivo* experiments reinforcing the conclusions from previous *in vitro* ones[9] that the sephadex test is sensitive and responds to changes in the BR-binding status. In the present and previous work it was also demonstrated that the test responds to the effects on BR binding of such factors as imma-turity (Table I, Fig. 3), age (Fig. 4, and Refs. 10, 11) and seriousness of the overall clinical condition (Table VI, Fig. 6). In this respect the test goes further than the TBR levels, TBR/TPR ratio, or BR/albumin molar ratio. The reason why the later are of limited predictive value is the important effect on BR binding of exogenous[16, 17] and endogenous,[56] interferring or competing sub-stances. As far as the endogenous substances are concerned, their effect, as detected by the sephadex test, is more marked in the sick, more immature infants and during the first 4–5 days of life (present material and Refs. 10, 11, 56–58). This is in agreement with both experimental and clinical evidence[15] that these factors increase the risk of BR toxicity.

Of all the tests of BR binding evaluated in clinical material the sephadex gel filtration gave consistently positive results in well-documented cases of Ker-nicterus.[9–11, 59–61] Two more methods have passed this test on a limited scale—the red cell binding and the peroxidase tests.[62–64] The sephadex and peroxidase methods have been compared in the same material and gave results—in clinical terms—in close agreement in spite of being based on completely different principles (Ref. 65 and Wennberg, Alfors, and Valaes, unpublished material).

Sephadex G-25 gel filtration is the basis of a number of methods using elution of the adsorbed BR from the gel instead of the diazo-staining reaction used in the present material.[58–60, 66–69] Additions of BR to the native sera have been used to determine the "total BR-binding capacity" and from this the "reserve BR-binding capacity." Similarly additions of BR can be used in the sephadex column chromatography test (Kernlute). The need for such additions was based on the assumption that any amount of "free" BR adsorbed by the sephadex gel signified that the safe limit was already exceeded and that treatment had to be instituted before "free" BR could be demonstrated by the sephadex. Also it was assumed that the "total BR-binding capacity" remained constant in a given patient and, once determined, the BR level could be used to guide treatment. Both these assumptions were erroneous as theory and actual experience indicate. The adsorption of BR by the sephadex gel is a complex equilibrium phenomenon and should be used only as an index of the BR-binding characteristics of the serum. Thus the results, however, expressed—"free BR," "BR binding capacity," "reserve BR-binding capacity," "1 or 2+ positive," etc. —have no *a priori* significance in terms of BR toxicity. Whether the partition of BR between the serum and the sephadex gel reflects the *in vivo* partition of BR between serum and the central nervous system needs to be verified in clinical material. The present and previous experience with sephadex column chromatography provides ample evidence that BR adsorption that gives a 1+ positive result corresponds to a BR-binding status not associated with obvious BR toxicity. It should also be mentioned that comparison of the chromatography and elution methods proved that the 1+ result by chromatography was obtained with BR levels just below the levels corresponding to the "total BR-binding capacity" as determined by the elution technique. Moreover, an average rise of BR concentration by 10 mg/dl was needed to change a 1+ result to 2+.[70] In the practical application of the sephadex-binding tests additions of BR to determine the reserve BR-binding are not necessary. The straight chromatography test as used in the present work is simple, requires only 0.1 ml of plasma, and the result is read in 20 min. No complicated apparatus and no technical skills beyond the handling of a pipette are required. No unusual effort had to be made in order to perform thousands of tests and closely monitor the BR-binding status in our material.

The fraction of plasma BR actually measured by the sephadex gel filtration has not yet been fully elucidated. This should not be considered an impediment in the clinical application of the test. In any case we do not know which is the "toxic form" of BR. Is it the "free-unbound-diffusable BR," the BR displaced to the secondary binding sites, or the BR taken up by cell membranes (as by the red cells), or possibly other carriers, or all of these as expressed by the BR binding characteristics of the serum? Until we can answer this question it will be idle to discuss the theoretical merits of the different binding methods, however accurately they measure any one of the above. Their performance in clinical material or in animal models is the acid test of their value and at the same time the only way to answer the question of which is the "toxic species of BR."

For the first time a large group of newborns at high risk for BR toxicity has been managed on the basis of a BR-binding test. Our results indicate that overt

BR toxicity has been prevented while the risk/benefit ratio has been improved—fewer patients subjected to the risk of ET—in relation to the recommended management on the basis of TBR level and clinical characteristics. It will be much more difficult to answer the question whether the suspected more subtle manifestations of BR toxicity have also been prevented. Our material demonstrates that a number of components of the total clinical condition influence the BR-binding status (Table VI) while other undefined factors must also be important (Fig. 6). We anticipate that it will prove a Herculean statistical task to differentiate the effects on the long-term outcome of the clinical complications from those of BR toxicity. We believe that this should not prevent the application of the sephadex test for the management of neonatal hyperbilirubinemia. After all, none of the old or newer systems of management has been shown conclusively to have achieved this goal; moreover, the existence of such subtle effects of BR toxicity is still surrounded by uncertainties.

REFERENCES

1. Hsia D. Y. -Y., Allen, F. H., Gellis, S. S., and Diamond, L. K., Erythroblastosis fetalis: VIII. Studies of serum bilirubin in relation to Kernicterus. *N. Engl. J. Med.* **247,** 668 (1952).

2. Ackerman, B. D., Dyer, G. Y., and Leydorf, M. M., Hyperbilirubinemia and kernicterus in small premature infants. *Pediatrics* **45,** 918 (1970).

3. Stern, L., and Denton, R. L., Kernicterus in small premature infants. *Pediatrics* **35,** 483 (1965).

4. Gartner, L. M., Snyder, R. N., Chabon, R. S., and Bernstein, J., Kernicterus: high incidence in premature infants with low serum bilirubin concentrations. *Pediatrics* **45,** 906 (1970).

5. Odell, G. B., Storey, G. N. B., and Rosenberg, L. A., Studies in Kernicterus III. The saturation of serum proteins with bilirubin during neonatal life and its relationship to brain damage at five years. *J. Pediatr.* **76,** 12 (1970).

6. Johnson, L., and Boggs, T. R., Bilirubin Dependent Brain Damage: Incidence and Indications for Treatment, in *Phototherapy in the Newborn:An Overview*, Odell, B. G., Schaffer, R., and Simopoulos, Eds. Washington, National Academy of Sciences, 1974, pp. 122–149.

7. Scheidt, P. C., Mellits, E. D., Hardy, J. B., Drage, J. S., and Boggs, T. R., Toxicity to bilirubin in neonates: Infant development during first year in relation to maximum neonatal serum bilirubin concentration. *J. Pediatr.* **91,** 292 (1977).

8. Odell, G. B., The dissociation of bilirubin from albumin and its clinical implications. *J. Pediatr.* **55,** 268 (1959).

9. Blondheim, S. H., Kapitulnik, J., Valaes, T., and Kaufmann, N. A., Use of a sephadex column to evaluate the bilirubin binding capacity of the serum of infants with neonatal jaundice. *Israel J. Med. Sci.* **8,** 22 (1972).

10. Kapitulnik, J., Valaes, T., Kaufmann, N. A., and Blondheim, S. H., Clinical evaluation of sephadex gel filtration in estimation of bilirubin binding on serum in neonatal jaundice. *Arch. Dis. Child.* **49,** 886 (1974).

11. Valaes, T., Kapitulnik, J., Kaufmann, N. A., and Blondheim, S. H., Experience with sephadex gel filtration in assessing the risk of bilirubin encephalopathy in neonatal jaundice. In *Bilirubin Metabolism in the Newborn (II)*, Blondheim, S. H., and Bergsman, D., Eds. *Birth Defects* **12,** 215 (1976).

12. Michaelsson, M., Nosslin, B., and Sjolin, S., Plasma bilirubin determination in the newborn infant. A methodological study with special reference to the influence of hemolysis. *Pediatrics* **35,** 925 (1965).

13. Maisels, M. J., Bilirubin: On understanding and influencing its metabolism in the newborn infant. *Pediatr. Clin. North Am.* **19,** 447 (1972).

14. Pearlman, M. A., Gartner, L. M., Lee, K. S., Morecki, R., and Horoupian, D. S., Absence of Kernicterus in low-birth-weight infants from 1971 through 1976: Comparison with findings in 1966 and 1967. *Pediatrics* **62,** 460 (1978).

15. Diamond, I., Bilirubin Encephalopathy (Kernicterus), in *Scientific Approaches to Clinical Neurology*, Goldensohn, E.S., and Appel, S.H., Eds. Lea and Febiger, Philadelphia, 1977, pp. 1212–1233.

16. Silverman, W. A., Anderson, D. H., Blanc, W. A., and Crozier, D. N., A difference in mortality rate and incidence of Kernicterus among premature infants allotted to two prophylactic antibacterial regimens. *Pediatrics* **18,** 614 (1956).

17. Harris, R. C., Lucey, J. F., and MacLean, J. R., Kernicterus in premature infants associated with low concentrations of bilirubin in plasma. *Pediatrics* **21,** 875 (1958).

18. Johnson, L., Garcia, M. L., Figueroa, E., and Sarmiento, F., Kernicterus in rats lacking glucuronyl transferase II. Factors which alter bilirubin concentration and frequency of Kernicterus. *Am. J. Dis. Child.* **101,** 322 (1961).

19. Schmid, R., Diamond, I., Hammaker, L., and Gundersen, C. G., Interaction of bilirubin with albumin. *Nature* **206,** 1041 (1965).

20. Diamond, I., and Schmid, R., The pathogenesis of bilirubin encephalopathy: Experimental models in newborn and adult animals. *Trans. Am. Neurol. Assoc.* **90,** 38 (1965).

21. Lucey, J. F., Hibbard, E., Behrman, R. E., DeGallardo, F. O. E., and Windle, W. F., Kernicterus in asphyxiated newborn rhesus monkeys. *Exp. Neurol.* **9,** 43 (1964).

22. Mollison, P. L., and Cutbush, M., Haemolytic Disease of the Newborn, in *Recent Advances in Paediatrics*, Gairduer, D., Ed. Churchill, London, 1954, pp. 110–132.

23. Panagopoulos, G., Valaes, T., and Doxiadis, S. A., Morbidity and mortality related to exchange transfusions. *J. Pediatr.* **74,** 247 (1969).

24. Meyer, T. C., A study of serum bilirubin levels in relation to Kernicterus and prematurity. *Arch. Dis. Child.* **31,** 75 (1956).

25. Crosse, M. V., Wallis, P. G., and Walsh, A. M., Replacement transfusion as a means of preventing Kernicterus of prematurity. *Arch. Dis. Child.* **33,** 403 (1958).

26. Corner, B. D., Hyperbilirubinemia in premature infants treated by exchange transfusion. *Proc. R. Soc. Med.* **51,** 1019 (1958).

27. Keenan, M. Y., Perlstein, R. H., Light, I. J., and Sutherland, J. M., Kernicterus in small sick premature infants receiving phototherapy. *Pediatrics* **49,** 652 (1972).

28. Rapmund, G., Bowman, J. M., and Harris, R. C., Bilirubinemia in nonerythroblastic premature infants. *Am. J. Dis. Child.* **99,** 604 (1960).

29. Shiller, J. G., and Silverman, W. A., Uncomplicated hyperbilirubinemia of prematurity. *Am. J. Dis. Child.* **101,** 587 (1961).

30. Wishingrad, L., Cornblath, M., Takakuwa, T., Rozenfeld, I. M., Elegant, L. D., Kaufmann, A., Lasser, E., and Klein, R. I., Studies of non-hemolytic hyperbilirubinemia in premature infants. I. Prospective randomized selection for exchange transfusion with observation on the levels of serum bilirubin with and without exchange transfusion and neurologic evaluation one year after birth. *Pediatrics* **36,** 162 (1965).

31. Smallpiece, V., and Davies, P. A., Immediate feeding of premature infants with undiluted breast milk. *Lancet* **2,** 1349 (1964).

32. Wennberg, R. P., Schwartz, R., and Sweet, A. Y., Early versus delayed feeding of low birth weight infants: Effects on physiologic jaundice. *J. Pediatr.* **68,** 860 (1966).

33. Wu, P. Y. K., Terlmann, P., Gabber, M., Vaughan, M., and Metcaff, V., "Early" versus "late" feeding of low birth weight neonates: Effects on serum bilirubin, blood sugar and responses to glucagon and epinephrine tolerance tests. *Pediatrics* **39,** 733 (1967).

34. Cremer, R. J., Perryman, P. W., and Richards, D. H., Influence of light on the hyperbilirubinemia of infants. *Lancet* **1,** 1094 (1958).

35. Lucey, J. F., Phototherapy of Jaundice—1969, in *Bilirubin Metabolism in the Newborn, Birth Defects* **6**(2), 63–70 (1970).

36. Trölle, D., Decrease of total serum bilirubin concentration in newborn infants after phenobarbitone treatment. *Lancet* **2,** 705 (1968).

37. Valaes, T., Petmezaki, S., and Doxiadis, S. A., Effect of neonatal hyperbilirubinemia of phenobarbital during pregnancy or after birth: Practical value of the treatment in a population with high risk of unexplained severe neonatal jaundice, in *Bilirubin Metabolism in the Newborn*, Bersma, D. and Hsia, D.Y.-Y., Eds. *Birth Defects* **6**(2), 46–54 (1970).

38. Vert, P., Hermann, D., Royer, R. J., André, M., and Badonell, Y., Effect of Phenobarbital on Hyperbilirubinemia in Premature and High Risk Infants. in *Neonatal Intensive Care*, Stetson, J. B., and Swyer, P. R., Eds. Green, St. Louis, 1976, pp. 219–235.

39. Cashore, W. J., Free bilirubin and Kernicterus in pre-term infants. (abstract) *Pediatr. Res.* **13**, 491 (1979).

40. Vaughan, V. C., III, Allen, F. H., Jr., and Diamond, L. K., Erythroblastoesis fetalis: IV Further observations on Kernicterus. *Pediatrics* **6**, 706 (1950).

41. Van Praagh, R., Diagnosis of Kernicterus in the neonatal period. *Pediatrics* **28**, 870 (1961).

42. Claireaux, A. E., Haemolytic disease of the newborn. I A Clinical pathological study of 157 cases. II. Nuclear jaundice (Kernicterus). *Arch. Dis. Child.* **25**, 61 (1950).

43. Perlestein, M., Neurologic sequelae of erythroblastosis fetalis. *Am. J. Dis. Child.* **79**, 605 (1950).

44. Gerrard, J., Kernicterus. *Brain* **75**, 526 (1952).

45. Byers, R. K., Paine, R. S., and Crothers, B., Extrapyramidal cerebral palsy with hearing loss following erythroblastosis. *Pediatrics* **15**, 248 (1955).

46. Fenwick, J. D., Neonatal jaundice as a cause of deafness. *J. Laryngol. Otol.* **89**, 925 (1975).

47. Valaes, T., Kipouros, K., Petmezaki, S., Solman, M., and Doxiadis, S. A., Effectiveness and safety of prenatal phenobarbital for the prevention of neonatal jaundice. *Pediatr. Res.* **14**, 947–952 (1980).

48. Boggs, T. R., Jr., Hardy, J. B., and Frazier, T. M., Correlation of neonatal serum total bilirubin concentration and developmental status at age eight months. *J. Pediatr.* **71**, 553 (1967).

49. Hardy, J. B., and Peeples, M. O., Serum bilirubin levels in newborn infants. Distributions and associations with neurological abnormalities during the first year of life. *J. Hopkins Med. J.* **128**, 265 (1971).

50. Upadhyay, Y., A longitudinal study of full-term neonates with hyperbilirubinemia to four years of age. *J. Hopkins Med. J.* **128**, 273 (1971).

51. Scheidt, P. C., Mellits, E. D., Hardy, J. B., Drage, J. S., and Boggs, T. R., Toxicity to bilirubin in neonates: Infant development during first year in relation to maximum neonatal serum bilirubin concentration. *J. Pediatr.* **91**, 293 (1977) (and complete text provided by the authors).

52. Naeye, R. L., Amniotic fluid infections, neonatal hyperbilirubinemia and psychomotor impairment. *Pediatrics* **62**, 497 (1978).

53. Rubin, R. A., Balow, B., and Fisch, R. O., Neonatal bilirubin levels related to cognitive development at ages 4 through 7 years. *J. Pediatr.* **94**, 601 (1979).

54. Pope, K. E., Buncíc, R. S., Ashby, S., and Fitzhardinge, P. M., The status at two years of low-birth-weight infants born in 1974 with birth weights of less than 1001 gm. *J. Pediatr.* **92**, 253 (1978).

55. Culley, P. E., Powell, J., Waterhouse, J., and Wood, B., Sequelae of neonatal jaundice. *Br. Med. J.* **3**, 383 (1970).

56. Valaes, T., and Hyte, M., Effect of exchange transfusion on bilirubin binding. *Pediatrics* **59**, 881 (1977).

57. Kapitulnik, J., Horner-Mibashan, R., Blondheim, S. H., Kaufmann, N. A., and Russell, A., Increase in bilirubin-binding affinity of serum with age of infant. *J. Pediatr.* **86**, 442 (1975).

58. Cashore, W. J., Horwich, A., Karotkin, E. H., and Oh, W., Influence of gestational age and clinical status on bilirubin-binding capacity in newborn infants. *Am. J. Dis. Child.* **131**, 898 (1977).

59. Jirsová, V., Jirsa, M., Heringová, A., Koldovský, O., and Weirichová, J., The use and possible diagnostic significance of sephadex gel filtration of serum from icteric newborn. *Biol. Neonat.* **11**, 204 (1967).

60. Schiff, D., Chan, G., and Stern, L., Sephadex G-25 quantitative estimation of free bilirubin

potential in jaundiced newborn infant's sera: A guide to the prevention of Kernicterus. *J. Lab. Clin. Med.* **80,** 455 (1972).

61. Zamet, P., Nakamura, H., Perez-Robles, S., Larroche, J. C., and Minkowski, A., The use of critical levels of birth weight and "free bilirubin" as an approach for prevention of Kernicterus. *Biol. Neonat.* **26,** 274 (1975).

62. Bratlid, D., Reserve albumin binding capacity (HBABA method) salicylate saturation index and red cell binding of bilirubin in neonatal jaundice. *Arch. Dis. Child.* **48,** 393 (1973).

63. Jacobsen, J. and Wennberg, R. P., Determination of unbound bilirubin in the serum of newborns. *Clin. Chem.* **20,** 783 (1974).

64. Wennberg, R. P., Lau, M., and Rasmussen, L. F., Clinical significance of unbound bilirubin. *Pediatr. Res.* **10,** 434 (1976).

65. Cashore, W. J., Monin, P. J. P., and Oh, W., Serum bilirubin binding capacity and free bilirubin concentrations: A comparison between sephadex G-25 filtration and peroxidase oxidation techniques. *Pediatr. Res.* **12,** 195 (1978).

66. Kaufman, N. A., Kapitulnik, J., and Blondheim, S. H., The absorption of bilirubin by the sephadex and its relationship to the criteria for exchange transfusion. *Pediatrics* **44,** 543 (1969).

67. Chunga, F., and Lardinois, R., Separation by gel filtration and microdetermination of unbound bilirubin. I. *In vitro* albumin and acidosis effects on albumin bilirubin binding. *Acta Paediatr. Scand.* **60,** 27 (1971).

68. Trivin, F., Odievre, M., and Lemonnier, A., Faster estimation of reserve bilirubin binding capacity of serum from the neonate by thin-layer chromatography on sephadex. *Clin. Chem.* **23,** 541 (1977).

69. Du Pont, C., and Sarkozy, E., A simplified micromethod for a reserve bilirubin binding capacity. *J. Lab. Clin. Med.* **89,** 439 (1977).

70. Kaufmann, N. A., Kapitulnik, J., and Blondheim, S. H., Bilirubin binding affinity of serum: Comparison of qualitative and quantitative sephadex gel filtration methods. *Clin. Chem.* **19,** 1276 (1973).

8

Evidence of Minor Damage Occurring during Phototherapy: Photoinduced Covalent Binding of Bilirubin to Serum Albumin

FIRMINO F. RUBALTELLI, GIULIO JORI, and ELIANA ROSSI

Previous studies in our laboratory showed that visible light-irradiation of the 1:1 bilirubin-human serum albumin (HSA) complex induces the modification of specific amino acid residues; as a consequence, the protein undergoes a partial denaturation and displays a reduced affinity for bilirubin.[1,2] Moreover, bilirubin was not completely removed from irradiated HSA by gel filtration on Sephadex G-75 columns. The data presented in this study demonstrate that the latter phenomenon is due to the formation of a covalent photoadduct between human (HSA) and bovine (BSA) albumin and bilirubin (or its photoisomers and/or photoproducts).

The HSA and BSA bilirubin complexes (0.1 mM) were irradiated at pH 7.4 (0.5 M phosphate buffer) and at 20°C with an Osram 1250-W halogen lamp; a 50% aqueous acetone filter was used to remove wavelengths below 330 nm. The irradiance in the 440–470 nm range was 300 μW/cm^2/nm. Several experimental approaches were used to elucidate the photoinduced interaction between the protein and the tetrapyrrole moiety and the presence of bilirubin in the samples analyzed was monitored by fluorescence emission (λ_{ex} = 460 nm) and fluorescence excitation (λ_{em} = 530 nm) spectroscopy.

Evidence for the photoinduced formation of the covalent product was obtained by precipitation of the protein-bilirubin complex, before and after

Department of Pediatrics and C.N.R. Center for the Physiology and Biochemistry of Hemocyanins and Other Metallo-Proteins, Institute of Animal Biology, University of Padova, Padova, Italy.

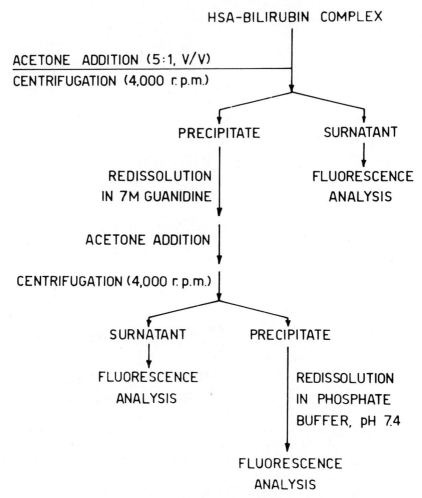

Fig. 1. Procedure for analysis of the serum albumin-bilirubin complex.

irradiation, through the addition of acetone in a fivefold excess over water (v/v) (Fig. 1). In unirradiated samples, a substantial fraction of bilirubin was extracted by acetone; complete removal was obtained only after redissolution in the presence of 7 M guanidine and acetone-induced reprecipitation. On the other hand, all irradiated protein samples retained a readily detectable amount of bound bilirubin even after addition of the denaturant. Kinetic studies indicated that the amount of bound bilirubin increased as a function of irradiation time and was higher when irradiations were performed in deoxygenated solutions.

Further insight into the nature of the bilirubin-BSA photoadduct was obtained by cleavage of the irradiated protein with cyanogen bromide according to the procedure of King and Spencer[3] and subsequent gel filtration on Sephadex G-75 (30% acetic acid as eluant).

Two fragments were obtained, fragment C and N, which correspond with the peptides 1–186 and 187–545, respectively, of bovine serum albumin.[3]

Fluorescence studies indicated that fragment C retained bound bilirubin, whereas fragment N was devoid of bound pigment. Cleavage of disulfide bonds of fragment C with dithiotreitol in a 60:1 molar excess over the peptide and subsequent gel filtration on Sephadex G-75 allowed us to isolate one bilirubin-containing peptide, whose amino acid composition was coincident within experimental error with that of albumin peptide 187–397. These findings would indicate that the formation of the bilirubin-albumin covalent photoadduct is characterized by a high degree of spatial selectivity; it appears reasonable to hypothesize that the photoinduced binding preferentially involves those amino acid residues which are adjacent to the binding site of albumin for bilirubin.

A similar spatially selective photoinduced binding was observed after irradiation of complexes between serum albumin and other dyes (e.g., fluorescein). In this case the authors suggested the occurence of a type I mechanism involving the formation of radical species from both the sensitizer and protein; recombination of the two radicals would lead to the formation of a dye-protein adduct.[4] The occurrence of such a mechanism in our system is also suggested by the fact that the photoreaction takes place with a higher yield in deoxygenated solutions. In the presence of oxygen, the formation of the photoadduct should be competitive with the deactivation of bilirubin by energy transfer to oxygen, followed by attack of singlet oxygen either on bilirubin itself or on human serum albumin (Fig. 2).

It is also possible that the aforesaid photoprocesses, that is, photoaddition and energy transfer to oxygen, occur with some photoisomers or photodegradation products of bilirubin; it is known that some of them can absorb the visible wavelengths used in our irradiation experiments.

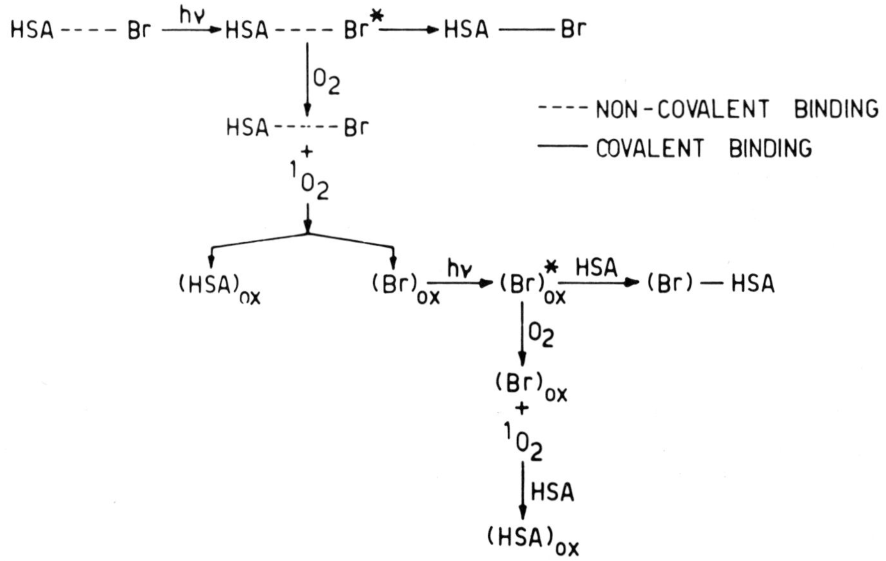

Fig. 2. Proposed scheme for the bilirubin-sensitized photomodification of human serum albumin.

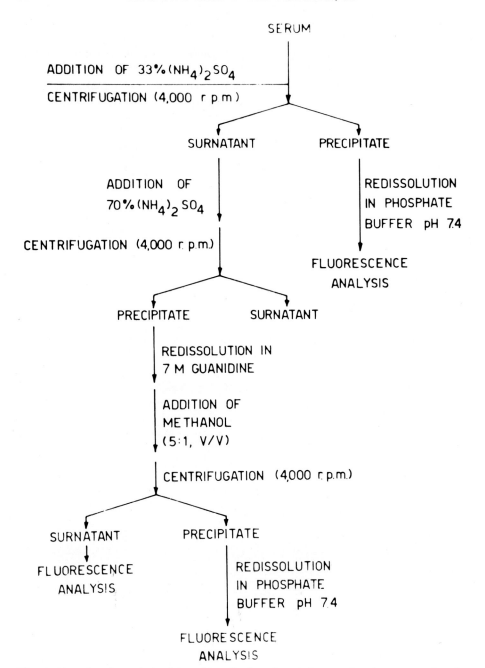

Fig. 3. Procedure for analysis of sera of jaundiced newborn infants used to demonstrate that the photoadduct specifically appears in the albumin fraction.

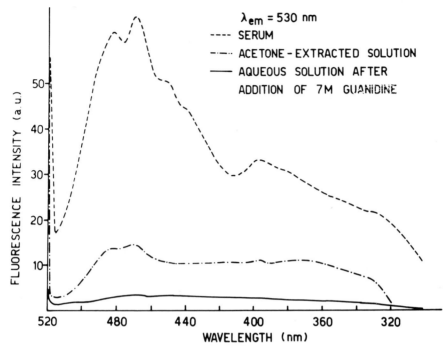

Fig. 4. Typical fluorescence excitation spectrum of bilirubin in sera of untreated jaundiced newborns and in their acetone extracts. The shape of the spectrum is coincident with that found for albumin bound bilirubin. After redissolution of the serum proteins in 7 M guanidine and acetone-induced reprecipitation, the typical fluorescence excitation is no longer detectable. The purity of the protein fraction was previously checked by monitoring the intrinsic fluorescence emission by the tryptophyl residues (λ_{ex} = 290 nm, emission λ_{max} = 348 nm).

It appeared of interest to investigate whether the above described photo-binding process also takes place as a consequence of the phototherapeutic treatment of jaundiced newborns. It has been generally assumed that no appreciable photodamage occurs during phototherapy, owing to the weak photosensitizing efficiency of bilirubin coupled with its high reactivity toward $^1O_2$.[5] In view of this, we have analyzed the sera of 29 full-term hyperbilirubi-nemic newborns before and after light treatment with a set of Superblue lamps. The intensity of the irradiation at the level of the infant was 22 $\mu W/cm^2$/nm in the 440/470 nm range. The experimental procedure adopted to ascertain the presence of the bilirubin-albumin photoadduct is the same as shown in Figure 1.

The formation of the photoadduct was clearly demonstrated by the acetone-induced precipitation method. Further demonstration of this was obtained by fractional precipitation with ammonium sulphate (Fig. 3); by this procedure, we were able to demonstrate that the photoadduct was specifically formed in the albumin fraction.

Figures 4 and 5 show the typical fluorescence excitation and emission spectra

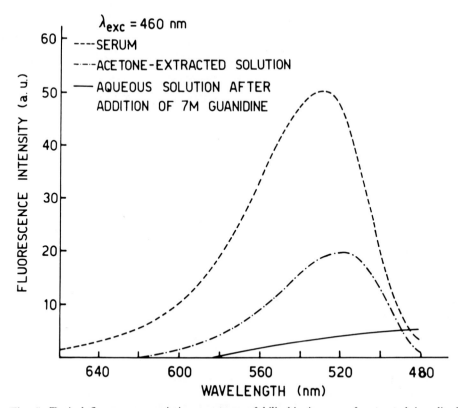

Fig. 5. Typical fluorescence emission spectrum of bilirubin in sera of untreated jaundiced newborns and in their acetone extracts. The shape of the spectrum is coincident with that found for albumin bound bilirubin. After redissolution of the serum proteins in 7 M guanidine and acetone-induced reprecipitation, the typical fluorescence emission is no longer detectable. The purity of the protein fraction was previously checked by monitoring the intrinsic fluorescence emission by the tryptophyl residues (λ_{ex} = 290 nm, emission λ_{max} = 348 nm).

of bilirubin in sera of jaundiced newborns and in their acetone extracts. After redissolution of the serum proteins in 7 M guanidine and acetone-induced reprecipitation, the typical fluorescence excitation and emission spectra of bilirubin are no longer detectable in the case of unirradiated infants. After phototherapy of the same infants, even after the aforesaid treatment, a detectable amount of serum protein-bound bilirubin is retained (Figs. 6 and 7).

A synthesis of our clinical studies is shown in Table I. Clearly, the formation of the photoadduct is detectable only after about 7–9 hr of phototreatment. In a few cases, we used white fluorescent lamps, which have a lower irradiance in the blue spectral region, and obtained similar results but after longer periods of exposure to light. The disappearance of the photoadduct at 15–20 days after the end of the phototreatment is in agreement with the normal turnover of the serum albumin.

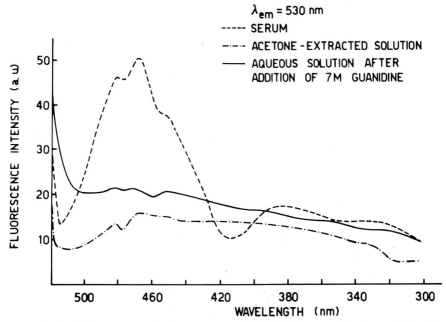

Fig. 6. Typical fluorescence excitation spectrum of bilirubin in sera of phototreated jaundiced newborns and in their acetone extracts. Even after redissolution of the serum proteins in 7 M guanidine and acetone-induced reprecipitation, a detectable amount of serum protein-bound bilirubin is retained. The purity of the protein fraction was checked by monitoring the intrinsic fluorescence emission by the tryptophyl residues (λ_{ex} = 290 nm).

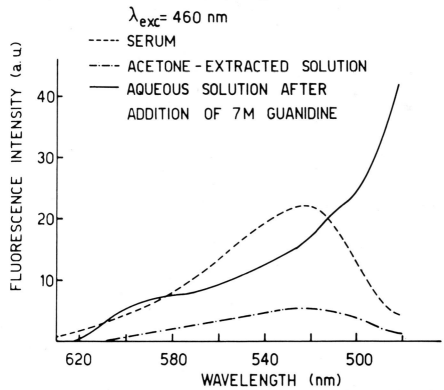

Fig. 7. Typical fluorescence emission spectrum of bilirubin in sera of phototreated jaundiced newborns and in their acetone extracts. Even after redissolution of the serum proteins in 7 M guanidine and acetone-induced reprecipitation, a detectable amount of serum protein-bound bilirubin is retained. The purity of the protein fraction was checked by monitoring the intrinsic fluorescence emission by the tryptophyl residues (λ_{ex} = 290 nm).

TABLE I

Number of investigated subjects: 29	Schedule of the phototreatment:	Summary of clinical studies:
Serum bilirubin levels at the beginning of the phototreatment: 10.8–15 mg/dl	Light source: four F20T12/BB Westinghouse Lamps l.c.·mu	Average irradiation time for appearance of the photoadduct: 7–9 hr
	Irradiance in the 440–470 nm range: 22 μW/cm^2/nm	Average time for the disappearance of the photoadduct: 15–20 days
	Type of treatment: continuous irradiation	

SUMMARY

The findings described in this paper demonstrate that the lack of complete removal of bilirubin or its photoproducts from serum albumin after *in vitro* irradiation with visible light is due to the formation of a covalent photoadduct between the protein and the tetrapyrrolic pigment. The same phenomenon takes place *in vivo*, demonstrating that some kind of biochemical damage is actually induced by phototherapy. The demonstration of the actual occurrence of *in vivo* phototherapy-induced damage stresses the importance of investigations aimed at avoiding overexposure of patients to the light sources.

ACKNOWLEDGMENTS

We would like to express our appreciation to the head nurse Mr. B. Giacon and to all the nursing staff of the Neonatal Intensive Care Unit for their continuous help.

This work was supported in part by CNR Grants No. 77.01550.64 and No. 78.01876.65 under the CNR-NSF cooperative research program.

REFERENCES

1. Rubaltelli, F. F., and Jori, G., Visible light irradiation of human and bovine serum albumin-bilirubin complex. *Photochem. Photobiol.* **29**, 991–1000 (1979).
2. Rubaltelli, F. F., Rossi, E., and Jori, G., Modification of serum albumin during phototherapy of jaundiced newborn babies. Lancet 2, 1295–1296 (1979).
3. King, T. P., and Spencer, M., Structural studies and organic ligand-binding properties of bovine plasma albumin. *J. Biol. Chem.* **245**, 6134–6148 (1970).
4. Jori, G., and Spikes, J. D., Mapping the three dimensional structure of proteins by photochemical techniques. *Photochem. Photobiol. Rev.* (edited by K. C. Smith), 193–275 (1978).
5. McDonagh, A. F., The photochemistry and photometabolism of bilirubin. *Phototherapy in the Newborn: An Overview.* Odell, G. B., Schaffer, R., and Simopoulos, A. P., Eds. National Academy of Sciences, Washington, D.C., 1974, pp. 56–73.

9

The Influence of Albumin Administration on the Effect of Phototherapy in Gunn Rats

LEONORE BALLOWITZ, GÜNTHER WIESE, and ARMIN STEIGERWALD

In 1972 Wong and co-workers[15] in two clinical trials compared the serum bilirubin decline under phototherapy with and without intravenous (IV) albumin administration prior to illumination. They found that the albumin-treated groups had higher and more prolonged jaundice than the groups given phototherapy alone. They concluded from their results that phototherapy is effective mainly on extravascular bilirubin, since IV-administered albumin withdraws bilirubin into the intravascular space, where it is probably beyond the reach of blue light.

In the course of studies with infant Gunn rats on the effects of stabilizers in commercial preparations of human albumin, we observed a bilirubin influx into areas where albumin was subcutaneously (SC) injected. The question arose as to whether albumin-caused SC bilirubin enrichment could bring more bilirubin within the reach of blue light.

Both observations induced us to investigate in more detail the influence of albumin on the phototherapy effect in Gunn rats. In the course of the investigations it became obvious that quantitative analyses of concentration/time-relations had to be carried out for convincing statements to be made.

MATERIALS AND METHODS

Homozygous Gunn rats 3–5 days old (without fur, weighing 6–11 g, ♂ and ♀) and 1 month old (with thick fur and weaned, weighing 80–120 g, ♀ only) were injected either IV or SC with different doses of human albumin or with equal volumes of 0.9% saline. The backs of the 1-month-old rats had previously been shaved over an area of about 4×8 cm. The SC doses were administered in the center of that area so that the resulting SC depot was under the shaved skin. In order to standardize the illuminated surface, the same kind of (dummy) shaving was done in the IV groups. After the injections some of the animals were kept in the dark, others under intense blue (Philips 20 W/52 BAM) or under daylight (Osram L20 W/19) phototherapy coming from two directions, as described in previous studies (Ballowitz, et al.[1-3]). On the animal level in the transparent macrolone cages the effective irradiance E_{bili} was 3.7 mW/cm^2 for BAM blue and 0.75 mW/cm^2 for daylight. (As for the radiometer used see also Ballowitz, et al.[1]) During the first 6 hr the 3–5-day-old rats were without dam. After 3 hr ≈0.1-ml glucose solution was given by gavage; after 6 hr the lactating mother rat remained with them (and suckled them) up to the end of the test. The dams provided a partial light trap for their youngsters. In blood taken from the cut tail serum bilirubin concentration was directly read on the American Optical Bilirubinometer,* prior to the albumin injection and there-after at fixed intervals (mostly 3, 6, 24, 48, 72 hr after the injection). In several animals, simultaneous protein analyses were done on biuret basis with centri-fichem autoanalyser (Roche) and agarose-gel-electrophoresis (see Siegert and Siemes[14]). The latter method allowed a clear-cut separation of the injected human albumin from the rats' own albumin.

Owing to our experience with the different stabilizers in commercial albumin preparations, we chose a 20% human albumin formulation which was not produced by the usual Cohn fractionation but by the heat ethanol method (Schneider, et al.[13]). In this procedure 4 mmol/liter Na caprylate were added before fractionation. The manufacturer declared that—in the final product—Na caprylate was not traceable at all by gas chromatography. The final product can be regarded as practically free of stabilizers.

DESCRIPTION OF THE CONCENTRATION/TIME-GRAPHS

In Figures 1–12 the measuring points obtained are given as symbols (□, ◇, or ▽). For visual reasons, only in some curves are standard deviations drawn. The lines were calculated with a computer by a least squares method (see below). After IV injection the *highest concentration of human albumin* in *the serum* of both age groups of rats was measured at the first check: 3 hr after the injection. In the following hours the concentration gradually declined, without significant differences as to both age groups (Figs. 1 and 2).

---

* *This instrument measures light transmission at 461 nm (and for hemoglobin compensation at 551 nm). In vitro addition of the human albumin preparation to sera of jaundiced infant rats induced a small decline (maximal 10%) of the readings beyond the effect of dilution. This is probably due to a shift of the absorption peak of bilirubin after increased albumin binding. (The shift did not occur in sera of adult rats.) This deviation was not corrected. It could be neglected, since both groups of animals—illuminated ones as well as controls in the dark—were equally affected.*

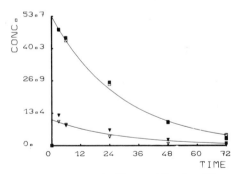

Fig. 1. In 1-month-old rats following IV injection.

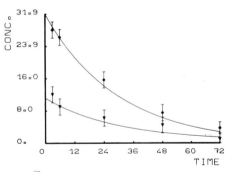

Fig. 2. In 3–5-day-old rats following IV injection.

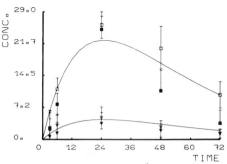

Fig. 3. In 1-month-old rats following SC injection.

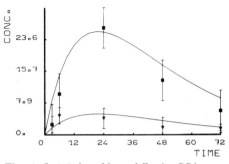

Fig. 4. In 3–5-day-old rats following SC injection.

Fig. 1–4. Concentration/time-functions for *human albumin* (in g/liter) injected into homozygous Gunn rats. (The drawn-out lines were calculated with a computer by a least squares program—Figs. 1–12.) Measuring Points: 8.0 g human albumin/kg ■ in the dark, □ under blue lights ($E_{bili} \approx 3.7$ mW/cm²); 4.0 g human albumin/kg ◆ in the dark, ◇ under blue lights; 0.8 g human albumin/kg ▼ in the dark, ▽ under blue lights.

In the serum of *1-month-old* (weanling) *rats* the highest human albumin concentration after SC application was measured 24 hr after the injection (Fig. 3). That does not mean, however, that this was the real peak. (No controls were made between 6 and 24 hr.) After 24 hr, serum concentration following IV or SC administration was about equal. No obvious differences were noticed in animals kept in the dark or under the lights (Figs. 1 and 3). Elimination of human albumin was not essentially influenced by phototherapy—in all probability not enhanced.

In *3–5-day-old* (infant) *rats*, the peak after SC injections (Fig. 8) was reached somewhat earlier than in the 1-month-old rats. That means, equilibration came on faster in the younger animals. But proportions between the two (three) doses tested (and the primary concentration following IV injections) were similar in both age groups.

In the dark serum bilirubin levels markedly increased after the albumin injections. The slope depended on the albumin dose and the age of the animal, and after IV injection was steepest during the first hours. With *small doses*

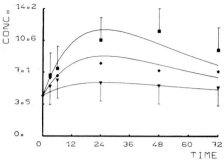

Fig. 5. In 1-month-old rats following IV injection of human albumin.

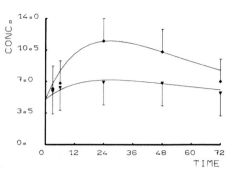

Fig. 6. In 3–5-day-old rats following IV injection of human albumin.

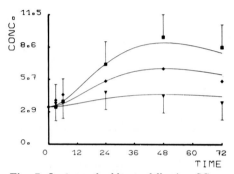

Fig. 7. In 1-month-old rats following SC injection of human albumin.

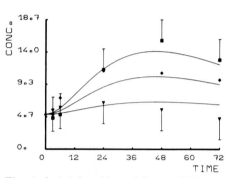

Fig. 8. In 3–5-day-old rats following SC injection of human albumin.

Figs. 5–8. For animals kept *in the dark*.
Figs. 5–12. Concentration/time-function for *serum bilirubin* (in mg/100 ml). (For better synopsis the functions were shifted in parallel so that the starting point for the lines in each graph became equal.) The symbols correspond to those of Figures 1–4.

(0.8 g albumin/kg), the peak was reached earlier than with *higher doses* (4–8 g albumin/kg).

A *comparison* of the graphs following *IV and SC application* shows an immediate serum bilirubin increase after IV, but—as could be expected—a delayed increase after SC application. In most SC-injected animals, there was initially a small decline from the starting level (not visible in the computer graphs)—lasting 3–6 hr. The sharp increase only occurred between 6 and 24 hr. This initial decline can partly be interpreted as (a small) bilirubin influx into the SC depot. But, since a similar decline occurred after SC saline injections (and here no bilirubin influx into the SC depot was visible), a volume effect needs also to be considered. In the computer graphs the volume effect was arithmetically compensated. The larger reflux into the circulation occurred only after the distribution of the SC injected albumin into the whole body of the rat (circulation included) had progressed. Correspondingly, the peak was postponed and somewhat broader compared to IV injection (Figs. 5, 7 and 6, 8).

Even after SC injections the serum *bilirubin peak* and the following decline were delayed compared to the *peak* and the elimination *of human albumin* in the rat serum (Figs. 3, 7 and 4, 8).

Infant rats had higher serum bilirubin starting levels than *weanling rats.* With corresponding albumin doses the absolute and the percentage increase was greater in the younger animals. This agrees with the well-known age related differences in bilirubin and protein metabolism of homozygous Gunn rats: i.e., high bilirubin and low albumin in infant, and low bilirubin and high albumin in weanling rats.

It is astonishing that in albumin injected animals, *under blue light photo-therapy serum-bilirubin* sharply declines (Figs. 9–12). Especially in those animals receiving a high albumin dose IV, there must occur a sharp competition between the bilirubin attraction of the circulating excess albumin and the simultaneous photodecomposition of the pigment.

A *comparison* of the graphs following the *different* IV and SC *doses* covers a somewhat steeper slope during 24 hr (at least) with the smaller albumin dose—in infant as well as in weanling rats. This points to a slight reduction of the phototherapy effect by the albumin-induced bilirubin influx into the circulation. But by no means, is all of the bilirubin drawn into the vascular space by the injected albumin beyond the reach of the lights.

With the same albumin dose the initial slope is somewhat steeper after *SC*

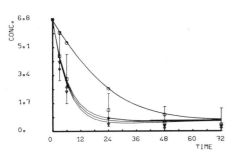

Fig. 9. In 1-month-old rats following IV injection of human albumin.

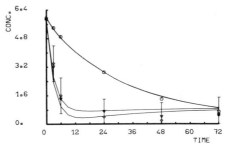

Fig. 10. In 3–5-day-old rats following IV injection of human albumin.

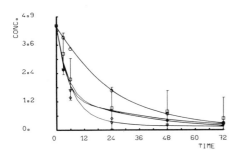

Fig. 11. In 1-month-old rats following SC injection of human albumin.

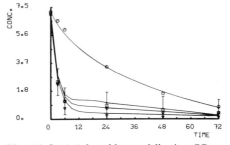

Fig. 12 In 3–5-day-old rats following SC injection of human albumin.

Figs. 9–12. For animals *under blue lights* ($E_{bili} \approx 3.7$ mW/cm^2). $\square$ = the bilirubin decrease in dummy (saline) injected rats.

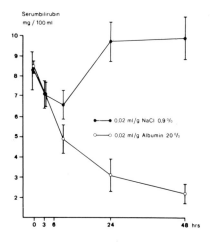

Fig. 13. (Not computer curves!) Serum bilirubin in 3–5-day-old homozygous Gunn rats under daylight phototherapy ($E_{bili} \approx 0.75$ mW/cm^2), following IV injection of 4.0 g human albumin/kg or equal volumes of 0.9% NaCl solution. (Mean values and SD of seven or eight animals, respectively.)

than after *IV injection*. That may point to the postulated bilirubin trapping effect of the albumin deposited in the skin.

In *dummy* (saline)-*injected* animals (lines at the tops of Figs. 9–12), bilirubin decline under blue phototherapy is slower than in *albumin-injected* rats (even with the largest doses IV or SC). This allows us to conclude that *albumin enhances the phototherapy effect*. The calculations described in the following pages were mainly carried out to test this hypothesis.

As an addition *white light phototherapy* (with an effective irradiance of about ¼ of the blue lights) was given to infant and weanling rats after IV injection of 4 g albumin/kg (the intermediate dose) or appropriate volumes of 0.9% NaCl solution. In the *1-month-old* rats, after saline injection, serum bilirubin slowly declined in accordance with the low effective irradiance applied. Three hours after albumin injection, serum bilirubin had increased under low-dose phototherapy almost in the same range as in control animals in the dark. A light-induced decline could only be seen after 6 hr of illumination. At 24 hr the level of the saline injected animals was reached, and at 48 and 72 hr serum bilirubin in albumin-injected rats was even somewhat lower than in saline injected.

In *infant rats* this phenomenon was still more marked. In dummy-injected 3–5-day-old rats serum bilirubin rose under (low-dose) illumination after 6 hr when the mother rat (a light trap) was placed with the infants. (This is in agreement with former investigations done by Hampel[8] in our hospital.) But, in albumin-injected rats it gradually decreased although more slowly than under blue lights (Fig. 13). The results of these additional tests strengthen the above-mentioned hypothesis.

CALCULATIONS

For the quantitative evaluation of the measured concentration of human albumin and bilirubin, respectively, in dependence on time after the IV or SC application, it is necessary to calculate the theoretical concentration/time-function.

a. The Concentration/Time-Function for Human Albumin after IV Application

If
y = intravascular concentration of human albumin (in g/liter),
t = time after IV administration of human albumin (in hr),
k_{2A} = elimination constant of human albumin (in hr^{-1}), the elimination rate is given by

$$\frac{dy}{dt} = -k_{2A} \cdot y. \tag{1}$$

Thus, one obtains for the concentration/time-function

$$y = \frac{D}{V} e^{-k_{2A} \cdot t} = a \cdot e^{-k_{2A} \cdot t} \tag{2}$$

where
D = dose of human albumin (in g),
V = distribution volume of human albumin after IV application (in liters),
a = D/V the theoretical concentration of human albumin for the moment, $t = 0$ (in g/liter).

The half-life of the human albumin by elimination out of the distribution volume can be calculated as

$$t_{1/2} = \frac{\ln 2}{k_{2A}}.$$

b. The Concentration/Time-Function for Human Albumin after SC Application

If the elimination rate of the human albumin from the subcutaneous depot is equal to the invasion rate into the intravascular volume, one can formulate

$$\frac{dy}{dt} = a \cdot k_{1A} \, e^{-k_{1A} \cdot t} \tag{3}$$

where k_{1A} = invasion constant of human albumin (in hr^{-1}).

The elimination rate being

$$\frac{dy}{dt} = -k_{2A} \cdot y, \tag{4}$$

hence, for the total change of the human albumin concentration one receives

$$\frac{dy}{dt} = a \cdot k_{1A} \, e^{-k_{1A} \cdot t} - k_{2A} \cdot y. \tag{5}$$

After integration of this equation one obtains

$$y = \frac{ak_{1A}}{k_{2A} - k_{1A}} (e^{-k_{1A} \cdot t} - e^{-k_{2A} \cdot t}). \tag{6}$$

c. *The Concentration/Time-Function of Bilirubin after IV Application of Human Albumin (without Phototherapy)*

If the invasion rate of the bilirubin is proportional to the concentration of human albumin, and the elimination rate of bilirubin is proportional to the concentration of intravascular bilirubin, the total change of the bilirubin concentration is

$$\frac{dy}{dt} = k_{1B} \cdot a \cdot e^{-k_{2A} \cdot t} - k_{2B} \cdot y, \tag{7}$$

where
y = intravascular concentration of bilirubin (in mg/100 ml),
k_{1B} = invasion constant of bilirubin (in hr^{-1}),
k_{2B} = elimination constant of bilirubin (in hr^{-1}).
Thus, one obtains after integrating

$$y = y_0 + \frac{a \cdot k_{1B}}{k_{2B} - k_{2A}} (e^{-k_{2A} \cdot t} - e^{-k_{2B} \cdot t}), \tag{8}$$

where y_0 = concentration of bilirubin in the intermediate steady state (in mg/100 ml).

d. *The Concentration/Time-Function of Bilirubin after SC Application of Human Albumin (without Phototherapy)*

The invasion of bilirubin into the intravascular volume is proportional to the concentration of human albumin. Using Eq. (6), the invasion rate of bilirubin will be

$$\frac{dy}{dt} = \frac{a \cdot k_{1A} \cdot k_{1B}}{k_{2A} - k_{1A}} (e^{-k_{1A} \cdot t} - e^{-k_{2A} \cdot t}). \tag{9}$$

The elimination rate of bilirubin out of the distribution volume is proportional to the concentration of bilirubin

$$\frac{dy}{dt} = -k_{2B} \cdot y. \tag{10}$$

In this case the total change of bilirubin concentration becomes

$$\frac{dy}{dt} = \frac{a \cdot k_{1A} \cdot k_{1B}}{k_{2A} - k_{1A}} (e^{-k_{1A} \cdot t} - e^{-k_{2A} \cdot t}) - k_{2B} \cdot y. \tag{11}$$

For the concentration/time-function we arrive at

$$y = y_0 + K_1 \cdot e^{-k_{1A} \cdot t} + K_2 \cdot e^{-k_{2A} \cdot t} + K_3 \cdot e^{-k_{2B} \cdot t}, \tag{12}$$

where

$$K_1 = \frac{a \cdot k_{1A} \cdot k_{1B}}{(k_{2A} - k_{1A})(k_{2B} - k_{1A})},$$

$$K_2 = \frac{a \cdot k_{1A} \cdot k_{1B}}{(k_{2A} - k_{1A})(k_{2A} - k_{2B})},$$

and

$$K_3 = \frac{a \cdot k_{1A} \cdot k_{1B}}{(k_{2a} - k_{2B})(k_{1A} - k_{2B})}.$$

e. The Concentration/Time-Function of Bilirubin after IV Application of Human Albumin with Phototherapy

By differentiating Eq. (8), one obtains for the change of the bilirubin concentration in darkness

$$\frac{dy}{dt} = \frac{a \cdot k_{2A} \cdot k_{1B}}{k_{2B} - k_{2A}} \cdot e^{-k_{2A} \cdot t} + \frac{a k_{1B} \cdot k_{2B}}{k_{2B} - k_{2A}} \cdot e^{-k_{2B} \cdot t}. \tag{13}$$

For the elimination rate of bilirubin by phototherapy

$$\frac{dy}{dt} = -k_{3B} \cdot y, \tag{14}$$

where k_{3B} = elimination constant of bilirubin by phototherapy.

After summation of Eqs. (13) and (14) and integration, one obtains

$$y = y_0 + K_4(e^{-k_{1A} \cdot t} - e^{-k_{3B} \cdot t}) + K_5(e^{-k_{2A} \cdot t} - e^{-k_{3B} \cdot t}), \tag{15}$$

where

$$K_4 = \frac{a \cdot k_{2A} \cdot k_{2B}}{(k_{2B} - k_{2A})(k_{2A} - k_{3B})}, \qquad K_5 = \frac{a \cdot k_{1B} \cdot k_{2B}}{(k_{2B} - k_{2A})(k_{3B} - k_{2B})}.$$

f. The Concentration/Time-Function of Bilirubin after SC Application of Human Albumin with Phototherapy

The change of the bilirubin concentration in darkness is obtained by differentiating eq. (12):

$$\frac{dy}{dt} = -K_1 \cdot k_{1A} \cdot e^{-k_{1A} \cdot t} - K_2 \cdot k_{2A} \cdot e^{-k_{2A} \cdot t} - K_3 \cdot k_{2B} \cdot e^{-k_{2B} \cdot t}. \tag{16}$$

Hence, one will obtain from Eqs. (14) and (16) after integration

$$y = y_0 \cdot e^{-k_{3B} \cdot t} + K_6(e^{-k_{1A} \cdot t} - e^{-k_{3B} \cdot t})$$
$$+ K_7(e^{-k_{2A} \cdot t} - e^{-k_{3B} \cdot t}) + K_8(e^{-k_{2B} \cdot t} - e^{-k_{3B} \cdot t}),$$

(17)

where

$$K_6 = K_1 \cdot \frac{k_{1A}}{k_{1A} - k_{3B}},$$

$$K_7 = K_2 \cdot \frac{k_{2A}}{k_{2A} - k_{3B}},$$

$$K_8 = K_3 \cdot \frac{k_{2B}}{k_{2B} - k_{3B}}.$$

Equations (2), (6), (8), (12), (15), and (17) allow us to calculate the characteristic parameters a, k_{1A}, k_{2A}, k_{1B}, k_{2B}, and k_{3B} with a computer by a least-squares program. The results are represented in Table I and illustrated in Figs. 1–12, respectively.

Altogether 1230 measuring points were taken into account for $k_{1A} - k_{3B}$. The amount of effective irradiance reaching the 3–5-day-old rats was reduced 6 hr after the start of the illumination when the lactating mother rat joined them. The degree of this reduction certainly varied. In respect of this the photolysis results obtained in 1-month-old rats may be mathematically more reliable.

RESULTS

Since albumin administration evokes shifting between the extra- and intra-vascular bilirubin pool, it is impossible to assess the degree of a simultaneous photolysis by evaluating serum bilirubin concentration alone.

Invasion and elimination constants for human albumin (injected into Gunn rats) and for bilirubin are within the same dimensions for infant and weanling animals with the exception of k_{1A} = the invasion constant for albumin. Invasion is faster in infant rats. This can be expected because of the underlying physicochemical processes, with only minor age-related differences.

$t_{1/2}$ for human albumin injected into Gunn rats was $\approx$20 hr.

A dose of 8 g albumin/kg must be regarded as an overdose, since about 50% of such an IV dose leaves the circulation of the animal very soon—long before our first check: 3 hr after the injection. 3–4 g albumin/kg can be taken as an optimum.

Light or darkness have no significant influence on invasion or elimination of human albumin in both groups of rats. Under the selected conditions there are two exits for intravascular bilirubin. k_{2B} stands for exit 1: effective in the dark (= physiological excretion + shifting induced by the progressive elimination of

TABLE I

	a (g/liter)	V (%)	k_{1A} (hr^{-1})	k_{2A} (hr^{-1})	$t_{1/2}$ (hr)	k_{1B} (hr^{-1})	k_{2B} (hr^{-1})	k_{3B} (hr^{-1})	$k_{3B \text{ NaCl}}$ (hr^{-1})
1-month-old rats	107.41 ±1.7	12.2 ±0.2	0.0457 ±0.005	0.0346 ±0.0034	20.0	0.0146 ±0.003	0.0438 ±0.004	0.149 ±0.003	≈0.04
3–5-day-old rats	106.42 ±8.8	13.0 ±1.1	0.0609 ±0.008	0.0339 ±0.006	20.45	0.0208 ±0.005	0.0412 ±0.004	0.321 ±0.004	≈0.03

a = albumin concentration in distribution volume.
V = distribution volume.
k_{1A} = invasion constant for albumin.
k_{2A} = elimination constant for albumin.
k_{1B} = invasion constant for bilirubin.
k_{2B} = elimination constant for bilirubin.
k_{3B} = photolysis constant (after albumin injection).
$k_{3B \text{ NaCl}}$ = photolysis constant [after NaCl injection—calculated by an equation analog to the Eq. (2)].

the added albumin). k_{3B} stands for exit 2: induced by phototherapy. In illuminated rats k_{3B} and k_{2B} are working simultaneously.

k_{3B}—the photolysis constant for bilirubin—is not reflected by zero. The bilirubin decline cannot be explained alone by to and fro diffusion; it cannot be characterized by k_{2B}—the elimination constant for bilirubin.

k_{3B} is smaller in weanling than in infant rats. This means: phototherapy is less effective in weanling (only partially shaved) rats than in infant rats (without fur).

k_{3B} is distinctly smaller in saline-injected than in albumin-injected rats. Photolysis must be enhanced by the addition of albumin.

A different influence of IV- or SC-administered albumin on the phototherapy effect is just about noticeable during the first few hours. But—on the whole—is of no major concern.

DISCUSSION

The prominent (primarily not expected) result of this study points to a marked enhancement of the phototherapy effect in Gunn rats following the administration of human serum albumin. It was about four times ($k_{3B}/k_{3B \text{ NaCl}}$ ≈ 4) in 1-month-old rats under blue lights. Compared to rat albumin, bilirubin-binding capacity of human albumin is markedly higher (Schmid and co-workers[12]). The injected human albumin obviously attracts bilirubin and provokes shifting from its original deposits in the animal. It can be postulated that under the selected experimental conditions, more albumin-bound (and less free or lipid- and cell-attached) bilirubin originated in the rats during (most of) the time phototherapy was applied.

In vitro tests comparing photodegradation of free and albumin-bound bilirubin have not yielded uniform results. In some investigations, albumin accelerated an initial component of bilirubin decay, but after 3 or more hr of illumination, the decay of free bilirubin was more progressive than that of the albumin-bound (Ostrow and v. Branham[10]). In other tests, catalyzed by peroxidase (see Pedersen, et al.[11]), free bilirubin was readily photooxidized, whilst the process was prolonged when the pigment was bound to native albumin. The photoisomerisation of IX α (Z) bilirubin to the IX α (E) isomer takes place on albumin-bound bilirubin (Brodersen[4]). Moreover, Ostrow and v. Branham described an anaerobic photodegradation of bilirubin taking place in vitro only in the presence of albumin. It is here that our in vivo observations connect.

The Gunn rat was used as a mathematical model to calculate the influence of IV and SC albumin injections on the phototherapy effect. With only minor simplifications, it was possible to describe the whole complex [intravascular albumin invasion and following bilirubin influx (equilibration): albumin elimination, bilirubin reflux, bilirubin elimination by photolysis] in one formula [Eq. (17)].

$t_{1/2}$ of the injected human albumin could be evaluated with this formula as well. It is obviously shorter than $t_{1/2}$ of homologous albumin.

The animal studies have clearly demonstrated once again that the application of albumin into jaundiced rats raises the intravascular fraction of bilirubin as it does in newborn infants (Odell,[9] Fette[6]). Thereafter, it is no longer possible to assess the phototherapy effect by estimating the plasma bilirubin concentration alone. It becomes necessary to take the countershifting of the pigment into consideration. The clinician may be impressed when a comparatively small effective irradiance and high albumin doses are administered, because, in that case, the albumin induced bilirubin influx into the plasma can superimpose the decrease by phototherapy (probably mainly during the first hours—as was seen in 1-month-old Gunn rats under daylight phototherapy). We assume that the data published by Wong and colleagues[15] can be interpreted in this way.

Although animal tests are not directly transferable to humans, the observations point to the usefulness of combining phototherapy with albumin injections. It is not only that the injected albumin brings about additional binding capacity, but it obviously also accelerates photodecomposition of bilirubin in vivo.

What about the optimal doses? In the Gunn rats the highest tolerable dose was about 8 g albumin/kg. But, after IV injection of such a high dose about 50% of the human albumin very soon left the circulation of the animal, being—most likely—promptly excreted in the urine (see Gardiner, et al.[7]): 4 g albumin/kg rendered the best results; here only 15–20% must have left the circulation soon after IV administration.

In newborn infants the danger of volume overloading has to be carefully considered, 1–1.5–(2) g albumin/kg may represent a sensible approach. Only albumin formulations with the smallest possible content of stabilizers should be used in the nurseries (see Brodersen and Hansen,[5] Ballowitz, et al.[1-3]).

ACKNOWLEDGMENTS

We wish to thank Mrs. E. Goitia, Mrs. R. Ludwig, and Mr. B. Behrens for technical assistance. The human albumin was a gift from SCHURA Blutderivate (Krefeld-Germany). The pherogram analysis was carried out in the laboratories of Arbeitsgruppe für Klinische und Experimentelle Plasmaproteinforschung, Berlin 33.

REFERENCES

1. Ballowitz, L., Geutler, G., Krochmann, J., Pannitschka, R., Roemer, G., and Roemer, I., Phototherapy in Gunn rats. *Biol. Neonat.* **31,** 229 (1977).
2. Ballowitz, L., Geutler, G., Goebel, A., and Krochmann, J., Dose-Response Relationships in Phototherapy, in *Intensive Care in the Newborn* II. Stern, L., Oh, W., and Friis-Hansen, B. Eds., New York, 1978, pp. 317–325.
3. Ballowitz, L., Schmid, J., Siegert, M., and Steffen, B., Effects of stabilizers in preparations of human serum albumin on the serum bilirubin in Gunn rats. *Acta Paediatr. Scand.* **67,** 505 (1978).
4. Brodersen, R., Prevention of kernicterus, based on recent progress in bilirubin chemistry. *Acta Paediatr. Scand.* **66,** 625 (1977).
5. Brodersen, R., and Hansen, P., Bilirubin displacing effect of stabilizers added to injectable preparations of human serum albumin. *Acta Paediatr. Scand.* **66,** 133 (1977).
6. Fette, J.: Die Wirkung von intravenösen Albumingaben bei Neugeborenen mit Hyperbilirubinaemie. *Inaug. Diss. FU Berlin* (1971).
7. Gardiner, M. E., Finlay-Jones, J. -M., and Morgan, E. H., Catabolism and urinary excretion of albumin and transferrin before and after intravenous injection of albumin in the rat: With observations on the urinary excretion of IgG globulin. *Biochem. Med.* **8,** 287 (1973).
8. Hampel, C., Die Wirkung verschiedener Leuchtstofflampen aus das Serumbilirubin in vivo und in vitro. *Inaug. Diss. FU Berlin* (1975).
9. Odell, G. B., Studies in kernicterus I. The protein binding of bilirubin. *J. Clin. Invest.* **38,** 823 (1959).
10. Ostrow, J. D., and v. Branham, R., Photodecay of bilirubin in vitro and in the jaundiced (Gunn) rat. *Birth Defects Orig. Art. Ser.* **6**(2)**,** 93 (1970).
11. Pedersen, A. O., Schønheyder, F., and Brodersen, R., Photooxydation of human serum albumin and its complex with bilirubin. *Eur. J. Biochem.* **72,** 213 (1977).
12. Schmid, R., Diamond, I., Hammaker, L., and Gundersen, C. B., Interaction of bilirubin with albumin. *Nature* (*Lond*) **206,** 1041 (1965).
13. Schneider, W., Wolter, D., and McCarty, L. J.: Technical improvements in heat-ethanol isolation of serum albumin. *Blut* **33,** 275 (1976).
14. Siegert, M., and Siemes, H., Agarose-gel-electrophoresis of cerebral spinal fluid protein and analysis of pherogram profiles by analog computer. *J. Clin. Chem. Clin. Biochem.* **15,** 635 (1977).
15. Wong, Y. K., Shuttleworth, G. R., and Wood, B. S. B., Effect of albumin administration on phototherapy for neonatal jaundice. *Arch. Dis. Child.* **47,** 241 (1972).

10

Mathematical Derivation of Dose-Response Relationship Calculations in Phototherapy

G. WIESE and L. BALLOWITZ

In connection with our studies on the effect of phototherapy and simultaneous administration of human albumin in Gunn rats, we recalculated the data of one of our previous publications (Ref. 3), and we were able to develop some generally valid mathematical formulas. In the experiments under discussion 1-month-old homozygous female Gunn rats were injected IV with 4.0 mg bilirubin/100 g body weight. After equilibration, bilirubin clearance under phototherapy with different fluorescent tubes was compared with the prolonged spontaneous elimination in the dark.

A. For the serumbilirubin concentration after elimination of "a" mg bilirubin, one gets the equation

$$c_a = \frac{(B - b) \cdot (x - a)}{x} \tag{1}$$

where
b = serum bilirubin concentration (in mg/dl) in the steady state before additional bilirubin was injected,
x = amount of bilirubin injected in mg/100 g body weight,
B = serum bilirubin concentration after bilirubin injection and equilibration (in mg/dl),
a = amount of bilirubin in mg by which the incorporated bilirubin shall be decreased (proceeding from the starting level B).

Childrens Hospital, Free University, Berlin

The elimination by phototherapy can be described by the following equation (Ref. 2)

$$c = c_0 \cdot e^{-k \cdot E_{bili} \cdot c_0 \cdot t} \tag{2}$$

where

c_0 = serum bilirubin concentration at the starting point (in mg/dl),
k = elimination constant (under our experimental conditions $k = 0.001732$),
E_{bili} = effective irradiance in mW/cm^2,
t = time of illumination (in hr).

Inserting Eq. (1) into Eq. (2) one gets

$$\frac{(B - b) \cdot (x - a)}{x} = B \cdot e^{-k \cdot E_{bili} \cdot B \cdot t}. \tag{3}$$

Solving the equation towards t gives that *time* which is necessary to eliminate "a" mg bilirubin using the effective irradiance E_{bili}

$$t = \frac{1}{B \cdot k \cdot E_{bili}} \cdot \ln \frac{x \cdot B}{(B - b) \cdot (x - a)} \tag{4}$$

B. Calculation of the effective radiant exposure $H_{bili} = \int E_{bili} \cdot dt$ necessary to eliminate 1 mg bilirubin.

By multiplication of Eq. (4) with E_{bili} one gets

$$E_{bili} \cdot t = H_{bili} = \frac{1}{B \cdot k} \cdot \ln \frac{x \cdot B}{(B - b) \cdot (x - a)}. \tag{5}$$

Under our experimental conditions one obtains

$$H_{bili} = 16.6 \text{ mWhr/cm}^2.$$

This value one easily gets by multiplying column 1 and 2 from Table I.

C. The *spontaneous* bilirubin elimination in the dark (*without* phototherapy)

TABLE I

Type of Fluorescent Tube Used	Effective Irradiance (E_{bili} in mW/cm^2)	t (in hr) for		
		$a = 1$ mg	$a = 2$ mg	$a = 3$ mg
Osram L 20 W/70 uv	0.30	55.4	94.4	161.0
Osram L 20 W/63 green	0.41	40.5	62.1	117.9
Osram L 20 W/19 daylight	0.77	21.6	36.8	62.8
Westinghouse F20 T12 BB special blue	3.75	4.4	7.6	12.9
Philips 20 W/52 BAM blue	4.15	4.0	6.8	11.6

Where $B = 20$ mg/dl; $b = 5$ mg/dl; $x = 4.0$ mg/100 g body weight.

can also be calculated. Under the condition that the spontaneous bilirubin elimination also follows an *e*-function

$$c = c_0 \cdot e^{-k_n \cdot t},$$

one receives

$$c = c_0 \cdot e^{-0.0115 \cdot t} \text{ that means } k_n = 0.0115 \pm 0.003. \tag{6}$$

Provided that the elimination rate in the dark also depends on the starting level (a fact that has not been previously examined) one gets the c_0-*independent* elimination rate k_n (for $B = 25$ mg/dl $k_n = 0.00046$). Taking this into consideration the elimination constant for phototherapy only (without the spontaneous elimination) can be calculated

$$k^+ = 0.001732 \cdot E_{\text{bili}} - 0.00046.$$

This is the concentration-time-function for the phototherapy induced bilirubin decrease:

$$c = c_0 \cdot e^{-k^+ \cdot c_0 \cdot t}. \tag{7}$$

The time which is necessary to eliminate 1 mg bilirubin by phototherapy alone can be calculated with these k^+ values and the respective hours are given in column 3 of Table II. It reveals that some of the lamps (uv and green) have almost no useful effect.

D. The measuring points of our former studies follow this equation (Fig. 4, Ref. 3):

$$c = c_0 \cdot e^{-k \cdot c_0 \cdot H_{\text{bili}}}. \tag{8}$$

They can be described by the line equation

$$y = \ln c = -m \cdot H_{\text{bili}} + d \tag{9}$$

TABLE II

Type of Fluorescent Tube Used	$0.001732 \cdot E_{\text{bili}}$	k^+	t (in hr) for $a = 1$ mg
Osram L 20 W/70 uv	0.0005196	0.000060	479.5 (55.3)[a]
Osram L 20 W/63 green	0.0007101	0.000250	115.1 (40.5)
Osram L 20 W/19 daylight	0.0013336	0.000874	32.9 (21.6)
Westinghouse F20 T12 BB special blue	0.0064950	0.006035	4.8 (4.4)
Philips 20 W/52 BAM blue	0.0071878	0.006728	4.3 (4.0)

[a] The value in parenthesis give the time for the *combined* (spontaneous and phototherapy induced) elimination of 1 mg bilirubin.

where

$$m = k \cdot c_0 \quad \text{and} \quad d = \ln c_0 \tag{10}$$

E) The measuring points in the former studies also follow this equation (Fig. 6, Ref. 3):

$$a = x \cdot \left(1 - \frac{B}{B - b} \cdot e^{-k \cdot B \cdot H_{\text{bili}}} \right). \tag{11}$$

For

$$H_{\text{bili}} = \frac{1}{k \cdot B} \cdot \ln \frac{B}{B - b} \tag{12}$$

Eq. (11) will result in zero.

If, for example, $B = 20$, $b = 5$, and $k = 0.001732$, one will receive $(H_{\text{bili}})_{\text{min}} = 8.3$. That means effective radiant exposures of less than 8.3 mWhr/cm^2 have no phototherapy effect *indepent* of the type of tubes used. Taking into account the spontaneous bilirubin elimination (in the dark), $(H_{\text{bili}})_{\text{min}}$ will only change insignificantly.

These formulas complete the statement of the former publication (Ref. 3). The new calculations do not uncover substantial contradictions to the former conclusions with the exception of those which derive from Fig. 6. in Ref. 3.

REFERENCES

1. Ballowitz, L., Geutler, G., Krochmann, J., Pannitschka, R., Roemer G., and Roemer, I., Phototherapy in Gunn Rats. *Biol. Neonate* **31**, 229–244 (1977).
2. Wiese, G., and Ballowitz, L., Phototherapy in Gunn Rats II. Further Calculations on the Effectivity of Different Irradiances (E_{bili}). *Biol. Neonate* (in press).
3. Ballowitz, L., Geutler, G., Goebel, A., and Krochmann, G., Dose Response Relationships in Phototherapy. In *Intensive Care in the Newborn* II, Stern. L. Oh., W., and Friis Hansen, B. Eds. Masson, New York, 1978, pp. 317–325.

11

Bilirubin Interaction with Albumin and Tissues

ROLF BRODERSEN, Ph.D.

Bilirubin is an important substance in neonatology because of its toxicity to the central nervous system. In the healthy organism, bilirubin is tightly bound to albumin in blood plasma whereas it is partially transferred to nerve cells in cases of kernicterus. It has been claimed that the toxic substance is free bilirubin anion in equilibrium with albumin-bound bilirubin and that transfer to biirubin from albumin to nerve cell takes place *via* free bilirubin anion. It is possible that this is correct; but it has not yet been finally demonstrated and methods for determination of free bilirubin concentration in plasma are not available nor is it possible to prove the existence of free bilirubin anion in plasma at acidotic pH values.[1, 2] Other possible mechanisms are direct transfer of bilirubin from the complex with albumin and transfer by means of a carrier vehicle of an unknown chemical nature (Fig. 1).

It is consequently better to avoid referring to free bilirubin as the toxic substance, and it is possible to establish a model of the toxic mechanism which is valid irrespective of the actual mode of transfer if we refer only to the transport of bilirubin from the complex with albumin to the membrane of the target cell. The equilibrium of this transport is governed by the affinities of bilirubin for albumin and for the target cell and these affinities are independent of whether or not free bilirubin exists.

Let us first consider the affinity of binding of bilirubin to the cell. In kernicterus, bilirubin is taken up by certain parts of the brain. The affinity of bilirubin for nervous tissue has been explained by assuming that bilirubin is lipophilic or lipid soluble. It has been said that unconjugated bilirubin is apolar

Professor of Medical Biochemistry, Institute of Medical Biochemistry, University of Aarhus, Denmark

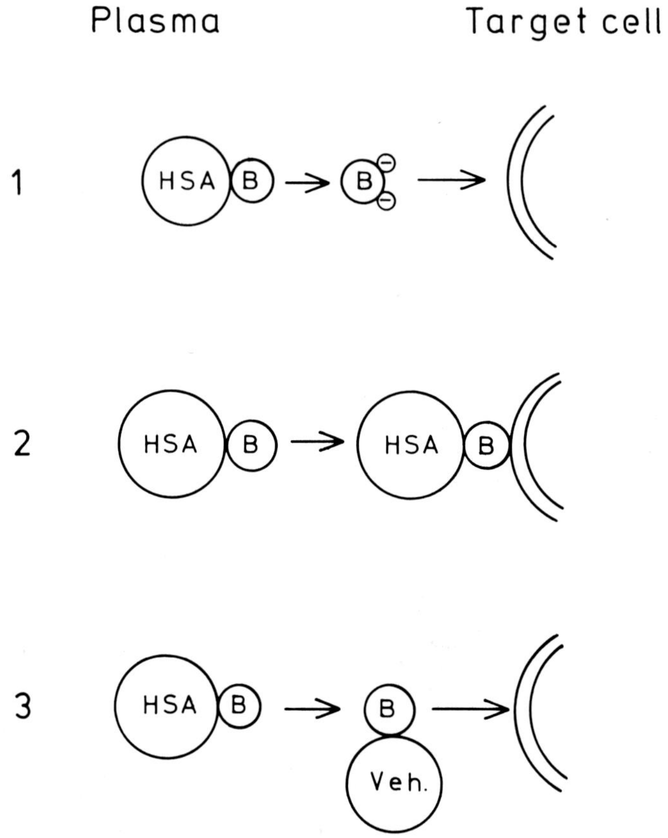

Fig. 1. Various hypothetical mechanisms for transfer of bilirubin from plasma albumin to nerve cells.

and lipophilic and therefore is neurotoxic while bilirubin conjugates are polar and hydrophilic and therefore not toxic to nervous tissue. If we look at the chemical structure, Figure 2a, it appears that bilirubin is a polar substance. The four pyrrole, two lactam, and two carboxyl groups, are polar, and altogether this molecule appears as quite soluble in water. The lipophilic parts are small and should not outweigh the strong polar forces. We have therefore tested the solubility in a wide range of solvents.[3] Some of the results are seen in Figure 3. Bilirubin is insoluble in lipid solvents and has a low solubility in fat. The solubility increases with increasing polarity of the solvent and becomes very high in formamide and dimethyl sulfoxide, solvents which are more polar than water and which do not dissolve fat. These results are consistent with the chemical structure and are in no way surprising to the chemist. It appears as if the old concept of bilirubin lipophilicity needs to be reconsidered.

How, then, could such a misconcept originate and be established to such an extent that it is found in textbooks and in many reviews on bilirubin metabolism? There are probably two main reasons for this: first, that bilirubin acid is insoluble in water and, second, that bilirubin combines with lipid membranes

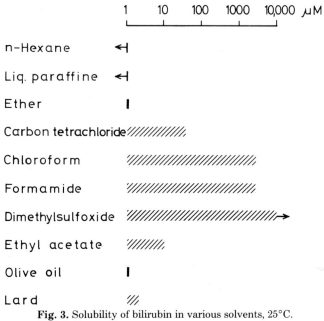

Fig. 2. Bilirubin IX-α(Z,Z), the main isomer of bilirubin and the toxic species, in this paper simply named *bilirubin*. In b the intramolecular hydrogen bonds are indicated.

	1	10	100	1000	10,000 μM

n-Hexane

Liq. paraffine

Ether

Carbon tetrachloride

Chloroform

Formamide

Dimethylsulfoxide

Ethyl acetate

Olive oil

Lard

Fig. 3. Solubility of bilirubin in various solvents, 25°C.

in the tissues. The insolubility in water, however, is due to formation of intramolecular hydrogen bonds[4] (Fig. 2b) and has little to do with lipophilic characteristics. Many polar substances are insoluble in water, such as calcium carbonate, but are not lipophilic.

The second aspect is more interesting: Bilirubin can combine with polar lipids in membranes. It has been known for many years that bilirubin forms complexes with phospholipids, the so-called ether-soluble bilirubin.[5] Binding of bilirubin to polar lipid membranes was first studied by Mustafa and King,[6] who demonstrated that the toxic effect of bilirubin on mitochondria is caused by binding of bilirubin to lipids, not to proteins, in the mitochondria. Bilirubin is bound to polar groups in the lipid-water interphase and is not dissolved in the fat. Formation of such a complex does not mean that bilirubin is lipophilic or apolar. Complexes of bilirubin with polar lipids have lately been studied by Nagaoka and Cowger[7] by Tipping, *et al.*[8] and by workers in our group.[9] Our results indicate that bilirubin can be attached to phospholipid membranes in two ways (Fig. 4), as the anion, and as aggregated bilirubin acid. It is conceiv-

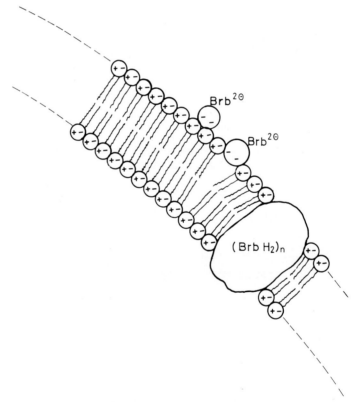

Fig. 4. Model of bilirubin binding to a phospholipid membrane. Two types of binding seem to take place, as bilirubin anions, and as aggregates of bilirubin acid. The latter causes profound changes of membrane permeability.

able that binding of single bilirubin anions is rather harmless to the membrane whereas incorporation of bilirubin acid aggregates causes profound changes in the membrane and may be considered as the toxic mechanism. There are no strong chemical forces between the membrane lipids and the aggregated bilirubin acid, and we believe that the process is a simple precipitation of bilirubin acid in the membrane. Such precipitation may take place when the concentration of dissolved bilirubin in the medium surpasses the limit of solubility. If the bilirubin concentration in the medium is higher than the solubility, aggregation of bilirubin acid may take place, followed by precipitation and attachment to the membrane. *Conversely*, if the concentration of bilirubin in the medium is below the solubility, dissolution of aggregates will occur. It is therefore interesting to study the solubility of bilirubin in water.

The process of reversible bilirubin precipitation and dissolution is

$$\text{Bilirubin}^{2-} + 2\text{H}^+ \rightleftharpoons \text{Bilirubin H}_2 \downarrow.$$

The solubility product is

$$[\text{Bilirubin}^{2-}] \times [\text{H}^+]^2 = K.$$

We would accordingly expect that the solubility should be inversely proportional to the square of the hydrogen ion concentration. By studying the solubility in a tris buffer at constant ionic strength we have found that this is indeed so (Fig. 5).[3] This finding is in good agreement with the clinical experience that kernicterus is aggravated by acidosis.[10]

The actual values of solubility are very low, especially at acidotic pH's, where the solubility is too low to be measured by present means but can be calculated from the expected curve. In blood plasma, the solubility is considerably increased by binding of bilirubin to albumin. This explains the well-known detoxifying effect of albumin. The efficiency of albumin in this respect depends upon the amount of available bilirubin binding sites, i.e., bilirubin solubility increases with increasing concentration of albumin and decreases with the presence of other substances which occupy the bilirubin binding site on albumin. The bilirubin toxicity of plasma thus depends upon the concentration of bilirubin, the pH of the plasma, and the amount of available binding sites (reserve albumin). Toxicity increases with the concentration of bilirubin, decreases with increasing pH, and decreases with increasing reserve albumin. The concentration of bilirubin can be measured by conventional methods for determination of unconjugated bilirubin in plasma, the pH can be measured, but the determination of available binding sites, reserve albumin, has caused considerable difficulties.

Some idea of the amount of available sites can be obtained by determination of the binding capacity for an added dye, such as hydroxy-benzene-azo-benzoic acid (HBABA)[11] and this method has proved its clinical utility.[12] The weak point is that the dye is bound also to other sites on the albumin molecules, and

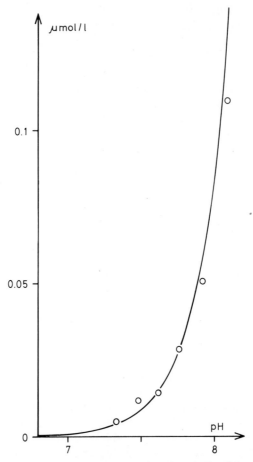

Fig. 5. Solubility of bilirubin in aqueous buffer as a function of pH, 37°C, tris buffer, ionic strength 0.15 *M* (0.1 *M* NaCl, 0.05 *M* tris hydrochloride).

that the sample is diluted to a considerable degree so that the effect of loosely bound competitors, such as sulfa drugs, is missed. Also, a strict determination of available sites should be carried out at 37°C not at room temperature. Other methods are based upon addition of bilirubin to saturation. Since bilirubin is bound with high affinity, one would expect that other competitors would be displaced by this procedure and their effect would be underestimated.

Two methods for determination of reserve albumin have been developed lately. Both are based on addition of a trace amount of a new ligand, bound with relatively low affinity, to the undiluted plasma followed by determination of the binding equilibrium. The added ligand must bind selectively to the bilirubin site alone and should be used in small quantity so that the binding equilibrium with other ligands is not shifted. This principle could be named the *selective trace-ligand* (STL) principle.[13] On theoretical grounds it is hardly possible to imagine any other possible for strict determination of reserve albumin than some form of the STL principle.

One STL method for determination of reserve albumin has been developed by Hsia in Toronto.[14] He utilizes a spin-labeled ligand and the determination of free and bound concentrations in equilibrium is carried out by electron spin resonance spectrography, a complicated but very useful technique, not yet available outside specialized laboratories. The method uses 10–25 μl of infant serum in a "sample-in, read, sample-out" procedure and is at present under clinical trial.

The other method[15] used mono-acetyl-diamino-diphenyl-sulfone (MADDS) as the selective trace ligand and is an adaptation of a previously reported method from our laboratory,[16] designed for use on small samples of infant sera, about 60 μl per single test. The MADDS method is also under clinical trial.

Through these or other forthcoming procedures it will be possible to measure the concentration of reserve albumin. Together with determinations of unconjugated bilirubin and pH, this should describe the bilirubin toxicity of the blood plasma in the newborn. If we consider the equilibria involved in the toxic process, we may understand that the toxicity is proportional to

$$\frac{B}{p} \times [\text{H}^+]^2,$$

where B is the concentration of unconjugated bilirubin and p is reserve albumin concentration. For the sake of easy handling we can take the logarithm of this,

$$\log \frac{B}{p} - 2p\text{H}.$$

Since we know the solubility of bilirubin at a fixed pH, and since we know the binding constant of bilirubin to albumin, we can calculate that precipitation of bilirubin can take place if the numerical value of this expression is more than -15.5.[1] For convenience we therefore add 15.5 and obtain an *index of plasma bilirubin toxicity*,

$$I = \log \frac{B}{p} - 2p\text{H} + 15.5.$$

The *index* is determined as follows. Unconjugated bilirubin, B (μmol/liter), is measured by conventional means, reserve albumin, p (μmol/liter), is determined by an STL technique, and the plasma pH is measured. I is calculated from the formula.

If the *index* turns out to be negative, bilirubin cannot precipitate, and toxic effects of bilirubin are probably excluded. If the *index* is positive, precipitation of bilirubin and damage to the central nervous system is thermodynamically and theoretically possible. In the limited clinical experience so far obtained,[17] a negative *index* is present in plasma from adults and healthy infants, *index*-value between 0 and 1 are usually found in icteric newborns, even though they present no acute signs of bilirubin toxicity, and values between 1 and 2 are found in affected infants (Table I).

Until now, clinical experience seems to confirm theoretical expectations. The reasons why no signs of toxicity are observed at *index*-values between 0 and 1 in spite of an imminent precipitation of bilirubin are probably the following,

1. Precipitation of bilirubin at moderately positive *index*-values may be slow and a small amount of precipitated bilirubin may redissolve after improvement of the condition with conversion of the *index* to negative values.

2. An oxidative enzyme system, *bilirubin oxidase*, is present in brain and other tissues and is capable of handling considerable amounts of bilirubin after entry into the cells.

3. Neurologic impairment may be minor and may not be detectable until later in life.

If, on the other hand, *index*-values increase above 1 (accurate limit to be determined by further clinical experience), precipitation of bilirubin occurs rapidly and the danger of manifest toxicity becomes acute.

Available means for keeping the *index* of plasma bilirubin toxicity low, preferably negative, include *exchange transfusion* (whereby bilirubin, B, is diminished and reserve albumin, p, is increased), *phototherapy* (keeping B low), *regulation of plasma pH* by proper ventilation and alkali therapy (keeping pH high), and finally by *avoiding drugs or other substances which would occupy bilirubin binding sites on albumin* (keeping p high). This evidently is not new to the clinician, as all these are well-established means of preventing brain damage in neonatal jaundice. What is new, is its quantitative formulation. We have thereby attempted to assign a certain weight to each of the three parameters, the unconjugated bilirubin concentration, the pH, and the reserve albumin concentration. The practical utility of doing so may become obvious from a few examples (Table II).

TABLE I

Approximate Ranges of *Index of Plasma Bilirubin Toxicity*. Precise Limits Need to be Fixed by Further Clinical Experience

−1.5–0: Adults and healthy infants
0–1: Icteric infants, not acutely affected
1–2: Acutely affected infants

TABLE II

Examples of *Index of Plasma Bilirubin Toxicity*

	Unconj. Bilirubin		pH	Reserve Albumin (μmol/liter)	Index
	(mg/dl)	(μmol/liter)			
Healthy adult	0.3	5	7.40	500	−1.3
Healthy infant	3.0	50	7.40	300	−0.1
Icteric infant	18	300	7.40	300	0.7
Acidotic and icteric infant	18	300	7.10	300	1.3
Icteric infant with occupied albumin	18	300	7.40	50	1.5
Combined type	9	150	7.10	50	1.8

REFERENCES

1. Brodersen, R., Binding of bilirubin to albumin. *Critical Reviews in Clinical and Laboratory Sciences*, **11**, 305 (1980).
2. Brodersen, R., Cashore, W., Wennberg, Ahlfors, C. E., Rasmussen, L. F., and Shusterman, D., Kinetics of bilirubin oxidation with peroxidase, as applied to studies of bilirubin-albumin binding. *Scand. J. Clin. Lab. Invest.* **39**, 143 (1979).
3. Brodersen, R., Bilirubin solubility and interaction with albumin and phospholipids. *J. Biol. Chem.* **254**, 2354 (1979).
4. Bonnett, R., Davies, J. E., and Hursthouse, M. B., Structure of bilirubin. *Nature* **262**, 326 (1976).
5. Howe, R. B., and Pinto, S. de T., Ether-soluble bilirubin. *Medicine (Baltimore)* **45**, 523 (1966).
6. Mustafa, G., and King, T. E., Binding of bilirubin with lipid. A possible mechanism of its toxic reaction in mitochondria. *J. Biol. Chem.* **245**, 1084 (1970).
7. Nagaoka, S., and Cowger, M. L., Interaction of bilirubin with lipids studied by fluorescence quenching method. *J. Biol. Chem.* **253**, 2005 (1978).
8. Tipping, E., Ketterer, B., and Christodoulides, L., Interaction of small molecules with phospholipid bilayers. *Biochem. J.* **180**, 327 (1979).
9. Eriksen, E. F., Danielsen, H., and Brodersen, R., Bilirubin-Liposome Interaction. Submitted for publication.
10. Stern, L., Doray, B., Chan, G., and Schiff, D., Bilirubin Metabolism and the Induction of Kernicterus, in *Bilirubin Metabolism in the Newborn II*, Bergsma, D., and Blondheim, S. H. Eds. Excerpta Medica, Amsterdam, 1976, pp. 255–263.
11. Porter, E. G., and Waters, W. J., A rapid micromethod for measuring the reserve albumin binding capacity in serum from newborn infants with hyperbilirubinemia. *J. Lab. Clin. Med.* **67**, 660 (1966).
12. Johnson, L., and Boggs, T. R., Bilirubin-Dependent Brain Damage, in *Phototherapy in the Newborn: An Overview*, Odell, G. B., Schaffer, R., and Simopoulus, A. P. Eds. Natl. Acad. Sci., Washington, D.C., 1974, p. 122.
13. Brodersen, R., Binding of Bilirubin and Other Ligands to Human Serum Albumin, in *Albumin Structure, Biosynthesis, Function, FEBS 11th Meeting, Copenhagen 1977*, Peters, T., and Sjöholm, I., Eds. Pergamon Press, Oxford, 1978, p. 61.
14. Hsia, J. C., Kwan, N. H., Er, S. S., Wood, D. J., and Chance, G. W., Development of a spin assay for reserve bilirubin loading capacity of human serum. *Proc. Natl. Acad. Sci. USA* **75**, 1542 (1978).
15. Brodersen, R., Andersen, S., Jacobsen, C., Sønderskov, O., Ebbesen, F., Cashore, W. T., and Larsen, S., Determination of Infant Serum Reserve Albumin for Binding of Bilirubin, Using a Selective Trace-Ligand. Submitted for publication.
16. Brodersen, R., Determination of the vacant amount of high-affinity bilirubin binding site of serum albumin. *Acta Pharmacol. Toxicol.* **42**, 153 (1978).
17. Ebbesen, F., to be published.

12

Effects of 1.25-Dihydroxycholecalciferol on Calcium, Phosphorus, and Magnesium Balance, and on Circulating Parathyroid Hormone and Calcitonin in Preterm Infants

JACQUES SENTERRE, M.D.,[1] LOUIS DAVID, M.D.[2] and BERNARD SALLE, M.D.[3]

From the results of chemical analysis of human fetal bodies, it has been calculated that the mean accumulation of calcium (Ca) and phosphorus (P) is about 140 mg and 75 mg/kg body weight/day respectively during the last trimester of gestation.[18, 43] On the other hand, low positive or even negative Ca balances[3-6, 40-43] and signs of osteopenia[21, 27, 30, 31, 47] have been reported frequently in low birth weight infants fed on milk with a wide range of Ca content. A number of factors such as Ca:P ratio in the milk,[2, 34] fat malabsorption,[3, 7, 42, 44, 46, 52, 53] fecal loss of endogenous Ca,[6, 41, 45] intake and metabolism of vitamin D,[3, 12, 21, 27, 30, 42, 43] and postnatal age[43] have all been implicated in poor Ca absorption by infants. In particular recent advances in the understanding of the metabolism of vitamin D have revealed the importance of dihydroxylated derivates in the control of Ca absorption.[8, 16, 23] We previously reported[42] that

[1] Maître de Recherches of the National Foundation for Scientific Research, Department of Pediatrics, State University of Liège, Hôpital de Bavière, Liège, Belgium

[2] Associate Professor, Department of Pediatrics, Hôpital Edouard Herriot, Lyon, France

[3] Professor of Pediatrics, Chief of Neonatal Department, Hôpital Edouard Herriot, Lyon, France

usual prophylactic doses of vitamin D did not improve Ca balance in preterm infants, and we suggested that the poor Ca absorption in these infants might be due to an impaired metabolism of vitamin D. A decreased rate of 25-hydroxylation of vitamin D in low birth weight infants was suspected by Hillman and Haddad,[24] but recent studies[22, 25, 54] did not support this view. By contrast, little is known about the capacity of the kidney of immature infants to convert 25-hydroxycholecalciferol (25-HCC) into the most active metabolite 1,25-dihydroxycholecalciferol (1,25-DHCC). However, an impaired production of this metabolite has been suggested in the pathogenesis of early neonatal hypocalcemia[1, 12, 25, 29] and in the development of defective skeletal mineralization[21, 27, 42, 43, 47] in low birth weight infants. The present study was undertaken in order to evaluate the effects of the substitution of 1,25-DHCC for vitamin D_3 on mineral balances and Ca homeostasis in preterm infants.

MATERIALS AND METHODS

Patients and Design of Study

Twenty 3-day balance studies were carried out in 10 healthy male preterm infants who were appropriate for gestational age: mean birth weight: 1810 g (range: 1520–2060 g); mean gestational age: 33 weeks (range: 30–35 weeks). The infants were fed on an adapted formula (NAN, Nestlé, Switzerland) from birth until the end of the study. This formula contained 400 mg/liter of Ca, 330 mg/liter of P, 40 mg/liter of magnesium (Mg), and 440 iu/liter of vitamin D_3. A daily oral dose of 30 μg (1200 iu) of vitamin D_3 was added from birth to day 15. It was replaced by a daily oral dose of 0.5 μg of 1,25-DHCC from day 16 to day 20. Capsules of 0.5 μg of 1,25-DHCC in lipid suspension were kindly supplied by Hoffman-Laroche, USA; the capsules were opened just before use and the suspension was mixed with a small amount of milk and given by tube feeding.

Two nitrogen, fat, Ca, P, and magnesium (Mg) balances were carried out on each infant. The first balance was performed between day 12 and 15 (D_3 period) and the second between day 17 and 20 (1,25-DHCC period). Parental consent had been given, and no objection was made to repeating the metabolic balances. The infants were nursed in incubators and were tube fed every 3 hr. The metabolic balances were performed as previously described.[39] The infant was loosely restrained on a hammock-shaped metabolic bed with a hole cut out to collect the feces into a metal basin. Urine was collected by introducing the penis into a small cylinder drained by a large tubing passed through a hole in the canvas into a bottle kept on ice outside the incubator. Two ml of capillary arterialized blood were drawn by heel puncture in all infants at day 12, 15, 17, and 20 for determination of serum levels of Ca, P, Mg, immunoreactive parathyroid hormone (iPTH), and calcitonin (iCT).

Laboratory Methods

From aliquots of prepared milk, fecal homogenate, and urine, total nitrogen was determined by the classical method of microkjeldahl, fat by the method of

Van de Kamer, et al.,[49] Ca and Mg by the method of Tisdall and Kramer,[48] and P by the method of Briggs.[11] Urinary excretion of total and free proline and hydroxyproline were measured by the method of Nusgens and Lapière.[33] Urinary creatinine was determined by the method of Owen, et al.[35]

The blood samples were centrifuged immediately after collection and the sera were stored at $-28°C$ until analysis in the same series of assays to avoid interassay variation. Serum Ca, inorganic P and Mg were determined by an automatic Technicon analyzer. Serum iPTH levels were measured by radioimmunoassays with carboxy-terminal recognition, using methods and antiserum described elsewhere.[38] The lower limit of sensitivity of the assay was 25 μlEq/ml and mean $\pm$ SD serum value in normal children was 63 $\pm$ 18 μlEq/ml. Serum iCT levels were determined by radioimmunoassay using the technique and the antiserum previously described.[38] The lower limit of sensitivity of the assay was 150 pg/ml, and serum values in normal children and adults were undetectable.

Calculation and Statistical Analysis

All the results were expressed as mean $\pm$ SD. Paired tests, student tests, and regression analysis were performed by submitting the data to an Olivetti computer.

RESULTS

Metabolic Balance Studies

Data of metabolic balances are gathered in Table I. There was no significant change in nitrogen and fat balances between both balance periods. The intake

TABLE I

Nitrogen, Fat, Calcium, Phosphorus, and Magnesium Balance Data (Mean $\pm$ SD) in 10 Preterm Infants Receiving Either 30 μg of Vitamin D_3 or 0.5 μg of 1.25-Dihydroxycholecalciferol

	Nitrogen	Fat	Calcium	Phosphorus	Magnesium
Vitamin D_3 Period					
Intake (mg/kg/day)	564 ± 68	6732 ± 620	79 ± 12	66 ± 8	7.8 ± 1.2
Feces (mg/kg/day)	65 ± 16	1561 ± 834	65 ± 15	5 ± 3	3.4 ± 0.8
Urine (mg/kg/day)	181 ± 51		2 ± 1	35 ± 16	0.8 ± 0.6
Retention (mg/kg/day)	318 ± 39		12 ± 9	26 ± 8	3.6 ± 1.5
Absorption (%)	88 ± 3	77 ± 14	18 ± 12	92 ± 5	56 ± 9
Retention (%)	56 ± 6		15 ± 12	39 ± 14	46 ± 14
1.25-DHCC Period					
Intake (mg/kg/day)	553 ± 52	6650 ± 695	79 ± 14	66 ± 7	7.7 ± 1.3
Feces (mg/kg/day)	51 ± 18	1131 ± 741	43[a] ± 11	4 ± 4	2.8 ± 0.6
Urine (mg/kg/day)	191 ± 47		5[a] ± 2	28 ± 15	1.0 ± 0.4
Retention (mg/kg/day)	311 ± 40		31[a] ± 11	34 ± 11	3.9 ± 1.2
Absorption (%)	91 ± 3	83 ± 12	46[a] ± 9	94 ± 5	64[b] ± 8
Retention (%)	56 ± 8		39[a] ± 9	52 ± 16	51 ± 11

[a] Significant difference ($P < 0.01$).
[b] Significant difference ($P < 0.05$) in comparison with vitamin D_3 period.

of minerals was not modified. A low Ca absorption was observed during the vitamin D_3 period: from a mean Ca intake of 79 mg/kg/day, the mean coefficient of Ca net absorption was only 18%. Substitution of 1,25-DHCC for vitamin D_3 resulted in a marked improvement of the Ca balance; there was a decrease in fecal loss of Ca, and the coefficient of Ca net absorption increased in all infants (Fig. 1), the mean value reaching 46%. In parallel there was an increase in the urinary excretion of Ca from 2 ± 1 to 5 ± 2 mg/kg/day. On the whole, there was a 150% increase in daily Ca retention during the 1,25-DHCC period (31 ± 11 vs. 12 ± 9 mg/kg/day).

Intestinal P absorption was high during the vitamin D_3 period: from a mean P dietary intake of 66 mg/kg/day, 92% was absorbed. The changes affecting the P balance under 1,25-DHCC were not significant. However, the results indicate a trend toward an increased retention of P (34 ± 11 vs. 26 ± 8 mg/kg/

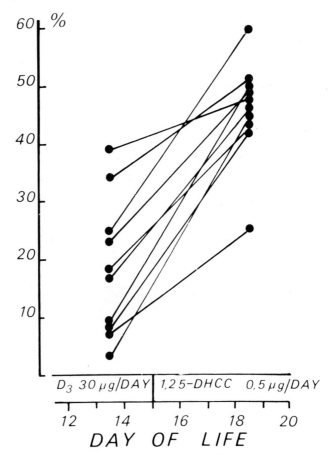

Fig. 1. Coefficients of net calcium absorption in preterm infants when daily oral dose of 0.5 µg of 1,25-dihydroxycholecalciferol was substituted for 30 µg of vitamin D_3.

day) together with a decrease in urinary P excretion (28 ± 15 vs. 35 ± 16 mg/kg/day).

A moderate but significant increase in Mg net absorption was observed under 1,25-DHCC (64 ± 8% vs. 56 ± 9%). In parallel there was a small but not significant decrease in fecal Mg and very little change in daily urinary Mg excretion.

Urinary Hydroxyproline

As shown in Table II, no significant changes took place in the urinary excretion of creatinine and of total or free proline and hydroxyproline.

Serum Levels

Data of serial serum levels of Ca, P, Mg, iPTH, and iCT are gathered in Table III. During the vitamin D_3 period, mean serum Ca and Mg levels were normal and, as usually observed in infants fed with cow's milk based formula, mean P level was elevated (8.2 ± 1.3 mg/100 ml). Within 5 days of treatment with 1,25-DHCC, mean serum Ca level increased from 9.8 ± 1.3 to 10.8 ± 0.4 mg/100 ml; two infants who had a level between 7 and 8 mg/100 ml reached normal range serum Ca levels (9.7–10.9 mg/100 ml) and three infants who were normocalcemic surpassed an 11 mg/100 ml serum Ca level. By contrast mean

TABLE II

Urine Volume and Urinary Excretion (Mean ± SD) of Creatinine and of Total and Free Proline and Hydroxyproline in the 10 Preterm Infants during Both Balance Periods

	Vitamin D_3 Period	1.25-DHCC Period
Diuresis (ml/kg/day)	135 ± 14	135 ± 11
Creatinine (mg/kg/day)	12.9 ± 2.0	12.4 ± 2.5
Total hydroxyproline (mg/kg/day)	16.2 ± 3.7	16.5 ± 3.4
Free hydroxyproline (mg/kg/day)	7.4 ± 2.5	8.1 ± 2.0
Total proline (mg/kg/day)	14.9 ± 2.3	16.4 ± 5.7
Free proline (mg/kg/day)	5.8 ± 2.5	6.2 ± 2.5

TABLE III

Serial Serum Levels (Mean ± SD) of Calcium, Phosphorus, Magnesium, Immunoreactive Parathyroid Hormone (iPTH) and Immunoreactive Calcitonin (iCT) in the 10 Preterm Infants during Both Balance Periods

Postnatal Age	Vitamin D_3 Period		1.25-DHCC Period	
	12 Days	15 Days	17 Days	20 Days
Ca (mg/100 ml)	9.9 ± 1.4	9.8 ± 1.3	10.6 ± 0.7	10.8^a ± 0.4
P (mg/100 ml)	8.0 ± 1.1	8.2 ± 1.3	7.9 ± 1.0	7.7 ± 0.5
Mg (mg/100 ml)	2.3 ± 0.4	2.4 ± 0.5	2.5 ± 0.6	2.4 ± 0.5
iPTH (μlEq/ml)	175 ± 103	174 ± 75	127 ± 79	89^a ± 74
iCT (pg/ml)	<150, $n = 4$	<150, $n = 4$	<150, $n = 6$	<150, $n = 7$
	165–220, $n = 6$	160–210, $n = 6$	150–190, $n = 4$	165–185, $n = 3$

[a] Significant difference ($P < 0.05$) in comparison with vitamin D_3 period.

serum levels of P and Mg were not significantly modified. Most infants were found with above normal range serum iPTH levels during the vitamin D_3 period (mean $\pm$ SD: 174 $\pm$ 75 μlEq/ml). By the end of the 1,25-DHCC period there was a marked decrease in serum iPTH levels and the majority of the infants reached normal range values (mean $\pm$ SD: 89 $\pm$ 74 μlEq/ml). There were no significant change in serum iCT levels; however, in view of the increase in serum Ca levels toward hypercalcemic range values under 1,25-DHCC, it is noteworthy that no infant demonstrated an increase in serum iCT levels and that, on the contrary, the number of infants with undetectable serum iCT levels increased from four to seven by the end of the 1,25-DHCC period.

DISCUSSION

In the present study Ca intestinal absorption and Ca retention were low in preterm infants receiving 30 μg (1200 IU) of vitamin D_3 daily and increased when these infants were given 0.5 μg of 1,25-DHCC per day for 5 days. Since its discovery, 1,25-DHCC has become recognized as the major, if not sole, physiologically active metabolite of vitamin D involved in the regulation of intestinal calcium transport.[16] It also enhances the rate of parahormone-mediated bone resorption.[36] Both effects raise the mineral ion product of the extracellular fluids and thereby increase the rate of bone mineralization. Low Ca intestinal absorption in preterm infants despite vitamin D_2 or D_3 administration has been reported,[42, 43] and several factors which may affect the metabolism of vitamin D have been considered as possible etiological factors of this resistance to vitamin D. This might be caused by a malabsorption of vitamin D resulting from inadequate synthesis of bile salts in preterm infants[50], however, from our results this seems unlikely as the fat balances showed a satisfactory net absorption of triglycerides. An impairment of the 25-hydroxylation of the vitamin D which might hamper the activation of vitamin D has been suggested by Hillman and Haddad[24] based on the observation that plasma levels of 25-HCC were low in the preterm infant. However, the recent study of Glorieux, et al.[22] showing that in preterm infants the plasma levels of 25-HCC increase according to the vitamin D intake tends to indicate that a limitation of this hepatic step in the vitamin D activation is not likely to be a major factor in the lack of effect of vitamin D in these infants. Our results rather suggest that this lack of effect might be related to an impaired conversion of 25-HCC into 1,25-DHCC as has been observed in newborn rats.[51] Yet, any definitive conclusions regarding the activity of this renal step will be only possible from measurements of plasma 1,25-DHCC levels. One cannot exclude from our study the possibility that the Ca malabsorption in preterm infants might result from an intestinal resistance to physiological levels of plasma 1,25-DHCC which could be overcome by giving pharmacologic amounts of 1,25-DHCC. Based on the report from the literature showing that a daily dose of 0.01 μg/kg of 1,25-DHCC can cure the biochemical and radiological abnormalities of vitamin D resistant ricket in infancy,[19] it is indeed likely that the daily dosage of 0.5 μg given to our infants was pharmacological. This is further substantiated by the fact that serum Ca level rose rapidly above normal range values in several infants and was accompanied by a marked increase in daily urinary Ca excretion. It is noteworthy that no change in daily urinary excretion of hydroxyproline was observed which would indicate that this hypercalcemic effect of 1,25-DHCC was not dependent upon an increased bone resorption but essentially resulted from a stimulation of the intestinal Ca absorption.

As indicated by the results of the Ca balances, the hypercalciuric effect of 1,25-DHCC was observed for a daily Ca retention of approximately 30–40 mg/ kg/day, which is far from the 140 mg/kg of Ca that these infants would have received daily *in utero*.[18, 43] This suggests that 1,25-DHCC had little effect in increasing the mineralization process in our infants. It also agrees with the experimental data suggesting that vitamin D derivatives other than 1,25-DHCC may be directly involved in the mineralization process.[9, 16, 28]

Phosphate intestinal absorption was high under vitamin D_3 and was not modified by the administration of 1,25-DHCC despite the clear-cut increase in Ca absorption. This observation indicates that the P intestinal transfer pathway in preterm infants is independent of the Ca transport process, which is in agreement with the current concept of P intestinal transport mechanism.[20, 37] However, it is at variance with the experimental data in adult man[10] and in rats,[13] showing that 1,25-DHCC stimulate intestinal absorption of inorganic P; age or species differences may account for these differences. On the other hand, serum P concentration plays an important regulatory role in the metabolism of 1,25-DHCC, and it is possible that the hyperphosphatemia present in our infants suppressed the 1 α-hydroxylase activity.[16]

Vitamin D is probably of little physiological importance in the regulation of Mg intestinal absorption. Yet experimental data indicates that the administration of vitamin D^{32} or 1,25-DHCC[15] to rats results in a moderate but definite increase in Mg intestinal absorption. Therefore, although the exact physiological significance of this finding is ill-defined, it is of interest that preterm infants similarly demonstrate a moderate significant increase in Mg absorption during 1,25-DHCC administration.

The great majority of the infants were found with elevated serum iPTH levels and normal serum Ca levels during the vitamin D_3 period. Several factors may have contributed to this secondary hyperparathyroidism, namely the low Ca absorption, the high P intake together with the resulting hyperphosphatemia, and, in view of the possible direct effect of 1,25-DHCC upon parathyroid secretion,[14] a lack of 1,25-DHCC. Treatment with 1,25-DHCC resulted in a marked decrease in serum iPTH levels in most infants within 5 days; the absence of parallel changes in either P absorption or serum P levels indicates that these factors were probably not determinant in the etiology of the secondary hyperparathyroidism; on the other hand no clear answer can be given as to whether a direct effect of 1,25-DHCC rather than the suppressive action of the elevated serum Ca levels contributed to the reduction of the parathyroid activity. It remains that a secondary hyperparathyroidism is present by the end of the second week of life in preterm infants fed with cow's milk based formula and supplemented with vitamin D. Recent observations in our laboratory indicate that this secondary hyperparathyroidism may persist for weeks or even months, and it is likely that it contributes to the defective skeletal development frequently seen in preterm infants.

In our study, 2-week-old preterm infants displayed mildly elevated to non-detectable (<150 pg/ml) levels of serum iCT. This contrasts with the markedly elevated serum iCT levels found during the first 48 hr of life, particularly in preterm infants,[7, 25, 26, 38] therefore indicating, contrary to the observations of Hillman[27] that neonatal hypercalcitoninemia is a rapidly regressive phenomenon. It is of interest that, despite the increase in serum Ca levels, there was no increase, and on the contrary in several infants a decrease, in serum iCT levels during the 1,25-DHCC administration period; whether this might result from a direct inhibitory effect of 1,25-DHCC upon calcitonin secretion or rather corresponds to the spontaneous evolutionary pattern of calcitonin metabolism in preterm infants during the third week of life cannot be answered from our data.

SUMMARY

An impaired metabolism of vitamin D has been proposed to explain the poor digestive absorption of calcium in preterm infants. In order to investigate this point, 20 nitrogen, fat, calcium, phosphorus, and magnesium balance studies were carried out in 10 preterm infants who were given a daily oral dose of 30 μg of vitamin D_3 from birth until the end of the first balance period (day 12 to day 15); thereafter, 0.5 μg of 1,25-dihydroxycholecalciferol (1,25-DHCC) until the end of the second balance period (day 17 to day 20). In each infant, serum Ca, P, Mg, immunoreactive parathyroid hormone (iPTH), and calcitonin (iCT) were determined at days 12, 15, 17, and 20. In addition, urinary excretion of creatinine and of total and free proline and hydroxyproline was measured during both balance periods.

There were no significant differences in the nitrogen and fat balances between both balance periods. Intakes of Ca (79 ± 13 mg/kg/day), of P (66 ± 8 mg/kg/day), and of Mg (8 ± 1 mg/kg/day) were not modified. However, when 1,25-DHCC was substituted for vitamin D_3, there was a significant increase in Ca net absorption (from 18 ± 12 to 46 ± 9%), in Ca retention (from 12 ± 9 to 31 ± 11 mg/kg/day), and in urinary Ca excretion (from 2 ± 1 to 5 ± 2 mg/kg/day). There was no significant change in mean P absorption (93 ± 4%); P retention rose slightly but not significantly from 26 ± 8 to 34 ± 11 mg/kg/day. Mean Mg absorption increased from 56 ± 9 to 64 ± 8%. Within 5 days of administration of 1,25-DHCC, mean serum Ca level increased from 9.8 ± 1.3 to 10.8 ± 0.4 mg/dl, whereas serum iPTH dropped from 174 ± 75 to 89 ± 74 μlEq/ml. Serum P, Mg and iCT levels and the urinary excretion of creatinine and of total and free proline and hydroxyproline was not modified.

This study indicates that oral administration of 0.5 μg of 1,25-DHCC instead of 30 μg of vitamin D_3 improves Ca absorption and retention in preterm infants. This is accompanied by a decrease in serum iPTH levels. However, it also results in a rapid increase in calcemia and calciuria. Further evaluation will be needed in order to determine the appropriate dosage and the effects of long-term treatment.

ACKNOWLEDGMENTS

This work was supported by The National Foundation of Medical Scientific Research of Belgium. We are grateful to all the nurses who took such care with the balances, to M. Cops for her expert technical assistance, and to Y. Vos de Wael for typing the manuscript.

REFERENCES

1. Barak, Y., Milbauer, B., Weisman, Y., Edelstein, S., and Spirer, Z., Response of neonatal hypocalcaemia to 1α-hydroxyvitamin D₃. *Arch. Dis. Child.*, **54**, 642 (1979).
2. Barltrop, D., and Oppe, T. E., Dietary factors in neonatal calcium homeostatis. *Lancet* **2**, 1333 (1970).
3. Barltrop, D., and Oppe, T. E., Absorption of fat and calcium by low birth weight infants from milks containing butterfat and olive oil. *Arch. Dis. Child.* **48**, 496 (1973).
4. Barltrop, D., and Oppe, T. E., Calcium and fat absorption by low birthweight infants from a calcium-supplemented milk formula. *Arch. Dis. Child.* **48**, 580 (1973).
5. Barltrop, D., Neonatal hypocalcemia. *Postgrad. Med. J.* **51** (*Suppl.* 3), 7 (1975).
6. Barltrop, D., Mole, R. H., and Sutton, A., Absorption and endogenous faecal excretion of calcium by low birthweight infants on feeds with varying contents of calcium and phosphate. *Arch. Dis. Child.* **52**, 41 (1977).
7. Barness, L. A., Morrow, G., III, Solverio, J., Finnegan, L. P., and Heitman, S. E., Calcium and fat absorption from infant formulas. *Pediatrics* **54**, 217 (1974).
8. Baele, M. C., Chan, J. C. M., Oldham, S. B., and DeLuca, H. F., Vitamin D: The discovery of its metabolites and their therapeutic applications. *Pediatrics* **57**, 729 (1976).
9. Bordier, P., Rasmussen, H., Marie, P., Miravet, L., Gueris, J., and Ryckwaert, A., Vitamin D metabolites and bone mineralization in man. *J. Clin. Endocrinol. Metab.* **46**, 284 (1978).
10. Brickman, A. S., Hartenbower, D. L., Norman, A. W., and Coburn, J. W., Action of 1 α-hydroxyvitamin D₃ and 1,25-dihydroxyvitamin D₃ on mineral metabolism in man. I. Effects on net absorption of phosphorus. *Am. J. Clin. Nutr.* **30**, 1064 (1977).
11. Briggs, A. P., A modification of the Bell-Doisy phosphate method. *J. Biol. Chem.* **53**, 13 (1922).
12. Chan, G. M., Tsang, R. C., Chen, I. W., DeLuca, H. F., and Steichen, J. J., The effects of 1,25(OH)₂ vitamin D₃ supplementation in premature infants. *J. Pediatr.* **93**, 91 (1978).
13. Chen, T. C., Castillo, L., Korycha-Dahl, M., and DeLuca, H. F., Role of vitamin D in phosphate transport of rat intestine. *J. Nutr.* **104**, 1056 (1974).
14. Chertow, B. S., Baylink, D. J., Wergedal, J. E., and Norman, A. W., Decrease in serum immunoreactive parathyroid hormone in rats and in parathyroid hormone secretion in vitro by 1,25-dihydroxycholecalciferol. *J. Clin. Invest.* **56**, 668 (1975).
15. Coburn, J., Personal communication.
16. DeLuca, H. F., The vitamin D system in the regulation of calcium and phosphorus metabolism. Nutrit. Rev., 37: 161 (1979).
17. Dirksen, H., and Anast, C., Interrelationships of serum immunoreactive calcitonin (iCT) and serum calcium in newborn infants (Abstr.). *Pediatr. Res.* **10**, 408 (1976).
18. Forbes, G. B., Calcium accumulation by the human fetus. *Pediatrics* **57**, 976 (1976).
19. Fraser, D., Kooh, S. W., Kind, H. P., Holick, M. F., Tanaka, Y., and DeLuca, H. F.: Pathogenesis of hereditary vitamin D-dependent rickets. *N. Engl. J. Med.* **289**, 817 (1973).
20. Garabedian, M., Pezant, E., Miravet, L., Fellot, C., and Balsan, S., 1,25-dihydroxycholecalciferol effect on serum phosphorus homeostasis in rats. *Endocrinology* **98**, 794 (1976).
21. Glasgow, J. F. T., and Thomas, P. S., Rachitic respiratory distress in small preterm infants. *Arch. Dis. Child.* **52**, 268 (1977).

22. Glorieux, F. H., Salle, B. L., Delvin, E. E., David L., and Senterre, J., Serum 25-hydroxyvitamin D levels following vitamin D administration during the first week of life in premature infants. *Pediatr. Res.* **13,** 475, (1979).

23. Haussler, M. R., and McCain, T. A., Basic and clinical concepts related to vitamin D metabolism and action. *N. Engl. J. Med.* **297,** 974 (1977).

24. Hillman, L. S., and Haddad, J. G., Perinatal vitamin D metabolism. II. Serial 25-hydroxyvitamin D concentrations in sera of term and premature infants. *J. Pediatr.* **86,** 928 (1975).

25. Hillman, L. S., Rojanasathit, S., Slatopolsky, E., and Haddad, J. G., Serial measurements of serum calcium, magnesium, parathyroid hormone, calcitonin, and 25-hydroxyvitamin D in premature and term infants during the first week of life. *Pediatr. Res.* **11,** 739 (1977).

26. Hillman, L. S., Hoff, N., Slatopolsky, E., and Haddad, J. G., Serial calcitonin serum concentrations in premature infant during first 12 weeks of life (Abstract). *Pediatr. Res.* **12,** 414 (1978).

27. Hoff, N., Tyrala, E., Haddad, J., and Hillman, L., 25-hydroxyvitamin D deficiency in osteopenia of the extreme premature (Abstract). *Pediatr. Res.* **10,** 410 (1976).

28. Kanis, J. A., Heynen, G., Russel, R. G. G., Smith, R., Walton, R. J., and Warner, G. T., Biological Effects of 24,25-Dihydroxycholecalciferol in Man, in *Vitamin D*, Norman, A. W., Ed. de Gruyter, Berlin, New York, 1977, p. 793.

29. Kooh, S. W., Fraser, D., Toon, R., and DeLuca, H. F., Response of protracted neonatal hypocalcaemia to 1α,25-dihydroxyvitamin D_3. *Lancet* **2,** 1105 (1976).

30. Lewin, P. K., Reid, M., Reilly, B. J., Swyer, P. R., and Fraser, D., Iatrogenenic rickets in low-birth-weight infants. *J. Pediatr.* **78,** 207 (1971).

31. McIntosh, N., Shaw, J. C. L., and Taghizadeh, A., Direct evidence for calcium and trace mineral deficits in the skeleton of preterm infants. *Pediatr. Res.* **8,** 896 (1974).

32. Meintzer, R. B., and Steenbock, H., Vitamin D and magnesium absorption. *J. Nutr.* **56,** 285 (1955).

33. Nusgens, B., and Lapière, Ch. M., The relationship between proline and hydroxyproline urinary excretion in human as an index of collagen catabolism. *Clin. Chim. Acta* **48,** 203 (1973).

34. Oppe, T. E., and Redstone, D., Calcium and phosphorus levels in healthy newborn infants given various types of milk. *Lancet* **1,** 1045 (1968).

35. Owen, J. A., Iggo, B., Scandrett, F. J., and Stewart, C. P., The determination of creatinine in plasma of serum and in urine; a critical examination. *Biochem. J.* **58,** 426 (1954).

36. Pechet, M. M., and Hesse, R. H., Metabolic and clinical effects of pure crystalline 1-hydroxyvitamin D_3 and 1,25-dihydroxyvitamin D_3. *Am. J. Med.* **57,** 13 (1974).

37. Rizzoli, R., Fleisch, H., and Bonjour, J. P., Role of 1,25-dihydroxyvitamin D_3 on intestinal phosphate absorption in rats with a normal vitamin D supply. *J. Clin. Invest.* **60,** 639 (1977).

38. Salle, B., David, L., Chopard, J., Grafmeyer, D., and Renaud, H., Prevention of early neonatal hypocalcemia in low birth weight infants with continuous calcium infusion: effect on serum calcium, phosphorus, magnesium and circulating immunoreactive parathyroid hormone and calcitonin. *Pediatr. Res.* **11,** 1180 (1977).

39. Senterre, J., Sodoyez-Goffaux, F., and Lambrechts, A., Metabolic balance studies in premature babies. I. Methodology. *Acta Paediatr. Belg.* **25,** 113 (1971).

40. Senterre, J., and Lambrechts, A., Nitrogen, fat and minerals balances in premature infants fed acidified or non-acidified half-skimmed cow milk. *Biol. Neonate* **20,** 107 (1972).

41. Senterre, J., Endogenous Faecal Calcium, Total Digestive Juice Calcium, Net and True Calcium Absorption in Premature Infants, in *Perinatal Medicine*, Stembera, Polacek, and Sabata, Eds. Thieme Edition, Stuttgart, 1976, p. 287.

42. Senterre, J., Calcium and Phosphorus Retention in Preterm Infants. in *Intensive Care of the Newborn. II*, Stern, L., Ed. Masson Publishers, New York, 1978, p. 205.

43. Shaw, J. C. L., Evidence for defective skeletal mineralization in low birthweight infants: the absorption of calcium and fat. *Pediatrics* **57,** 16 (1976).

44. Southgate, D. A. T., Widdowson, E. M., Smits, B. J., Cooke, W. T., Walker, C. H. M., and Mathers, N. P.: Absorption and excretion of calcium and fat by young infants. *Lancet* **1,** 487 (1969).

45. Sutton, A., Mole, R. H., and Barltrop, D., Urinary and faecal excretion of marker calcium (^{46}Ca) by low birthweight infants. *Arch. Dis. Child.* **52,** 50 (1977).

46. Tantibhedhyangkul, P., and Hashim, S. A.: Medium-chain triglyceride feeding in premature infants: effects on calcium and magnesium absorption. *Pediatrics* **61,** 537 (1978).

47. Thomas, P. S., and Glasgow, J. F. T., The "mandibular mantle"—a sign of rickets in very low birth weight infants. *Br. J. Radiol.* **51,** 93 (1978).

48. Tisdall, F. F., and Kramer, B., Methods for the direct quantitative determination of sodium, potassium, calcium and magnesium in urine and stools. *J. Biol. Chem.* **48,** 1 (1921).

49. Van de Kamer, J. H., Ten Bokkel Huinink, H. B., and Weijers, H. A., Rapid method for the determination of fat in feces. *J. Biol. Chem.* **177,** 347 (1949).

50. Watkins, J. B., Bile acid metabolism and fat absorption in newborn infants. *Pediatr. Clin. North Am.* **21,** 501 (1974).

51. Weisman, Y., Sapir, R., Harell, A., and Edelstein, S., Maternal-perinatal interrelationships of vitamin D metabolism in rats. *Biochim. Biophys Acta* **428,** 388 (1976).

52. Widdowson, E. M., Absorption and excretion of fat, nitrogen and minerals from "filled" milks by babies one week old. *Lancet* **2,** 1099 (1965).

53. Williams, M. L., Rose, C. S., Morrow, G., Sloan, S. E., and Barness, L. A., Calcium and fat absorption in neonatal period. *Am. J. Clin. Nutr.* **23,** 1322 (1970).

54. Wolf, H., Gräff, V., and Offermann, G., Influence of Vitamin D$_3$ on Calcium Metabolism of the Newborn Infant, in *Vitamin D*, Norman, A. W., Ed. de Gruyter, Berlin, New York, 1977, p. 855.

13

Vitamin D Metabolism in Preterm Infants: Its Relation to Early Neonatal Hypocalcemia

FRANCIS H. GLORIEUX[1], BERNARD SALLE[2], EDGARD E. DELVIN[1], and LOUIS DAVID[2]

Early neonatal hypocalcemia (ENH) is a frequent event during the first 24–48 hr of life in preterm infants (PI). Whether it represents an adaptive step to extrauterine life or expresses an imbalance of mineral (calcium and phosphorus) homeostasis is still a matter of major debate. Proposed mechanisms to explain ENH include inappropriate secretion of parathyroid hormone (PTH)[1] and calcitonin (CT)[2] as well as defective vitamin D absorption or activation.[3] We have elected to focus on the latter possibility and have evaluated whether, in PI, the enzymes responsible for the activation of vitamin D were active and responsive to their known inducing factors.[4] We have observed that, at 32 weeks of gestation, the activation pathway of vitamin D was reactive and sensitive to hypocalcemia and hyperparathyroidism. These findings preclude the pharmacologic use of vitamin D metabolites in ENH, and focus on the importance of an adequate supply of the parent vitamin, as well as of calcium.

VITAMIN D ACTIVATION

The present stage of knowledge[4] of the metabolic conversions undergone by vitamin D in order to fulfill its hormonal functions is depicted in Figure 1. Two sources of vitamin D are available to man. The first proceeds from the skin where, upon ultraviolet light irradiation (280–300 nm), 7-dehydrocholesterol is first photochemically converted to precholecalciferol, which by molecular

---

[1] McGill University, Shriners Hospital, Genetics Unit, Montréal, Canada
[2] Service de Néo-natologie, Hôpital Edouard-Herriot, Lyon, France

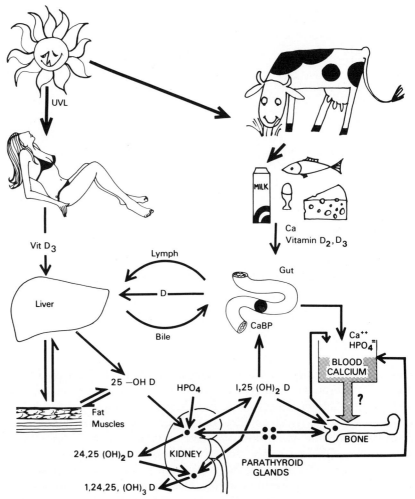

Fig. 1. Schematic overview of the current state of our knowledge on the activation pathway of vitamin D and its homeostatic control.

rearrangement yields cholecalciferol (vitamin D_3). This pathway is the natural source of antirachitic activity when exposure to sunlight is adequate. The second important source available to man is ergocalciferol (vitamin D_2), which arises from the ultraviolet irradiation of ergosterol present in plants. In the days when cattle were grazing on the green fields, it was available in milk and its by-products. Nowadays artificially fortified dairy products, multivitamin preparations, and fish liver oil have become, particularly in cold climates, the main dietary source of the vitamin. On a weight basis, 25 ng of vitamin D_2 has been designated as 1 international unit (IU) of antirachitic activity. It is estimated that 400 units are required per day to prevent rickets and osteomalacia. Since, in man, the biological activity of vitamin D_2 and vitamin D_3 are identical, they will be both hereafter referred to as vitamin D.

Endogenous and exogenous vitamin D are transported by a β-lipoprotein, through the lymphatic system, to the liver where it is hydroxylated to yield 25-hydroxyvitamin D(25-OHD).

This metabolite is the major circulating form of vitamin D as the parent substance is present at only a tenfold less concentration. Presumably vitamin D excess is mainly stored in the adipose and muscular tissues and skin. The production of 25-OHD is loosely product-feedback regulated, if at all, as large doses of vitamin D give rise to high circulating levels of 25-OHD. Therefore when there is no liver damage or enterohepatic cycle impairment, the serum level of 25-OHD may rightfully be regarded as an adequate index of vitamin D nutritional status in man.

Rapidly cleared from the liver, 25-OHD is transported to the kidney where it is further metabolized. In conditions of vitamin D depletion or in states of hypocalcemia and hyperparathyroidism it is enzymatically converted to $1\alpha,25$-dihydroxyvitamin D $[1\alpha,25\text{-}(OH)_2D]$. In experimental animals (rats and pigs), the extracellular phosphate ion concentration has also been shown to play a role in the regulation of $1,25\text{-}(OH)_2D$ synthesis. However at the present time there is no data confirming that such a mechanism prevails in man. By virtue of its synthesis (in the kidney) distal from its sites of action (gut and bone), its direct action on the target tissues, and its feedback regulation, $1,25\text{-}(OH)_2D$ can truly be considered as a hormone. Acting alone in intestine, it promotes calcium transport and phosphate absorption. Together with parathyroid hormone, it mediates the resorption and probably also accretion of bone.[5] In conditions of euparathyroidism, normocalcemia, and normophosphatemia, renal 1α, hydroxylase activity decreases and another enzyme, renal 25-hydroxyvitamin D-24-hydroxylase becomes predominantly active, yielding 24,25-dihydroxyvitamin D. The role of this metabolite is less understood. It has been shown to be present in and produced by the epiphyseal cartilage of rats.[6] It has also been suggested that it plays a role in calcification[4] and in the suppression of PTH secretion. However, further evidence will be required before a functional role could be assigned to this metabolite. Other metabolites like 1,24,25-trihydroxyvitamin D and 25,26-dihydroxyvitamin D (not shown in the figure) have been identified. Neither of these two hydroxylated derivatives have been definitively assigned a function, although measurable amounts of the latter product have been found in human serum. It is currently proposed that they are products of the excretory pathway of the vitamin rather than biologically active metabolites.

In the present study we have, in preterm infants, evaluated their vitamin D nutritional status and their capacity to absorb and metabolize the vitamin in liver and kidney. We have also assessed the effects of vitamin D supplementation upon serum levels of calcium.

MATERIALS AND METHODS

Subjects

All premature infants selected for the study were born after an uneventful pregnancy and immediately transferred to the newborn intensive care unit of the Edouard Herriot Hospital (Lyon, France). None had a history of maternal diabetes or toxemia. They all weighed between 1600 and 2500 g. The gestational age, as assessed by the Dubowitz scoring system,[7] ranged between 32 and 37 weeks. Blood pH was measured at birth and daily thereafter. No respiratory distress or infection episodes were noted during the time of the study. All infants were infused with a 10% glucose solution without calcium from 3 hr after birth. Being all of small birth weight, all prematures received the same amount of human milk. The daily ingestion evaluated according to the formula of Barltrop and Hillier,[8] varied from 82 to 111 mg for calcium and from 43 to 60 mg for phosphorus. Informed consent was obtained in all cases from the legal guardians.

To evaluate the extent of vitamin D absorption and liver and kidney metabolism capacities, the selected 14 premature infants were divided into two matched groups. The first group received a daily oral dose of 52.5 μg (2100 IU) of vitamin D_3 for 5 days. The second group serving as controls received no vitamin D_3 supplements.

Methods

The 4 ml venous blood samples, obtained from a scalp vein at 5 days of age, were spun within 1 hr and the serum frozen at $-20°C$ until shipment to Montreal on dry ice. Calcium and phosphorus were measured colorimetrically on a Technicon[r] Auto Analyzer (Tarrytown, N.Y.). When possible, the circulating immunoreactive parathyroid hormone (iPTH) was measured by radioimmunoassay using an antiserum reactive with the carboxy terminal fragments and intact PTH.[9] With this assay, the levels in normal children and adults ranged from 25 to 100 mlEq/liter.

For the measurement of 25-OHD and $1\alpha,25$-$(OH)_2D$, aliquots of serum, to which were added 25-hydroxy(26,27-^{3}H-methyl)cholecalciferol and $1\alpha,25$-dihydroxy(23,24-(n)-^{3}H)cholecalciferol (Amersham-Searle, Oakville, Ont., Canada) as tracers were extracted and chromatographed to separate the vitamin D metabolites. The fraction containing 25-OHD was assayed in triplicate according to the method of Haddad and Chyu.[10] The mean concentrations ($\pm$ SD) and range of concentration observed in samples collected from November to April in 40 healthy infants and children (8–36 months) are 20.2 $\pm$ 4.3 and 13.9–38.1 ng/ml, respectively. The serum fraction $1\alpha,25$-$(OH)_2D$ was assayed in triplicate using the competitive binding assay of Eisman, et al.,[11] modified by separating the bound from free hormone with a Dextran T-20 (5%) coated Nuchar charcoal (5%) suspension instead of a polyethylene glycol (PEG) solution.

The displacement curve obtained by incubating increasing concentrations of $1\alpha,25$-$(OH)_2D$ in the presence of a fixed amount of labeled hormone is shown in Figure 2. The intra- and interassay coefficients of variation are 8% and 10%, respectively. The mean concentration ($\pm$ SD), obtained from 13 healthy children of both sexes (7–15 years), is 44.0 $\pm$ 9.5 pg/ml and agrees with normal values reported by others.[12]

RESULTS

Table I shows that the administered vitamin D_3 is well absorbed by the gut since upon supplementation the serum levels rise from a mean of 7.8 ng/ml to 29.3 ng/ml ($p < 0.0005$). Furthermore, while the effect of supplementation is

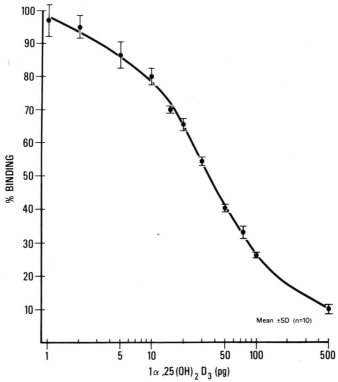

Fig. 2. Displacement curve of the radioactive tracer in the presence of increasing concentration of $1\alpha,25$-$(OH)_2D_3$, used in the determination of $1,25$-$(OH)_2D$ levels in serum.

TABLE I

Summary of the Biochemical Data of the Premature Control and Vitamin D_3-Supplemented Infants at the Age of 5 Days

	Ca (mg/dl)	Pi (mg/dl)	iPTH (lEq/l)	25-OHD (ng/ml)	1,25(OH)₂D (pg/ml)
C[a] (±S.D.)	7.4 ± 0.3	5.9 ± 0.3	160.3 ± 32.3	7.8 ± 1.8	56.4 ± 8.4
n[b]	(7)	(7)	(3)	(7)	(7)
+ D₃[c] (±S.D.)	8.2 ± 0.4	6.3 ± 0.4	167.7 ± 50.0	29.3 ± 2.7	154.5 ± 16.6
n[b]	(7)	(6)	(3)	(7)	(7)
p[d]	NS	NS	NS	<0.0005	<0.0005

The significance levels for the difference in means (p values) were calculated with the Student's t-test for paired variates (t_{dep}).

[a] C: control group.
[b] n: number of subjects per group.
[c] +D₃: vitamin-D₃-supplemented group (52.5 μg/d).
[d] NS: not significant.

marginal on the serum calcium levels ($p < 0.10$), not correcting the hypocalcemia, it has no effect either on the circulating iPTH or on the serum phosphorus levels. Although the 25-OHD levels are low in the control group, the 1,25-(OH)D levels are comparable to those observed in our control group of older children (44.0 ± 9.5 pg/ml). Supplementation with vitamin D_3 brings about a significant increase in the hormone circulating levels (154.5 ± 16.6 pg/ml, $p < 0.0005$).

When the serum 25-OHD concentrations are plotted against those of 1,25-(OH)$_2$D observed in the same sample (Fig. 3), a clear positive and highly significant correlation is observed ($r = 0.86$, $p < 0.001$), showing the direct relationship between the amount of substrate in circulation (25-OHD) and the product of the 1α-hydroxylation in kidney [1,25-(OH)$_2$D]. The relationship holds despite the relatively high serum phosphate concentration (Table I).

DISCUSSION

The data presented show that in preterm infants at 32 weeks of gestation vitamin D is well absorbed by the intestine and that it is properly hydroxylated

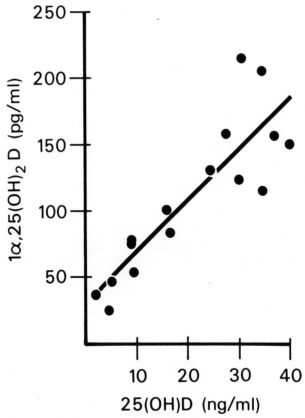

Fig. 3. Relation between circulating concentrations of 25-hydroxy D and 1α,25-(OH)$_2$D in premature infants at 5 days of age. Each dot ($n = 16$) represents one specimen. The regression analysis of the line was $y = 30.2 \pm 3.8\ x$, $r = 0.80$, $p < 0.005$.

in the liver to 25-OHD and in the kidney to 1,25-$(OH)_2$D. We have also shown that there is no transient hypoparathyroidism confirming earlier reports.[2] Furthermore, evidence is presented that the kidney responds adequately to the hyperparathyroid state probably secondary to the hypocalcemia by increasing the synthesis of 1,25-$(OH)_2$D. It is worth noting that, in the group studied, the levels of serum 25-OHD in the control group were well below the norms reported for North American populations.[10] Since serum 25-OHD has been shown to reflect vitamin D nutritional status in man,[4] we may therefore conclude that the infants studied were marginally vitamin D deficient. Moreover, since a direct relationship between the maternal serum 25-OHD levels and those of cord blood has been demonstrated,[13] it follows from our results that the mothers were also relatively vitamin D deficient.

Also of interest is the fact that although the serum 25-OHD levels are low in the control group, the levels of 1,25-$(OH)_2$D are within the normal range observed for older children.[12] However, it must be stressed that in the face of hyperparathyroidism and hypocalcemia, e.g., either direct or indirect stimuli for 1α-hydroxylase activity,[4] these levels may be regarded as abnormally low. One hypothesis that stems from those observations is that there might be a limitation in the substrate (25-OHD) available. This is reflected in the group receiving supplemental vitamin D since, in that group, the serum 1,25-$(OH)_2$D rose to levels threefold our normal mean, showing an excellent correlation between the levels of 25-OHD and those of 1,25-$(OH)_2$D (Fig. 3).

Finally we observed that despite high levels of 1,25-$(OH)_2$D neither the hypocalcemia nor the hyperparathyroidism seems to be corrected.

Our results rule out the hypotheses of transient hypoparathyroidism[1] and defects in absorption or activation of vitamin D^3 to explain ENH. However, it remains as an open possibility that an inadequate response of the intestine (end organ) to the hormone [1,25-$(OH)_2$D] would explain the higher than normal levels of the renal metabolite observed after 5 days of vitamin D_3 supplementation. From the calculated calcium and phosphorus intakes it may also be that despite adequate hormonal control these infants are placed in a state of calcium deficiency. Finally it must be stressed that the group studied seemed at first glance somewhat vitamin D deficient. Therefore, both factors may, together, play an important role in the etiology of ENH.

From our data, it may be concluded that the use of vitamin D metabolites, with the always existing risks of intoxication, is not warranted in premature infants after 32 weeks of gestation. Careful dosage of vitamin D in the mother during the pregnancy, together with increased calcium intake, may solve some of the problems causing ENH in the aftermath of a premature delivery.

ACKNOWLEDGMENTS

The authors are indebted to the staff of the Newborn Unit of the Hôpital Edouard Herriot, to Ms. A. Arabian, M. Dussault, and R. Travers for their technical contribution, and to Ms. D. Bissonnette for her expert secretarial assistance.

This work was supported by the Shriners of North America, Le conseil de la Recherche en Santé du Québec, and the France-Québec exchange program.

REFERENCES

1. Tsang, R. C., Light, I. J., Sutherland, J. M., and Kleinman, L. I., Possible pathogenetic factors in neonatal hypocalcemia of prematurity. *J. Pediatr.* **82,** 423 (1973).
2. Hillman, L. S., Rojanasathit, S., Slatopolsky, E., and Haddad, J. G., Serial measurements of serum calcium, magnesium, parathyroid hormone, calcitonin, and 25-hydroxy-vitamin D in premature and term infants during the first week of life. *Pediatr. Res.* **11,** 739 (1977).
3. Hillman, L. S., and Haddad, J. G., Perinatal vitamin D metabolism. II. Serial 25-hydroxyvitamin D concentrations in sera of term and premature infants. *J. Pediatr.* **86,** 928 (1975).
4. DeLuca, H. F., *Vitamin D Metabolism and Function*, Monographs on Endocrinology, Vol. 13, Gross F., Grumbach, M. M., Labhart, A., *et al.*, Eds. Springer-Verlag, New York, 1979.
5. Meunier, P. J., Edouard, C., Arlot, M., Lejeune, E., Alexandre, C., and Leroy, G., Effects of 1,25-Dihydroxyvitamin D on Bone Mineralization, in *Molecular Endocrinology*, MacIntyre, I., and Szelke, M., Eds. Elsevier/North-Holland Biochemical Press, New York, 1979, p. 283.
6. Garabedian, M., Bailly Du Bois, M., Corvol, M. T., Pezant, E., and Balsan, S., Vitamin D and cartilage. I. In vitro metabolism of 25-hydroxycholecalciferol by cartilage. *Endocrinol.* **102,** 1262 (1978).
7. Dubowitz, L. M. S., Dubowitz, V., and Goldberg, C., Clinical assessment of gestational age in the newborn infant. *J. Pediatr.* **77,** 1 (1970).
8. Barltrop, D., and Hillier, R., Calcium and phosphorus content of transitional and mature human milk. *Acta Paediatr. Scand.* **63,** 347 (1974).
9. Salle, B. L., David, L., Chopard, J. P., Grafmeyer, D. C., and Renaud, H., Prevention of early neonatal hypocalcemia in low birth weight infants with continuous calcium infusion: Effect on serum calcium, phosphorus, magnesium, and circulating immunoreactive parathyroid hormone and calcitonin. *Pediatr. Res.* **11,** 1180 (1977).
10. Haddad, J. G., and Chyu, K. J., Competitive protein binding radioassay for 25-hydroxycholecalciferol. *J. Clin. Endocrinol.* **33,** 992 (1971).
11. Eisman, J. H., Hamstra, A. J., Kream, B. E., and DeLuca, H. F., A sensitive, precise and convenient method for determination of 1,25-dihydroxyvitamin D in human plasma. *Arch. Biochem. Biophys.* **176,** 235 (1976).
12. Scriver, C. R., Reade, T. M., DeLuca, H. F., and Hamstra, A. J., Serum 1,25-dihydroxyvitamin D levels in normal subjects and in patients with hereditary rickets or bone disease. *N. Engl. J. Med.* **299,** 976 (1978).
13. Hillman, L. S., and Haddad, J. G., Human perinatal vitamin D metabolism I: 25-hydroxyvitamin D in maternal and cord blood. *J. Pediatr.* **84,** 742 (1974).

14

Extrauterine Adaptation of Renal Function in Full-Term and Preterm Newborn Infants

ANITA APERIA, OVE BROBERGER, PETER HERIN, and
ROLF ZETTERSTRÖM

Most previous studies in which renal function in preterm infants has been compared with the conditions in full-term infants have been carried out during the first postnatal days. In these studies several differences have been demonstrated between newborn preterm infants of a gestational age below 34 weeks and newborn full-term infants. It may thus be assumed that the conditions for renal functional adaptation to extrauterine life may vary with gestational age. In this paper the studies on renal functional development during the first month of life in preterm infants born before the 34th gestational week and those born at term will be reported. The results from the studies uniformly suggest that the renal functional capacity in preterm infants is related to postmenstrual rather than to postnatal age during the entire first month of life.

MATERIAL AND METHODS

The studies were performed in 45 preterm infants (gestational age 32–34 weeks) and 40 full-term infants (gestational age 39–41 weeks) at postnatal ages between 1 and 34 days. The full-term infants that were all healthy were studied in the obstetric wards or in the outpatient unit. The postnatal course for the preterm infants was considered uncomplicated for preterm babies. For the

Department of Pediatrics, Karolinska Institute, St. Göran's Children's Hospital, Stockholm, Sweden

evaluation of renal function, urine specimens were collected for an exact time of 8–10 hr and a capillary blood sample was taken during the time of urine sampling. Urine and serum were analyzed for creatinin using a modification of the Jaffe method, for beta-2-microglobulin using a radio immuno assay method (Pharmacia®, Phadeba), and for sodium and potassium with a flame photometer. The urine specimens were analyzed for aldosterone with a radio immuno assay method.

On the basis of the analytical results obtained, creatinin clearance, which was used as an index of glomerular filtration (GFR), fractional beta-2-microglobulin, and fractional excretion of sodium were calculated. Student's t test has been used for statistical analysis. p values less than 0.05 are considered to be significant.

RESULTS

At 2 days of age GFR was found to be slightly lower in preterm than in full-term infants (Fig. 1). In full-term infants there is a significant increase in GFR from the 2nd to the 4th postnatal day. From 4 to 30 days of age there is a less pronounced but still significant further increase in GFR. In contrast to full-term infants, preterm infants are unable to rapidly increase GFR immediately after birth. In preterm infants GFR thus relates linearly to age from 2 to 30 days. At 30 days after birth GFR is still somewhat lower than in full-term infants.

The renal handling of beta-2-microglobulin has been used as a marker of renal proximal tubular function. Beta-2-microglobulin, which has a molecular weight of around 12,000, is easily filtered and subsequently reabsorbed in the

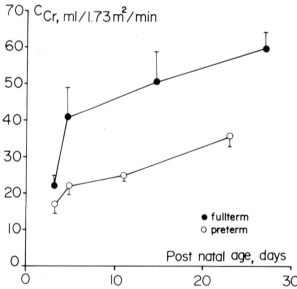

Fig. 1. Glomerular filtration rate in full-term and preterm newborn infants during the first month after birth. Each dot represents the average of 8–12 determinations, the bars SEM.

proximal tubule by pinocytosis. As is shown in Figure 2, the amount of filtered beta-2-microglobulin rises continuously with increasing gestational age. Despite that, the fractional reabsorption of beta-2-microglobulin is less efficient in preterm infants than in those born at term (Fig. 3). During the first 4

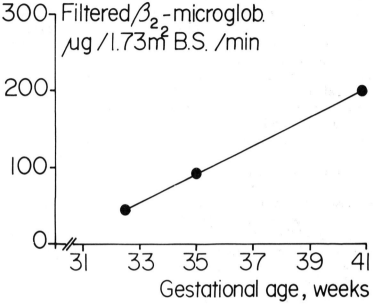

Fig. 2. Filtered beta-2-microglobulin (GFR × serum-beta-2-microglobulin) in relation to gestational age.

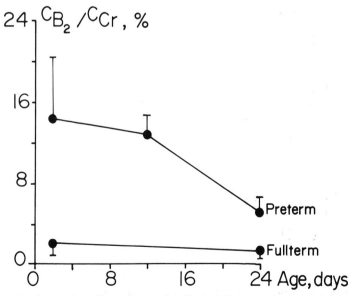

Fig. 3. Fractional excretion of beta-2-microglobulin in full-term and preterm infants during the first month after birth. Each dot represents the average of 8–12 determinations.

postnatal weeks fractional excretion of beta-2-microglobulin will decrease slowly in preterm infants and will at the age of 1 month still be higher than in full-term infants. The results demonstrate that the glomerular tubular imbalance at the level of the proximal tubule will in preterm infants persist during the first postnatal month.

In newborn full-term infants the urinary sodium excretion is low (Fig. 4). Sodium intake is relatively high during the first weeks since the sodium content of breast milk is then much higher than during later lactation. As is also shown in Figure 4 the intake of sodium will considerably exceed the urinary excretion. In preterm infants, the urinary excretion of sodium exceeds the intake during the first week after birth (Fig. 5), since the preterm infants have generally been fed mature breast milk with a low concentration of sodium. The marked negative sodium balance in preterm infants is not only due to higher urinary losses than in full-term infants but also to a lower intake of sodium. The relatively high sodium excretion in preterm infants is due to a lower sodium tubular reabsorptive capacity as indicated by a high fractional sodium excretion (Fig. 6).

Urine aldosterone excretion is high in preterm as well as in full-term infants during the first weeks of age and ranges from 18 to 105 μmol/1.73 m^2 BSA/day, which is higher than in adults, where the normal range in this laboratory is 5.5 to 33 μmol/1.73 m^2 BSA/day (Fig. 7). The postnatal pattern for aldosterone excretion is similar in preterm and full-term infants; the excretion generally is higher in preterm than in full-term infants, but the difference is never of more than borderline significance. It is well established that aldosterone

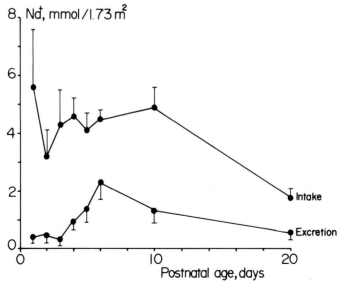

Fig. 4. Average hourly urinary sodium excretion and sodium intake in full-term infants aged 1–21 days fed breast milk from their mothers. Each filled circle represents the average of 5–7 observations. The bars represent SEM.

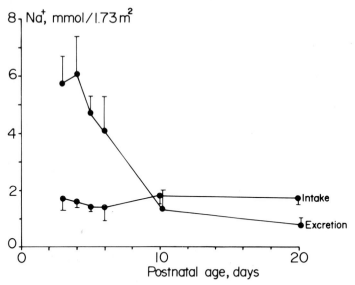

Fig. 5. Average hourly sodium intake and urinary sodium excretion in preterm infants aged 3–21 days that have been fed pooled mature breast milk. Each filled circle represents the average of 4–9 observations.

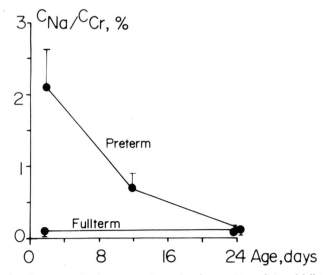

Fig. 6. Fractional sodium excretion in preterm (gestational age ≤ 34 weeks) and full-term infants at 2, 12, and 24 days after birth. Glomerular filtration rate was determined as the clearance of creatinine. Each filled circle represents the mean from 8–12 infants. The bars represent SEM.

affects sodium and potassium transport in opposite direction. An increase in the urinary potassium sodium quotient U_{K^+}/U_{Na^+} can therefore be interpreted as secondary to the effect of aldosterone on the tubular transport of those electrolytes. In newborn full-term infants there is a good correlation ($r = 0.84$)

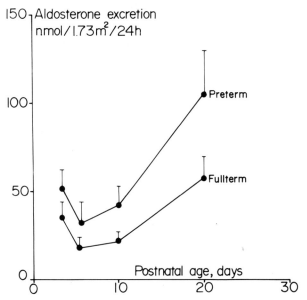

Fig. 7. Postnatal changes in aldosterone excretion in preterm (gestational age $\leq$ 34 weeks), and full-term infants. Each filled circle represents the average of 4–10 observations. The bars represent SEM.

between aldosterone excretion and U_{K^+}/U_{Na^+} as is shown in Figure 8a. The relationship is the same in infants aged 0–10 days as in those aged 12–21 days. In preterm infants aged 1–10 days there is no relationship between aldosterone excretion and U_{K^+}/U_{Na^+} (Fig. 8b). In preterm infants aged 10–20 days the urinary U_{K^+}/U_{Na^+} is higher than in newborn preterm infants, and there is a correlation between aldosterone excretion and U_{K^+}/U_{Na^+} quotient. These results suggest that newborn infants of a gestational age below 34 weeks do not respond adequately to aldosterone.

COMMENTS AND CONCLUSIONS

The results of the studies reported in this paper demonstrate that GFR as well as tubular function is less well developed before the 34th week of gestation than in infants born at term. It is also evident that renal functional development is not accelerated by birth to the same extent in preterm infants as in infants born at term.

The characteristics of renal function in newborn infants with a gestational age of less than 34 weeks have a number of clinical implications. Due to the very low GFR such infants are much more likely to develop azotemia than infants born at term. They are also much more susceptible to disturbances in fluid and electrolyte homeostasis than full-term infants. The kinetics of drugs which are excreted by the kidneys is different in preterm infants than in those born at term. The finding of a relatively low fractional reabsorption of beta-2-

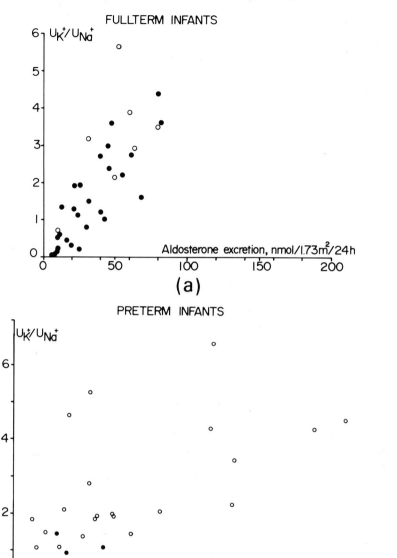

Fig. 8. Relationship between aldosterone excretion and urinary K^+/Na^+ ratio in full-term infants (a) and preterm infants of a gestational age ≤ 3 weeks (b). Filled circles represent infants aged 1–10 days and unfilled circles infants aged 12–21 days.

microglobulin in preterm infants suggests that infants of very low gestational age may have a considerable leakage of low molecular peptides like peptide hormone into the urine.

ACKNOWLEDGMENT

This study had been supported by a grant from the Swedish Medical Research Council (No. 3644).

REFERENCES

1. Aperia, A., Broberger, O., Thodenius, K., and Zetterström, R., Developmental study of the renal response to an oral salt load in preterm infants. *Acta Paediatr. Scand.* **63,** 517 (1974).
2. Aperia, A., Broberger, O., Herin, P., and Zetterström, R., Salt content in human breast milk during the three first weeks after delivery. *Acta Paediatr. Scand.* **68,** 441 (1979).
3. Aperia, A., Broberger, O., Herin, P., and Zetterström, R., Sodium excretion in relation to sodium intake and aldosterone excretion in newborn preterm and fullterm infants. *Acta Paediatr. Scand.* **68,** 813 (1979).
4. Aperia, A., and Broberger, U., Beta-2-microglobulin, an indicator of renal tubular maturation and dysfunction in the newborn. *Acta Paediatr. Scand.* **68,** 669 (1979).
5. Aperia, A., Broberger, O., Elinder, G., Herin, P., and Zetterström, R., Postnatal development of renal function in preterm and fullterm infants. *Acta Paediatr. Scand.,* in press.

15

Role of Neuraminidase-Producing Organisms in Necrotising Enterocolitis

G. DUC, M.D., P. JOLLER, Ph.D., and R. SEGER, M.D.

Necrotising enterocolitis (NEC) affects up to 7.5% of all premature infants admitted to intensive care units and still carries a mortality rate of 30–70%.[21] The cause of the disease remains unknown. Proposed etiologies have included infection, intestinal ischemia and hypoxia, and direct mucosal damage.[19]

The role of infection as a primary etiologic agent or secondary complication has been discussed extensively.[19] The signs and symptoms of the disease frequently mimic that of neonatal sepsis. Poor peripheral perfusion, temperature instability, lethargy, bradycardia, apnoea, gastric retention, and diarrhea are common both in sepsis and NEC.

In many institutions, NEC occurs as an epidemic disease. Cases have often been clustered in location and season[6, 9, 30, 49] with the association in some epidemics of a single organism in the stool.[11–13, 16, 40, 43, 45, 50] Institution of strict measures of control appears to limit the extent of epidemics.[6] Antibiotic treatment seems to be effective[34] and fresh breast milk protective, at least in the experimental NEC of the rats.[37] Among the possible bacteria implicated in the pathogenesis, anaerobes are the most discussed, particularly the Clostridia.

Epidemic, necrotising enterocolitis in newborn piglets[14] was associated with Clostridium perfringens, type C exotoxin[22] and in newborn lambs with Clostridium perfringens, Type B.[22] In piglets the epidemics can be stopped by administration of antitoxin or by vaccination of the sow followed by secondary production of colostrum antitoxin antibodies.[22]

"Darmbrand" is a form of NEC seen in adults in postwar Germany caused by Clostridium perfringens type F, enterotoxin.[52] A similar disease, the Pig bel, was observed in adult Highlanders of New Guinea after a pig feast and was

Department of Pediatrics and Obstetrics, University of Zurich

associated with Clostridium perfringens type C enterotoxin.[24, 25] The disease could be prevented by immunisation with clostridial toxoid.[25] In adults, clostridial gas gangrene of the gut can occur after intestinal ischemia and trauma.[42]

In newborn infants, Engel[8] suspected clostridial infection in three clustered cases of NEC, where postmortem specimens revealed histology similar to that in piglet enteritis, caused by Clostridium perfringens. Pedersen[36] reported six patients with NEC and histologic evidence of invasion of intestinal mucosa with gram-positive rods. Howard[15] implicated Clostridium butyricum as the cause of an outbreak of 12 cases of NEC. Kosloske, et al.[20] analysed the peritoneal fluid from cases of nonperforated NEC and found Clostridia in seven out of 17.

The mechanism of the penetration of Clostridia through intestinal walls remains unknown. Direct mucosal damage caused by hypertonic formula[5] or secondary to ischemia or hypoxia[41] has been postulated. But NEC has been observed in neonates receiving isotonic formulas (118 cases of 120 in Cleveland)[19] and also in infants without predisposing risk factors. Comparing infants with NEC with matched control groups, no differences were found in the incidence of respiratory distress syndrome, umbilical artery, or venous catheters,[51] low Apgar scores, hypothermia, hypotension, and exchange transfusion.[10]

Primary damage to the intestinal mucosa by Clostridia is very unlikely as Clostridia belongs to the normal neonatal intestinal flora, even in the breast fed. However, it is possible that neuraminidase-producing anaerobic bacteria play a major role in the genesis of the disease. Penetration of the intestinal walls by bacteria could be secondary to the effect of neuraminidase on the neuraminidic acid of the intestinal wall. It is the purpose of the present study to assess the role of anaerobes in patients with NEC using a serological test described by Thomsen as early as 1927,[46] which measures unmasking of Thomsen cryptantigen of the red cell by neuraminidase-producing anaerobes.[7, 28, 31]

METHODS

Study Population

Twenty-six newborns with NEC diagnosed on the grounds of abdominal distension and gastrointestinal bleeding were studied between October 1978 and August 1979. All but two patients had x-ray evidence of pneumatosis intestinalis. All affected babies were managed initially by nasogastric suction, intravenous fluids, and intravenous antibiotics (ampicillin, gentamycin, and chloramphenicol). Indication for operation was the appearance of pneumoperitoneum. A control group of 25 newborns without intestinal disease sampled at random in our neonatal intensive care unit was also studied.

Serological Methods

Thomsen-Antigen (T-Antigen) Test. This test described by Thomsen[46] is based on the effect of extracellular neuraminidase produced by some clostridia[7, 28] and bacterium fragilis[31] on the red cell membranes. Neuraminidase splits off N-acetylneuraminidic acid from the plasma membrane of red cells leading to exposure of a cryptantigen, the T-antigen.[46] Unmasking of this antigen can be demonstrated using anti-T-agglutinins from the common peanut (arachis hypogaea) at 20°C.[1, 46] Our arachis extract was standardized to contain an equivalent of 200 µg/ml of anti-Thomsen lectin purified by affinity chromatography on a D-galactose-Sepharose column[26] and available commercially (Serva, Heidelberg). The highest dilution of the arachis extract still agglutinating red cells is called the arachis titer. For indirect immunofluorescence tests a rabbit antipeanut globulin was raised which was coupled to rhodamine. The intensity of the fluorescence was graded from + to ++++.

Bacteriological Methods

Blood cultures were performed using separate aerobic (Brain Heart Infusion diphasic medium) and anaerobic media (Thiol Broth) under vacuum with added CO_2. Anaerobes were identified by biochemical analysis and by gas chromatography according to the VPI manual.

RESULTS

Nine of 26 newborns with NEC had positive arachis agglutination reactions (35%) and a positive arachis fluorescence (Table I). The immunofluorescence test showed 100% of unmasked cells. The intensity of the fluorescence correlated with the height of the agglutination titer. The blood cultures were positive only in one case, yielding colonies of C. perfringens. In another case C. butyricum was isolated from peritoneal fluid cultures obtained during surgery; gram stains revealed invasion of the resected intestinal wall by gram-positive rods. Culture filtrates of C. perfringens and C. butyricum exposed Thomsen-antigen on red cells of healthy adults after incubation for 1 hr at 37°C. In patients with NEC, but negative arachis agglutination reactions, blood cultures were positive in nine of 17 cases. They yielded mainly aerobic bacteria, namely Staph. albus or aureus (3/17), E. coli (3/17), Klebs. pneumoniae (2/17),

TABLE I

NEC: Thomsen-Ag-Positive Cases

Case	Arachis Aggl. Titre	Arachis Fluorescence	Blood Cultures	Clinical Complications	Final Outcome
1, 2, 3	<512	≤++	—	none	survived
4	512	+++	—	none	survived
5	512	++	—	perf.[a] (caecum)	survived
6	512	+++	—	perf. (colon ascend.)	survived
7	1024	++++	Cl. perfringens	perf. (ileum, transv.)	died
8	4096	++++	—[b]	perf. (colon transv.)	survived
9	4096	++++	—	none	survived

[a] perf. = perforation.
[b] Cl. butyricum in peritoneal fluid.

Butyrivibrio fibrisolvens (1/17). Culture filtrates of these organisms did not expose Thomsen-antigens on red cells of healthy adults.

In patients with positive arachis agglutination reactions the arachis titer seemed to correlate with the clinical course of the disease being highest when the patients were most ill. In two patients aggravation of the symptoms coincided with a further rise in the arachis titer, attaining maximal levels at the height of the disease.

The survival of Thomsen-antigen positive red cells was traced in four of the nine infants. Survival times ranged from 31 to 61 days with a mean of 43 days and are thus within the normal range for premature infants.

Four of the nine patients with positive arachis agglutination reactions were further studied to differentiate the original T-antigen unmasked by neuramin-idase from two other recently described Thomsen-antigens, called Tk- and Th-antigens.[2, 4] Two cases had classical T-activation alone, a third patient had classical T-activation and Tk-activation, and a fourth had Th-activation alone.

As antibodies against Thomsen-antigen may normally be present in adult blood, potential hazards from transfusion of whole blood were evaluated by crossmatching the red cells of the nine patients with positive arachis reactions with adult human sera, containing antibodies against Thomsen-antigens. The red cells of three patients with low arachis titers showed no reaction while the red cells of six patients with high titers were agglutinated by about 50% of adult sera.

DISCUSSION

As summarised in the introduction, there is increasing evidence that anaer-obic bacteria, especially Clostridia, play a central role in the pathogenesis of NEC.[6, 9, 11-13, 16, 30, 40, 43, 45, 49, 51] The identification of anaerobic bacterial invasion in NEC is possible using appropriate anaerobic cultures from peritoneal fluid[20] and from blood.[19] However, these are technically demanding and the results are only available after 48 hr at the earliest. In the present study, the usefulness of a rapid and reproducible serological test, the T-antigen determination, was evaluated in order to estimate the role of anaerobes in patients with NEC. The test first used by Van Loghem[47, 48] in clostridial infection was proposed in NEC by Fischer[9] and Poschmann.[39] Demonstration of unmasking T-antigen on the red cells of patients with NEC is indirect evidence of bacterial invasion through neuraminidase producing organisms. The usefulness of the test was confirmed in the present study: nine of 26 patients with NEC had positive T-antigen reactions. Neuraminidase responsible for the positive T-antigen reaction may have reached the blood stream in two ways: production by anaerobes in the gut lumen and absorption through a compromised intestinal mucosa or pro-duction of the enzyme by anaerobes which have already invaded the gut wall or the blood.

When evaluating the usefulness of the arachis reaction as a diagnostic aid in NEC, we checked its clinical, serological, and microbiological specificity. Ar-achis reactions were all negative in 25 newborns without intestinal disease, sampled at random in our intensive care unit. However, in addition to NEC, positive arachis reactions have also been reported in infants with intestinal necroses from other causes, namely strangulated inguinal hernia,[3] volvulus,[35] milk curd obstruction syndrome,[39] and Hirschsprung's disease.[35] The arachis reaction is positive only with the T-antigen exposed by neuraminidase with two exceptions. There are two other cryptantigens also showing a positive reaction with arachis lectin, namely Tk[35] and Th-antigens.[4] They are exposed by still unknown enzymes differing from neuraminidase, but again probably released by anaerobic bacteria. T, Tk, and Th are differentiated from each other by the use of additional plant agglutinins.[4]

Unmasking of T-antigens has also been described in infections caused by pneumococci, influenza, and parainfluenza viruses.[38] In our nine cases with unmasked Thomsen-antigens pneumococcal infections could be excluded by standard bacteriological methods. Although viral infections could not be completely ruled out,[23] convalescent sera showed no increase in complement fixation titer for the viruses mentioned. Aerobic bacteria frequently isolated in NEC, like Staph. aureus, E. coli, Klebs. pneumoniae, are not known to produce extracellular neuraminidase in significant amounts.[32]

The role of neuraminidase-producing microorganisms in the pathogenesis of NEC has not been established.[18, 27] It is possible that these microorganisms invade the peritoneal cavity and blood stream through an intestinal mucosa already compromised by unknown causes or that these organisms (probably Clostridia and bacteroides species) may be primary pathogens, causing NEC as observed in animals[14] and New Guineans,[25, 33] in which case neuraminidase may then have the task of facilitating the action of other more important toxins on the intestinal mucosa. Such a synergism has been described for cholera neuraminidase and enterotoxin.[44]

In spite of our ignorance of the exact pathogenetic role of neuraminidase-producing microorganisms in NEC, a positive arachis reaction test will influence management of newborns with necrotising enterocolitis in two ways. Therapy should include antibiotics active against anaerobes, such as chloramphenicol[19] or metronidazole.[17] The known polyagglutinability of arachis positive cells should be considered before blood transfusions.[47, 3, 29] Transfusion reactions can be avoided by giving either packed or washed red cells.

CONCLUSION

With a new diagnostic aid, we are able to show unmasking of T-antigen on the red cells in nine of 26 cases with clinical signs of NEC. The titers of these patients seem to correlate with the severity of the disease and the clinical course. In two of these cases, a neuraminidase-producing Clostridium perfringens and butyricum could be isolated. Unmasked Thomsen-antigen can lead to severe reactions upon transfusions of whole blood. These reactions are best avoided by the routine agglutination test with arachis lectin and by transfusion of packed or washed red cells to arachis positive cases.

Despite the high incidence of neuraminidase producing organisms in NEC,

further studies are necessary to answer the following questions:
Do neuraminidase producing organisms cause NEC?
Are they secondary to the disease or associated by chance?
Are neuraminidase producing organisms in NEC more pathogenic and could
they explain some pathophysiologic aspects of the disease?

REFERENCES

1. Bird, G. W. G., Anti-T in peanuts. *Vox Sang.* **9,** 748 (1964).
2. Bird, G. W. G., and Wingham, J., Tk: A new form of red cell polyagglutination. *Br. J. Haematol.* **23,** 759 (1972).
3. Bird, T., and Stephenson, J., Acute haemolytic anaemia associated with polyagglutinability of red cells. *J. Clin. Pathol.* **26,** 868 (1973).
4. Bird, G. W. G., Wingham, J., Beck, M. L., Pierce, S. R., Oates, G. D., and Pollock, A., Th, a new form of erythrocyte polyagglutination. *Lancet* **1,** 1215 (1978).
5. Book, L. S., Herbst, J. J., Atherton, S. O., and Jung, A. L., Necrotising enterocolitis in low-birth-weight infants fed on elemental formula. *J. Pediatr.* **87,** 602 (1975).
6. Book, L. S., Overall, J. C., Jr., Herbst, J. J., *et al.,* Clustering of necrotising enterocolitis. Interruption by infection-control measures. *N. Engl. J. Med.* **297,** 984 (1977).
7. Caselitz, F. H., and Stein, G.: Experimentelle Beiträge zum Problem der Haemagglutination nach Thomsen. *Z. Immunitätsforsch.* **110,** 165 (1953).
8. Engel, R., Report of the Sixty-Eighth Ross Conference on Pediatric Research, 1974, p. 66.
9. Fischer, K., Personal communication.
10. Frantz, I. D., L'Heureux, P., Engel, R. R., *et al.,* Necrotising enterocolitis. *J. Pediatr.* **86,** 259 (1975).
11. Hathaway, W., Report of the Sixty-Eighth Ross Conference on Pediatric Research, 1974, p. 86.
12. Henderson, A., Maclaurin, J., and Scott, J. M., Pseudomonas in a Glasgow baby unit. *Lancet* **2,** 316 (1969).
13. Hill, H. R., Hunt, C. E., and Matsen, J. M., Nosocomial colonization with klebsiella, type 26, in a neonatal intensive care unit associated with an outbreak of sepsis, meningitis, and necrotising enterocolitis. *J. Pediatr.* **85,** 415 (1974).
14. Hogh, P., Dr. Med. Vet. thesis, Royal Veterinary and Agricultural University, Copenhagen, 1974.
15. Howard, F. M., Flynn, D. M., Bradley, J. M., Noone, P., and Szawatkowski, M., Outbreak of necrotising enterocolitis caused by Clostridium butyricum. *Lancet* **2,** 1099 (1977).
16. Johnson, F. E., Crnic, D. M., Simmons, M. A., *et al.,* Association of fatal coxsackie B$_2$ viral infection and necrotising enterocolitis. *Arch. Dis. Child.* **52,** 802 (1977).
17. Khan, O., and Nixon, H. H.: The management of neonatal necrotising enterocolitis 1977: a preliminary report. *Z. Kinderchir.* **25,** 196 (1978).
18. Kindley, A. D., Roberts, P. J., and Tulloch, W. H., Neonatal necrotising enterocolitis. *Lancet* **1,** 649 (1977).
19. Kliegman, R. M., Neonatal necrotising enterocolitis, implications for an infectious disease. *Pediatr. Clin. North Am.* **26,** 327 (1979).
20. Kosloske, A. M., Ulrich, J. A., and Hoffman, H.: Fulminant necrotising enterocolitis associated with clostridia. *Lancet* **2,** 1014 (1978).
21. *Lancet* Editorial: Necrotising enterocolitis. *Lancet* **1,** 459 (1977).
22. *Lancet* Editorial: Clostridia as intestinal pathogens. *Lancet* **2,** 1113 (1977).
23. Lake, A. M., Lauer, B. A., and Clark, J. C., Enterovirus infections in neonates. *J. Pediatr.* **89,** 787 (1976).
24. Lawrence, G., and Walker, P. D., Pathogenesis of enteritis necroticans in Papua New Guinea. *Lancet* **1,** 125 (1976).
25. Lawrence, G., Shann, F., Freestone, D. S., and Walker, P. D., Prevention of necrotising enteritis in Papua New Guinea by active immunisation. *Lancet* **1,** 227 (1979).

26. Lotan, R., Skutelsky, E., Danon, D., and Sharon, N.: The purification, composition, and specificity of the anti-T lectin from peanut (Arachis hypogaea). *J. Biol. Chem.* **25,** 8518 (1975).

27. Mata, L. J., and Urrutia, J. J., Intestinal colonization of breast-fed children in rural area of low socioeconomic level. *Ann. N.Y. Acad. Sci.* **176,** 93 (1971).

28. McCrea, J. F., Modification of red-cell agglutinability by Cl. welchii toxins. *Austr. J. Exp. Biol. Med. Sci.* **25,** 127 (1947).

29. Mollison, P. L., *Blood Transfusion in Clinical Medicine.* Blackwell, Oxford, 1979, p. 408.

30. Moomjian, A. S., Packham, G. J., Fox, W. W., et al., Necrotising enterocolitis-endemic vs epidemic form. *Pediatr. Res.* **12,** 530 (1978).

31. Müller, H. E., and Werner, H., In vitro-Untersuchungen über das Vorkommen von Neuraminidase bei Bacteroides-Arten. *Microbiol.* **36,** 135 (1970).

32. Müller, H. E., Neuraminidase of bacteria and protozoa and their pathogenetic role. *Behring Inst. Mitt.* **55,** 34 (1974).

33. Murrell, T. G. C., Roth, L., Egerton, J., et al., Pig-bel: Enteritis necroticans. *Lancet* **1,** 217 (1966).

34. Nelson, J. D., Report of the Sixty-Eighth Ross Conference on Pediatric Research 1974, p. 80.

35. Obeid, D., Bird, G. W. G., and Wingham, J.: Prolonged erythrocyte T-polyagglutination in two children with bowel disorders. *J. Clin. Pathol.* **30,** 953 (1977).

36. Pedersen, P. V., Hansen, F. H., Halveg, A. B., and Christiansen, E. D., Necrotising enterocolitis of the newborn—is it gas gangrene of the bowel? *Lancet* **2,** 715 (1976).

37. Pitt, J., Barlow, B., and Heird, W. C., Protection against experimental necrotising enterocolitis by maternal milk. I. Role of milk leucocytes. *Pediatr. Res.* **11,** 906 (1977).

38. Poschmann, A., Fischer, K., Grundmann, A., and Vongjiirad, A.: Neuraminidase-induzierte Haemolyse. *Monatsschr. Kinderheilkd.* **124,** 15 (1976).

39. Poschmann, A.: Blutaustauschtransfusion bei einem Säugling mit Hämolyse infolge Gasbrandinfektion, in *Praktische Transfusionsmedizin,* Zöckler, H., Ed. Gräfelfing, 1977. p. 18–27.

40. Roback, S. A., Foker, J., Frantz, I. F., et al., Necrotising enterocolitis. *Arch. Surg.* **109,** 314 (1974).

41. Santulli, T. V., Schullinger, J. N., Heird, W. C., et al., Acute necrotising enterocolitis in infancy: A review of 64 cases. *Pediatrics* **55,** 376 (1975).

42. Sawyer, R. B., Sawyer, K. C., and List, J. E.: Infectious emphysema of the gastrointestinal tract in the adult. *Am. J. Surg.* **120,** 579 (1970).

43. Speer, M. E., Taber, L. H., Yow, M. D., et al., Fulminant neonatal sepsis and necrotising enterocolitis associated with a "nonenteropathogenic" strain of Escherichia coli. *J. Pediatr.* **89,** 91 (1976).

44. Stärk, J., Ronneberger, H. J., and Wiegandt, H.: Neuraminidase, a virulence factor in Vibrio cholerae infection? *Behring Inst. Mitt.* **55,** 145 (1974).

45. Stein, H., Beck, J., Solomon, A., et al., Gastroenteritis with necrotising enterocolitis in premature babies. *Br. Med. J.* **2,** 616 (1972).

46. Thomsen, O., Ein vermehrungsfähiges Agens als Veränderer des isoagglutinatorischen Verhaltens der roten Blutkörperchen, eine bisher unbekannte Quelle der Fehlbestimmungen. *Z. Immunol. Forschr.* **52,** 85 (1927).

47. Van Loghem, J. J., Van der Hart, M., and Land, M. E., Polyagglutinability of red cells as a cause of severe haemolytic transfusion reaction. *Vox Sang.* **5,** 125 (1955).

48. Van Loghem, J. J., Some comments on autoantibody induced red cell destruction. *Ann. N.Y. Acad. Sci.* **124,** 465 (1965).

49. Virnig, N. L., and Reynolds, J. W., Epidemiological aspects of neonatal necrotising enterocolitis. *Am. J. Dis. Child.* **128,** 186 (1974).

50. Waldhausen, J. A., Herendeen, T., and King, H., Necrotising colitis of the newborn. Common cause of perforation of the colon. *Pediatr. Surg.* **54,** 365 (1963).

51. Yu, V. Y. H., and Tudehope, D. I.: Neonatal necrotising enterocolitis. II. Perinatal risk factors. *Med. J. Austr.* **1,** 688 (1977).

52. Zeissler, J., and Rassfeld-Sternberg, L., Enteritis necroticans due to clostridium welchii type F. *Br. Med. J.* (Feb.), **12,** 267 (1949).

16

Fresh Human Milk in the Prevention of Necrotising Enterocolitis in Very Low Birth Weight Infants

E. D. BURNARD[1] and D. B. THOMAS[2]

INTRODUCTION

The experimental studies of Santulli, Heird, and their colleagues[1, 11] aroused speculation that fresh mother's milk might have protective value against necrotising enterocolitis (NEC) in the human infant. They discuss the various possibly protective mechanisms, and attach a good deal of importance to the cellular elements, which are likely to be damaged, though to a variable extent, by processing.[4, 10]

Although it has been stated that fresh milk is "widely" used in the feeding of premature infants,[5] we are unaware of any report of its value in the context of NEC.

Pooled and processed human milk has been in general use for many years for feeding preterm babies, more so in European than in North American countries, and there has been an impression, often voiced but nowhere documented, that NEC was less common in nurseries following the practice than in those using formula feeds. That has not been our experience.

Our hospital has for many years used pooled human milk, collected from donors in the wards, frozen for storage, and then brought briefly to the boil before feeding, for smaller preterm babies. For the purpose of this study we

The Women's Hospital (Crown Street), Sydney, Australia
[1] Senior Research Fellow, Children's Medical Research Foundation, Royal Alexandra Hospital for Children; Director of Neonatal Intensive Care, The Women's Hospital (Crown Street)
[2] Neonatologist, The Women's Hospital (Crown Street)

have directed attention to those at most risk, i.e., below 1500 g birthweight, and for them we had an incidence of NEC of 12% for the years 1973–1976. The reported incidence for babies admitted to intensive care nurseries ranges from 7% to over 20%, and any general comparison is hard to draw. However, there are two series in the weight range below 1500 g. In one,[17] with formula feeding, incidence was 10%. The second,[7] in which the incidence was 20%, is of additional interest in that it failed to show an advantage for refrigerated and stored, but otherwise fresh breast milk.

Not only was our incidence of NEC with pooled and processed breast milk as the feed no better than that of nurseries using other feeding methods, but the case survival rate also was poor, below 25% for the years 1974–1976. Thus it was decided to see whether benefit might result from feeding fresh, unprocessed human milk.

METHODS AND MATERIALS

The study was confined to babies of 600–1500 g birth weight. Since oral feeding and colonisation of the bowel are preconditions for NEC,[2] babies who died for other reasons without receiving a feed were excluded from the totals. Feeding was started within 6 hr of birth to give quantities of 60, 90, and 120 ml/kg/day for the first 3 days, rising to 150 and later 180, by a fine orogastric or in larger babies by nasogastric tube. Volumes were small and given at frequent intervals. The regime was flexible and varied according to incidental complications, e.g., feeding was reduced or suspended during periods when nasal continuous positive pressure was required. Fluid requirements were supplemented parenterally as circumstances dictated. Electrolytes were monitored regularly and supplemented as required.

As far as possible the mother's own milk was fed to her baby but fresh donor milk had also to be used. Hand expression[8] was the preferred method of collection, but some mothers found a breast pump easier to work with especially when the supply was large. On leaving hospital she continued expressing into a sterile plastic container, stored the sample in the domestic refrigerator, and brought or sent it in daily (most mothers were spending an hour or two beside their infant each day). Bacteriological checks were made at weekly or more frequent intervals depending on the flora grown. Colony counts were not done.

For an initial period of 6 months while the system was being established, babies were preferentially fed fresh milk, but some received pooled, processed milk which as mentioned above has been the standard practice. We then began an alternate case study (a blind one was not feasible in circumstances where nursing staff was involved in collection and distribution).

Diagnosis of NEC. We were dissatisfied with the survival record in the previous years, and inclined to attribute the poor result to delay in waiting for intramural gas in the x-ray before instituting fully energetic treatment. Intramural gas can be difficult to identify. Although it was a feature of all patients in the interesting report of Richmond and Mikity,[14] it had not been recognised in some of our cases which came later to autopsy. We therefore now accepted a distended loop or loops of the bowel in the abdominal x-ray which remained fixed for 24 hr or longer as radiographic evidence of affected bowel (Figs. 1, 2, and 3, K. M. de Silva, personal communication).

RESULTS

During the initial period of establishing the system (in early 1977) 18 babies received fresh milk without incident. Seven were fed the processed product, of whom two developed NEC. The illness was treated early, on x-ray evidence as described as well as the usual clinical features, and they survived.

Results of the alternate case study are shown in Table I. They were analysed

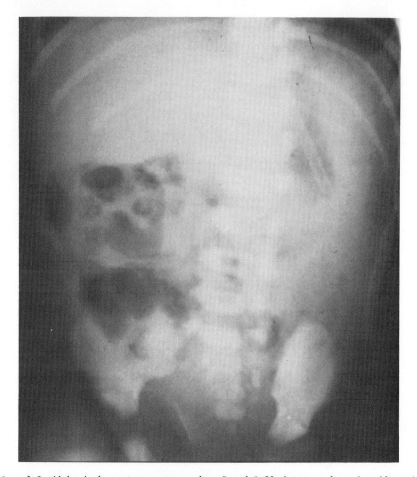

Figs. 1 and 2. Abdominal roentgenogram on days 5 and 6. No intramural gas is evident. A distended loop of gut with a reverse C configuration is consistently present in right upper quadrant. (By courtesy of Dr. M. de Silva.)

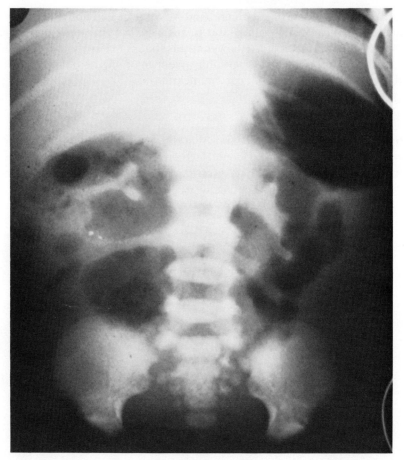

Fig. 2

after 18 months at a point when the nurses who, as has already been remarked, inevitably had prior knowledge were convinced of the advantage of fresh milk. They were disturbed not only because of what they felt was an unnecessary death toll but also because they observed a lower incidence of lesser gastrointestinal problems with fresh milk which fell outside any specific diagnostic category and are difficult to document precisely.

The value for probability in the alternate case study (Table I) fell just short of significance.

However, when the previous 6 months' experience was added (Table II), a significant difference was apparent.

There were no important differences between the groups in Table II in factors which are believed to predispose to bowel ischemia. In birth history (Table III) they were well matched for gestational age and birth weight; there was a slight predominance of females in those fed pooled milk. Serious asphyxia at birth, as indicated by the need for active intervention, was equally spread.

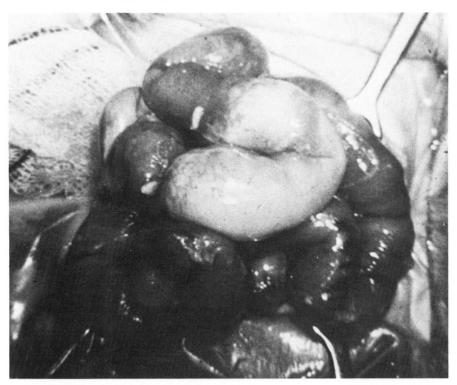

Fig. 3. Operation photograph to show corresponding ischaemic area of bowel; recovery followed its resection. (By courtesy of Dr. M. de Silva.)

TABLE I

Alternate Case Study[a]

	Fresh	Pooled
n	27	26
NEC	1 (lived)	5 (3 deaths)

[a] $P = 0.077$ (Fisher's exact test).

TABLE II

All Patients[a]

	Fresh	Pooled
n	45	33
NEC	1	7

[a] $P = 0.008$ (Fisher's exact test).

The only statistically significant difference was in the antenatal administration of steroid to mothers; interpretation is dubious but in principle it might be expected to have led to less anoxic insult in the babies after birth, and to have favoured the pooled-fed group in this respect.

In the neonatal history (Table IV) the only significant difference was in the

TABLE III

Birth Experience, All Cases

	Fresh	Pooled
n	45	33
Male	23	12
Female	22	21
Gestation (weeks)	29.4	29.2
Birth weight (g)	1145	1250
Active resuscitation	16	11
Maternal steroid	21	23[a]

[a] $P = 0.024$; other differences not significant (Fisher's exact test).

TABLE IV

Neonatal Experience, All Cases

	Fresh	Pooled
n	45	33
Arterial catheter	33	17[a]
Exchange T	0	1
Patent ductus	12	5
Theophylline/nasal CP	21	11
Hyaline membrane disease	6	5
Small for dates	5	5
Proved infection	7	4
Respirator	10	3

[a] $P = 0.027$, other differences not significant (Fisher's exact test).

TABLE V

Bacteriology of Expressed Breast Milk

	Percent
S. aureus	10
S. albus	16
S. Faecalis	4
E. Coli	10
Klebsiella	6
Proteus	6
Mixed growth	36
No growth	16

greater frequency of arterial catheters in the fresh-fed babies. Exchange transfusion, a recognised predisposing cause for NEC, was performed only once. Patent ductus arteriosus, which has also been proposed as predisposing to bowel ischemia, was rather more common in the fresh-fed group; in two of the babies fed processed milk it was contemporaneous with the development of NEC. Apnea serious enough to indicate treatment with theophylline, a small continuous pressure by nasal prongs, or both, was about equally distributed in the two groups. Hyaline membrane disease, as judged by the x-ray and results of the shake test on gastric aspirate, had a surprisingly low incidence in these very immature babies. This was probably attributable in part to the antepartum administration of steroids and also to the fact that many were the subjects of intrauterine stress from prolonged rupture of membranes, chronic antepartum haemorrhage, and in a few cases severe toxemia usually with intrauterine growth retardation. There were some small-for-dates babies, rather more in the pooled-fed group. A higher proportion of fresh-fed infants required mechanical respiratory support, for hyaline membrane disease or apnea. Infection was a difficult element to assess. Potential pathogens were cultured from nearly all the babies. At the same time, most of them received antibiotics in the early days, with repeat courses in some, and the line between colonisation and significant infection was hard to draw.

Summarising the data in Tables III and IV, the odds would appear to have been somewhat stacked against the fresh-fed babies, though a more sophisticated analysis would be needed to show that the two apparently significant differences had the same weight when measured against the other factors predisposing to NEC.

The degree of bacterial contamination in our fresh milk specimens is indicated in Table V. As mentioned under "Methods," we did not undertake colony counts, and so cannot compare the material against the standards whereby pasteurisation might be thought desirable.[4, 16]

The trial was terminated without an entirely satisfactory statistical result, under some duress for reasons already indicated. However, we can report that, in the 6 months since, none of the 30 babies fed fresh milk have developed the clinical signs of NEC.

DISCUSSION

Although there is some doubt as to the nutritional suitability of human milk for the immature infant,[3] there is very little about its protective value against infection in babies of any gestational age.[6, 12, 15] The maternally transmitted immune globulins are conceded to have the principal role in the general case. However, in the special context of NEC in the preterm infant, it is possible that the leucocytes, which are vulnerable to processing, are primarily important.[1, 11]

The trial was set up because we were dissatisfied with the results of a traditional belief that human milk after processing was "best" for preterm babies. It is open to criticism on several grounds. It was not blind. A statistical manipulation (Table II) may offend the purist. Also bacteriological control was less than optimal, but it is interesting that in a well-designed study of milk banking procedures two-thirds of the human specimens supplied were judged fit to be fed without processing.[16]

The results support the idea that fresh human milk has value in protecting preterm babies against NEC without great risk of other complications, though a warning with respect to group B streptococcal contamination, which we did not encounter (Table V), has been sounded.[9] It is not proposed as a panacea, for we did have one case among babies who received only fresh milk (Table I) and others are reported.[13]

REFERENCES

1. Barlow, B., Santulli, T. V., and Heird, W. C., An experimental study of acute necrotising enterocolitis—the importance of fresh breast milk. *J. Pediatr. Surg.* **9,** 587–596 (1974).
2. Brown, E. G., and Sweet, A. Y., Preventing necrotising enterocolitis in neonates. *J.A.M.A.* **240,** 2452–2454 (1978).
3. Fomon, S. I., Milk of the premature infant's mother: interpretation of data. *J. Pediatr.* **93,** 164 (1978).
4. Gibbs, J. H., Fisher, C., Bhattacharya, S., Goddard, P., and Baum, J. D., Drip breast milk: its composition, collection and pasteurization. *Early Hum. Develop.* **1,** 227–245 (1977).
5. Human milk in premature infant feeding: summary of a workshop, *Pediatrics* **57,** 741–743 (1976).
6. Jelliffe, E. F. P., Infant feeding practices: associated iatrogenic and commerciogenic diseases. *Pediatr. Clin. North Am.* **24,** 49–61 (1977).
7. Kliegman, R., Pittard, W., and Fanaroff, A., Necrotising enterocolitis in neonates fed breast milk. (Abstract), *Pediatr. Res.* **13,** 402 (1979).
8. Liehaber, M., Lewiston, N. J., Asquith, M. J., and Sunshine, P., Comparison of bacterial contamination with two methods of human milk collection. *J. Pediatr.* **92,** 236–237 (1978).
9. Lucas, A., and Roberts, C. D., Group B. streptococci in pooled human milk. *Br. Med. J.* **2,** 919–920 (1978) (corresp.).
10. Paxson, C. L., and Cress, C. C., Survival of human milk leucocytes. *J. Pediatr.* **94,** 61–63 (1979).
11. Pitt, J., Barlow, B., and Heird, W. C., Protection against experimental necrotising enterocolitis by maternal milk. I. Role of milk leucocytes. *Pediatr. Res.* **11,** 906–909 (1977).
12. Pittard, W. B., Breast milk immunology. *Am. J. Dis. Child.* **133,** 83–87 (1979).
13. Reisner, S. H., and Garty, B., Necrotising enterocolitis despite breast feeding. *Lancet* **2,** 507 (1977) (corresp.).
14. Richmond, J. A., and Mikity, V., Benign form of necrotising enterocolitis. *Am. J. Roentgenol. Radium Ther. Nucl. Med.* **123,** 301–306 (1975).
15. Welsh, J. K., and May, J. T., Anti-infective properties of breast milk. *J. Pediatr.* **94,** 1–9 (1979).
16. Williamson, S., Hewitt, J. H., Finucane, E., and Gamsu, H. R., Organisation of bank of raw and pasteurised human milk for neonatal intensive care. *Br. Med. J.* **1,** 393–395 (1978).
17. Yu, V. Y. H., Tudehope, D. I., and Gill, G. J., Necrotising enterocolitis: I. Clinical aspects. *Med. J. Austr.* **1,** 685–688 (1977).

17

The Significance of Fibrin Degradation Products in Normal Newborns

S. MARAGHI, M.D., A. SHAMS EL-DIN,[1] Ph.D.,[2] and
Y. ABU ZENT, D. Ch.[3]

Fibrinogen/fibrin degradation products (FDPs) may appear in the blood when plasmin digests fibrinogen and fibrin in the process of fibrinolysis; under physiological conditions intravascular thrombosis and fibrinolysis go on in strict harmony so that neither thrombosis nor free plasmin could normally be detected. The presence of FDPs in normal sera (less than 4/µg/ml serum) seems to verify this mechanism and confirms the theory of ongoing intravascular coagulation in the human body[1]; the microthrombi are, however, continuously removed by the fibrinolytic system: pathological levels of FDPs would be detected whenever the fibrinolytic system is overactive and plasmin is generated in excess. FDPs are known to have a deleterious effect on hemostasis.[2] Reports on serum FDPs in normal neonates are few and controversial.[3-7] Since the presence of FDPs in serum has been used as an indication of intravascular coagulation, this work was carried out to clarify the situation in normal newborns.

MATERIALS AND METHODS

The study was carried out on a series of 20 full-term nonasphyxiated infants born by vaginal delivery. Thirteen cases were males and seven were females; their gestational age varied from 38 to 41 weeks. Their birth weight ranged between 2800 and 4000 g. Cord blood samples were tested for the presence of

Departments of Pediatrics and Clinical Pathology, Cairo University, Cairo
[1] Professor of Pediatrics, Cairo University, Cairo
[2] Professor of Clinical Pathology, Cairo University, Cairo
[3] Research Fellow, Pediatric Children's Hospital, Cairo

serum FDPs and plasma fibrinogen level. Fibrinogen estimation was done by the determination of clotting time, referring to a special table for the estimation of fibrinogen concentration in mg/100 ml.* FDPs were demonstrated using the staphylococcal reagent. A macroscopically visible clumping of staphylococci occurs whenever this reagent is added to serum containing fibrin degradation products.[8]

RESULTS

The results of the present study are illustrated in Tables I and II.

Table I shows the results of fibrinogen and FDPs in all cases studied. The mean plasma fibrinogen level was 157 mg/100 ml (range 80–259). Serum FDPs were measurable in 11 infants (55%). The titres were low as FDPs were only detected in undiluted serum.

Table II illustrates the plasma fibrinogen levels in group I (11 cases with positive serum) and in group II (nine newborns with undetectable FDPs). The mean plasma fibrinogen was significantly lower (128.09 mg/100 ml) in group I compared to its corresponding level in group II (192.67 mg/100 ml), indicating a negative correlation between fibrinogen and its degradation products.

DISCUSSION

FDPs were demonstrated in 55% of the studied newborns. Reports on serum FDPs in normal neonates are controversial. Hathway claimed that serum of normal newborns does not contain FDPs. On the other hand Bonifaci, et al.[7] and Steihm, et al.[5] have found positive FDPs in 40% and 65% respectively of their series of normal newborns. Chessells,[3] who reported an incidence of 5% among her cases, criticized the findings by Stiehm, et al. and attributed their high incidence of FDPs to technical errors. It was repeatedly stressed that the technique markedly affects the results of FDP tests[7]; as mentioned, normal sera are reported to demonstrate minute amounts of FDPs not exceeding 4 μg/ml of serum.[1] As the minimal threshold for FDP detection of the reagent used in this work is 12 mg/ml of serum, it is thus evident that 55% of normal neonates of the series exhibit pathological levels for FDPs at birth.

The origin of serum FDPs is debatable. Our samples were drawn from cord blood, and it is likely that the FDPs are of placental origin. The fibrinolytic system in cord blood is overactive. This known lytic activity is a reflection of increased plasminogen activators. It results in a mild subclinical defibrination, which may partly account for the low fibrinogen observed.

In fact the mean plasma fibrinogen level (157 mg%) is below the figures previously reported in the neonatal period.[8] Other causes of hypofibrinogenemia are defective production by the neonatal liver comparable to hypothrombinemia in the newborn, as well as the presence of an abnormal molecule of fibrinogen, the so-called "fetal fibrinogen." This type of fibrinogen is not

---

* Behrinwerke test Kit (Modification of the Clauss Method, 1968)

TABLE I

Fibrinogen and Fibrinogen Degradation Products (FDP) in Cord Blood of Normal Newborns

Case Number	Fibrinogen (mg/100 ml)	Fibrinogen Degradation Products
1	140	+
2	148	+
3	129	+
4	159	+
5	138	+
6	138	+
7	129	+
8	206	−
9	189	−
10	172	−
11	229	−
12	122	+
13	179	−
14	189	−
15	80	+
16	159	−
17	259	−
18	80	+
19	138	+
20	159	−
Range	80–259	(+vef.d.p.s) = 11
Mean	157.15	
SD	43.77	55%
SE	9.79	

TABLE II

Plasma Fibrinogen Levels in Group I (Positive FDP) and Group II (Negative FDP)

Number	Fibrinogen (mg/100 ml)	
	Group I	Group II
1	148	206
2	148	189
3	129	172
4	159	229
5	138	159
6	138	159
7	129	159
8	122	172
9	80	189
10	80	
11	138	
Total number	11	9
Percentage	55%	45%
Mean	128.09	192.67
SD	25.90	33.63
SE	7.81	11.2
T	4.86	
P	0.001	

clottable or only slowly clottable by thrombin. According to Witt and Muller,[10] fetal fibrinogen may predominate in the neonatal period, a situation which is in a way comparable to fetal hemoglobin.

In the present work the fibrinogen was estimated by biological means, e.g., clotting of fibrinogen by thrombin. Fetal fibrinogen is thus expected to give low values. This further contributes to the hypofibrinogenemia observed. The wide range of variation and high standard deviation of plasma fibrinogen shown in the present as well as other studies using the same technique, may be explained by the different distribution and the variable amounts of fetal fibrinogen in individual cases.

Secondary fibrinolytic activity with increased FDPs may occur due to disseminated intravascular coagulopathy (DIC). However, there was no clinical evidence of disturbed hemostasis. The mere presence of serum FDPs in the perinatal period is not in itself an indication of a state of disseminated intravascular coagulation. Apart from low plasma fibrinogen, this disorder must be based on additional evidence; e.g., alterations in platelet count as well as depletion of the consumable coagulation factors.

Since FDPs are slowly cleared from the circulation ($T_{1/2}$ = 24–72 hr), serial estimation of serum FDPs may be of better prognostic or diagnostic value in the course of DIC.

SUMMARY

Twenty normal newborns were investigated for serum FDPs and plasma fibrinogen in cord blood. Eleven cases (55%) demonstrated FDPs in their sera. They were associated with highly significant low fibrinogen level (mean 128.09 mg/100 ml); nine cases had absent FDPs, and their mean fibrinogen was 192.67 mg/100 ml. A negative correlation between fibrinogen and its degradation products was present. Hypofibrinogenemia may be attributed to low production by neonatal liver, mild defibrination in cord blood as well as the presence of "fetal fibrinogen."

There was no clinical evidence of disturbed hemostasis. The mere presence of serum FDPs in the perinatal period is not in itself an indication of a state of disseminated intravascular coagulation (DIC); apart from low plasma fibrinogen, this disorder must be based on additional evidence, e.g., alterations in platelet count, as well as depletion of the consumable coagulation factors.

REFERENCES

1. Das, P. C., Allan, A. G. E., Woodfield, D. G., and Cash, J. D., Fibrin degradation products in sera of normal subjects. *Br. Med. J.* **4**, 718 (1967).
2. Hirsh, J., Fletcher, A. P., and Sherry, S., Effect of fibrin and fibrinogen proteolysis products. *Am. J. Physiol.* **209**, 415 (1965).
3. Chessells, J. M., The significance of fibrin degradation products in the blood of normal infants. *Biol. Neonate* **17**, 219 (1971).
4. Hathway, W. E., Fibrin split products in serum of newborn, possible technical errors. *Pediatrics* **45**, 154 (1970).

5. Stiehm, E. R., and Clatanoff, D. V., Split products of fibrin in the serum of newborns. *Pediatrics* **43,** 770 (1969).

6. Uttley, W. S., Fibrin/fibrinogen degradation products in sera of normal infants and children. *Arch. Dis. Child.* **44,** 761 (1968).

7. Bonifaci, E., Demonstration of split products of fibrinogen in the blood of normal newborns. *Biol. Neonate* **12,** 29 (1968).

8. Hawiger, J. *et al.*, Measurement of fibrinogen and fibrin degradation products in serum by staphylococcal clumping test. *J. Lab. Clin. Med.* **75,** 93–108 (1970).

9. Kline, B. S., Microscopic observation of the development of the placenta. *Am. J. Obst. Gynecol.* **61,** 1065 (1951).

10. Witt, I., and Muller, H., Evidence for the existence of fetal fibrinogen. *Thromb. Diath. Haemorrh.* **22,** 101 (1969).

18

Neonatal Group B Streptococcal Infection: Study of Serum Type Specific Antibody Levels

N. W. SVENNINGSEN,[1] K. K. CHRISTENSEN,[2] and P. CHRISTENSEN[3]

In recent years there has been a growing interest in the epidemiology and early detection of group B streptococci (GBS) infections in newborn infants.[2, 5, 11, 13, 17, 18] In our own neonatal intensive care unit we have also observed an increase in the incidence of early-onset GBS septicemia (Fig. 1).

The mortality rate in early onset GBS septicemia is high, although awareness and early diagnosis may influence the final outcome. However it has been reported that even in cases diagnosed early within a few hours after birth and treated with appropriate antibiotics the mortality will still be high.[4, 13] We have therefore focused our efforts for prevention and treatment not only on the newborn infant but increasingly on the pregnant woman.

The aim of our investigation was to study the following:

1. The rate of GBS-carriers in parturient women in a Swedish population.
2. The rate of GBS colonisation of the newborn infants in this population.
3. Perinatal data before and during delivery in GBS-carrier and non-carrier mothers.
4. The level of type-specific GBS-antibodies in the GBS-carrier mothers.

MATERIAL AND METHODS

A prospective study comprising 799 parturient women and their infants was carried out from November 1978 through February 1979. The design of the

[1] University Hospital, Lund, Sweden Neonatal Unit, Department of paediatrics
[2] Obstetrics and Gynecology
[3] Medical Microbiology

165

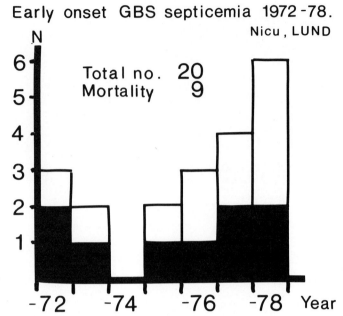

Fig. 1. Number of infants with early-onset GBS septicemia and the mortality rate in the Neonatal Intensive Care Unit from 1972 to 1978.

study is presented in Figure 2. Specimens for GBS culture were obtained from the urethra and cervix of each patient before or during labour. In newborn infants cultures were taken from the external auditory canal, throat, and umbilicus immediately after delivery and repeated on day 4 of life. Maternal type-specific GBS antibodies were measured before or at delivery.

The methodology for isolation, identification, and typing of GBS (serotypes Ia, Ib, Ic, II, and III) as well as the methods for type-specific GBS antibody quantitation have been described in detail elsewhere.[1, 7, 8, 9]

In addition to the prospective study we have also examined seven newborn infants with neonatal GBS infection and their mothers for GBS type and levels of type-specific GBS antibodies.[9]

The chi-square test was used for statistical evaluation (n.s. = not significant, i.e., $P > 0.05$).

RESULTS

Rate of GBS Colonisation

The number of GBS carriers and noncarriers in the parturient women in this population is presented in Table I. The maternal GBS-carrier rate was 16% and the GBS-colonisation rate among newborn infants at delivery was 10% in this material.

The GBS serotypes found in mothers and newborn infants are shown in

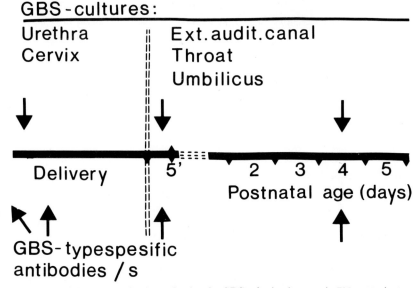

Fig. 2. Design of the prospective investigation for GBS colonisation rate in 799 parturient women and their infants.

TABLE I

Incidence of Maternal GBS Carriers (Urethra/Cervix) and of Newborn Infants Colonised with GBS in the Prospective Study from November 1978 through February 1979

Total number examined	799
GBS carrier parturient women	128 (16%)
Noncarrier parturient women	671
Newborn infants colonised with GBS at delivery	82 (10%)

TABLE II

Distribution of GBS Serotypes in Mothers and Newborn Infants Colonised at Delivery

Number	Mothers (128)	Infants (82)
GBS serotype		
Ia	23%	24%
Ib	7%	13%
Ic	1%	0%
II	29%	34%
III	40%	29%

Table II. These were mainly types Ia, Ib, II, and III, and the distribution was similar in mothers and newborn infants.

Certain changes in the rate of GBS colonisation in the newborn infants occurred during the first postnatal days (Table III). In infants of GBS-carrier mothers 64 of 128 (50%) were colonised at delivery, and 35 of these were colonised still at 4 days of age (27%). In infants of noncarrier mothers, only 18 of 671 (2.7%) were colonised at birth, and 11 of these remained colonised on

TABLE III

Changes in GBS Colonisation Panorama in Newborn Infants from Delivery to Day 4 of Life

Mothers	Number	Newborn Infants Colonised	
		At Delivery	On Day 4
Total	799	82	90
GBS carriers	128 ⟶ 64 ⟶ 35		46
		+11	
Noncarriers	671 ⟶ 18 ⟶ 11		44
		+33	

day 4 of life (1.6%). However, in both groups a certain number of initially non-GBS-colonised newly born infants became colonised between the day of birth and day 4, e.g., 11 infants of GBS-carrier mothers and 33 of noncarrier mothers. The 11 infants of GBS carriers on day 4 harboured the same GBS serotype as the one found in their respective mothers before or at delivery. The relative distribution of the different GBS subgroups was the same in the infants on day 4 as that found in mothers and infants colonised at birth (see Table II).

Site of GBS-Colonisation

In maternal GBS carriers 85 of 128 were both cervical and urethral GBS carriers. Amongst their infants 59% were colonised at birth in comparison to 27% of the infants whose mothers were colonised with GBS in the urethra only.

The sites of GBS colonisation in the infants at birth and on day 4 are shown in Table IV. At delivery there was a widespread colonisation rate in both the external auditory canal, throat, and umbilicus. On day 4 of life the main sites were throat and/or umbilicus. There was no predilection site for a particular GBS subgroup in the present investigation.

Perinatal Data of GBS Carriers and Noncarriers

Relevant perinatal data observed in the 128 GBS-carrier and the 671 noncarrier parturient women is presented in Table V. Neither in the incidence of previous abortions, breech presentation, duration of labour, or timing of rupture of the fetal membranes nor in the obstetrical management were any differences found between the two groups. It must be observed that the obstetrician in charge did not know whether the mother was a GBS carrier or not as this was designed as a prospective investigation.[10]

In 9% of GBS carriers the delivery took place after the 42nd week of gestation compared to only 3% in the noncarrier group ($P < 0.01$).

During the first stage of labour reliable fetal heart rate recordings were obtained with fetal scalp electrodes in 89% in both groups. These recordings were assessed later without knowledge of other obstetrical data including whether the mother was a GBS carrier or not. There was a statistically greater incidence of abnormalities in GBS carriers than in noncarriers. Similar results were found in the analyses of fetal scalp pH, with a significantly higher incidence of fetal acidemia in infants of GBS-carrier parturients ($P < 0.01$).

TABLE IV

Site of Neonatal GBS Colonisation at Birth and on Day 4 of Life

	At Birth	On Day 4
Number of colonised infants	82	90
External auditory canal	70	12
Throat	57	45
Umbilicus	67	60

TABLE V

Perinatal Data: Maternal GBS Carriers and Noncarriers

	GBS Carriers	Noncarriers	P value
Number	128	671	
Abortions			
legal	10%	12%	n.s.
spontaneous	14%	13%	n.s.
Breech presentation	3%	3%	n.s.
Duration of labour			
<12 hr	87%	91%	n.s.
12–24 hr	13%	8%	n.s.
>24 hr	0%	0.4%	n.s.
Rupture of membranes			
<12 hr	92%	96%	n.s.
12–18 hr	7%	3%	n.s.
>18 hr	1%	1%	n.s.
Obstetrical procedures:			
Amniotomy	61%	59%	n.s.
Fetal scalp electrode	92%	92%	n.s.
Intrauterine catheter	25%	26%	n.s.
Perineotomy	29%	23%	n.s.
Forceps/Vacuum extractor	7%	7%	n.s.
Cesarean section:			
acute	5%	5%	n.s.
elective	2%	2%	n.s.
Gestational age at delivery:			
28–36 weeks	3%	5%	n.s.
37–42 weeks	88%	92%	n.s.
>42 week	9%	3%	<0.01
Cardiotachographic registration	89% (114)	89% (596)	n.s.
a. Abnormal fetal heart rate baseline	15%	11%	n.s.
b. Abnormal decelerations	7%	5%	n.s.
a + b	5%	1%	<0.01
Fetal scalp blood pH	11% (14)	8% (53)	n.s.
pH < 7.20	5%	1%	<0.01

Thus there was a higher incidence of postmaturity and intrauterine fetal distress in infants of GBS-carrier mothers in this study.

Type-Specific GBS Antibody Levels

In addition to the prospective investigation of the GBS colonisation rate and the perinatal data of GBS-carrier parturients, we have also studied the occur-

TABLE VI

Clinical Data in Infants with Proved Neonatal Early-Onset and Late-Onset GBS Infection

Case	Delivery	Gest. Age (weeks)	GBS Infection	Onset	GBS Type
1. Boy	VD	36	Septicemia	Day 1	Ia
2. Boy	VD	42	Septicemia	Day 1	Ib
3. Girl	CS	34	Septicemia	Day 1	Ib
4. Boy	VD	30	Septicemia	Day 2	III
5. Boy	VD	40	Meningitis	Day 21	III
6. Girl	CS	34	Meningitis	Day 28	Ib
7. Girl	VD	40	Meningitis	Day 42	III

VD = Vaginal delivery, CS = Cesarean section.

rence of type-specific GBS antibody levels in seven cases of verified GBS infection (Table VI). There were four cases of early-onset GBS septicemia (cases no. 1–4) and three cases of late-onset GBS meningitis (cases no. 5–7) occurring 21, 28, and 42 days after delivery. There were four boys and three girls; three full-term and four preterm infants with five delivered vaginally and two delivered by Cesarean section. The GBS types found were Ib and III in three cases each and Ia in one infant with early-onset septicemia.

The maternal sera from each mother of cases 1–7 have been tested against the type of GBS carried by her and causing the GBS infection in her newborn infant. The levels of type-specific antibodies in these mothers are compared in Figure 3 to the type-specific antibody levels measured in maternal GBS carriers with infants colonised at birth but without symptoms or signs of early-onset or late-onset GBS disease. All but one (case no. 4) had antibody levels well below −2 SD and also below the range of type-specific GBS antibody levels found in mothers with colonised but noninfected newborn infants.

The exceptional finding in case no. 4 may be explained by the special clinical circumstances in this case. This boy, born in the 30th week of gestation with a birth weight of 1200 g and at delivery colonised with GBS type III in the umbilicus and throat, had severe Rh-immunisation. Repeated exchange transfusions were required, and because of severe hyaline membrane disease he had to be intubated and treated with a ventilator almost from birth. Through these procedures he probably underwent overwhelming invasion with GBS colonising the throat and umbilicus. This would explain his GBS septicemia in spite of the high maternal GBS antibody level as shown in Figure 3.

DISCUSSION

It is well known that GBS infection in newborn infants may occur either as an early-onset disease within the first 12–48 hr with signs of septicemic shock proceeding rapidly to death or as a late-onset meningitis with low mortality but increased risk of neurological sequelae.[4, 13, 18] Culture of pharyngeal aspirates at birth has been proposed as a screening measure for neonatal GBS septicemia.[17] A history of artificial premature or prolonged rupture of fetal membranes in preterm infants with low absolute neutrophil count, localized

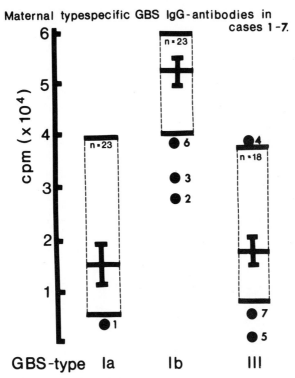

Fig. 3. Maternal type-specific antibody levels in seven cases with proven neonatal GBS infection in relation to levels (mean, standard deviation, and range) in GBS-carrier parturient women with colonised but noninfected infants. The antibody level expressed as the radioactive protein A in counts per minute (cpm) bound to bacteria after coating with serum.

pulmonary infiltrates on chest x-ray, and rapid progression of respiratory distress symptoms have been considered to be specific risk factors.[18] Yet it is apparent that the early-onset septicemia may develop without early warning signs and may lead rapidly to death in spite of appropriate administration of antibiotics in both preterm and full-term infants.[4, 5, 11, 12, 13]

The aim of our investigations has therefore been to study first the GBS-colonisation rate in our population. Secondly, we wanted to find out whether there was any correlation between maternal GBS antibody level and the colonisation rate and/or GBS infection in the newborn infant both with regard to early-onset and late-onset GBS disease. Finally we wanted to study the occurrence of any perinatal warning signs.

In 1973 Baker and Barrett[2] reported a GBS-colonisation rate in pregnant women of 25% and a colonisation rate of 26% in the newborn infants in Houston, Texas. The incidence of proven neonatal GBS infection was about 1–3 per 1000 live-born infants as also reported by others.[2, 12, 17] In the present investigation the colonisation rate in this Swedish population was 16% in parturient women and 10% of newborn infants at birth.

Klesius, et al.[14] have pointed out that at least three components are involved in the immune response to GBS: plasma factors, cellular phagocytosis, and type-specific antibodies.

Plasma factors, e.g., nonspecific opsonins for GBS serotypes Ib, Ic, II, and III, have been found in 95% of human sera but in only 10% for GBS type Ia. This may explain some cases of neonatal disease from GBS type Ia.[15]

It has also been shown that opsonisation needs type-specific antibodies and complement in addition to polymorphonuclear leucocyte ability to phagocytize GBS.[16]

From these observations it would seem a plausible hypothesis that newborn infants of women who are GBS carriers but deficient in transmissible GBS antibodies should be those at risk for GBS infection and not just GBS colonisation.

In 1976 Baker and Kasper[3] reported that sera from seven women giving birth to infants with invasive GBS type III infections all were deficient in GBS antibody. In our studies we have been able to verify those findings.[10] In addition we have shown maternal type-specific GBS-antibody deficiency for both GBS serotypes Ia, Ib and III (see Fig. 3). Maternal type-specific antibody deficiency was related not only to the early-onset GBS septicemia but in three cases also to late-onset GBS meningitis.

In our study of perinatal warning signs we found no differences between GBS-carrier and noncarrier parturient women as regards obstetrical management, mode of delivery, rupture of fetal membranes, or preterm delivery (see Table V). On the other hand we found a significantly higher rate of postmaturity and signs of intrauterine fetal distress and fetal acidemia in GBS carriers.

Neither the abnormalities indicating intrauterine asphyxia nor the higher incidence of postterm delivery could be related to any of the specific GBS serotypes. Some infants had moderately lowered Apgar scores after delivery, but none acquired neonatal GBS infection during the prospective study. The antibody levels in sera from mothers whose infants had shown signs of intrauterine fetal distress did not differ from those without these signs. Thus there was no definite correlation between deficient type-specific maternal GBS-antibody level and the occurrence of fetal distress.[10]

The exact mechanism whereby carriage or colonisation of GBS is related to the findings of fetal distress and postterm delivery cannot be determined from our data at present. Yet our findings may support the suggestion by others that early-onset GBS septicemia is already acquired *in utero*.[4] We have recently found widespread GBS infection at autopsy as the cause of death in an infant dying *in utero*, as has also been described by Bergquist, *et al.*[6]

In a new prospective study currently in progress we are now screening for maternal GBS carriers during pregnancy. The fetuses and newborn infants of those GBS-carrier pregnant women who in addition are shown to be deficient in type-specific GBS antibodies will be considered as those at risk for perinatal GBS infection. Preventive measures either with immunization of the mother with polysaccharide vaccine or intensive antibiotic treatment before, during, and after delivery will be considered only in these cases.

SUMMARY

The rate of GBS colonisation in a Swedish population has been studied in a prospective investigation. The rate of maternal GBS carriage was 16% and in newborn infants the colonisation rate at birth was 10%. In six of seven mothers of newborn infants with GBS infection the type-specific GBS-antibody levels were significantly lower than in colonised but noninfected cases. This was found not only in early-onset but also in late-onset GBS disease for both GBS serotypes Ia, Ib, and III. In GBS-carrier mothers there was a higher incidence of postmaturity and intrauterine fetal distress in their infants.

Our results support the hypothesis that low type-specific GBS-antibody levels in urogenital GBS-carrier parturient women implies a major risk for the development of neonatal GBS infection in their infants. Consequently the perinatal management for the prevention of GBS disease should comprise screening during pregnancy for GBS carriers with low type-specific GBS-antibody levels.

ACKNOWLEDGMENT

These studies were supported by grants from Malmöhus County Council Research Foundation.

REFERENCES

1. Baker, C. J., Clark, J., and Barnett, F. F. Selective broth medium for isolation of group B streptococci. *Appl. Microbiol.* **26,** 884 (1973).
2. Baker, C. J., and Barrett, F. F., Transmission of group B streptococci among parturient women and their neonates. *J. Pediatr.* **83,** 919 (1973).
3. Baker, C. J., and Kasper, D. L., Correlation of maternal antibody deficiency with susceptibility to neonatal group B streptococcal infection. *N. Engl. J. Med.* **294,** 753 (1976).
4. Baker, C. J., Clinical note: Early onset group B streptococcal disease. *J. Pediatr.* **93,** 124 (1978).
5. Bergquist, G., Hurvell, B., Malmborg, A. S., Rylander, M., and Tunell, R., Neonatal infections caused by group B streptococci. *Scand. J. Infect. Dis.* **3,** 157 (1971).
6. Bergquist, G., Holmberg, G., Rydner, T., and Vaclavinkova, V., Intrauterine death due to infection with group B streptococci. *Acta Obstet. Gynecol. Scand.* **57,** 127 (1978).
7. Christensen, K. K., Christensen, P., Mårdh, P. A., and Weström, L., Quantitation of serum antibodies to surface antigens of neisseria gonorrhea with radiolabelled protein A of staphylococcus aureus. *J. Infect. Dis.* **134,** 317 (1976).
8. Christensen, K. K., and Christensen, P., Typing of group B streptococci from the throat and urogenital tract of females. *Scand. J. Infect. Dis.* **10,** 209 (1978).
9. Christensen, K. K., Christensen, P., Dahlander, K., Faxelius, G., Jacobson, B., and Svenningsen, N. W., Quantitation of serum antibodies to surface antigens of group B streptococci types Ia, Ib and III. *Scand. J. Infect. Dis.* (1979) in press.
10. Christensen, K. K., Dahlander, K., Ingemarsson, I., Svenningsen, N. W., and Christensen, P., Relation between maternal urogenital carriage of group B streptococci and postmaturity and intrauterine asphyxia during delivery. *Scand. J. Infect. Dis.* (1979) in press.
11. Franciosi, R. A., Knostman, J. D., and Zimmerman, R. A., Group B streptococcal neonatal and infant infection. *J. Pediatr.* **82,** 707 (1973).
12. Howard, J. B., and McCracken, G. H., Jr., The spectrum of group B streptococcal infection in infancy. *Am. J. Dis. Child.* **128,** 815 (1974).

13. Jeffery, H., Mitchison, R., Wigglesworth, J. S., and Davies, P. A., Early neonatal bacteraemia: comparison of group B streptococcal, other gram-positive and gram-negative infections. *Arch. Dis. Child.* **52,** 683 (1977).

14. Klesius, P. H., Zimmerman, R. A., Mathews, J. H., and Krushak, D. H., Cellular and humoral immune response to group B streptococci. *J. Pediatr.* **83,** 926 (1973).

15. Mathews, J. H., Klesius, P. H., and Zimmerman, R. A., Opsonin system of group B streptococcus. *Infect. Immun.* **10,** 1315 (1974).

16. Shigeoka, A. O., Hall, R. T., Hemming, V. G., Alfred, C. D., and Hill, H. R., Role of antibody and complement in opsonization of group B streptococci. *Infect. Immun.* **21,** 475 (1978).

17. Slack, M. P., and Mayon-White, R. T.: Group B streptococci in pharyngeal aspirates at birth and the early detection of neonatal sepsis. *Arch. Dis. Child.* **53,** 540 (1978).

18. Vollman, J. H., Smith, W. L., Ballard, E. T., and Light, I. J., Early onset group B streptococcal disease: Clinical, roentgenographic and pathologic findings. *J. Pediatr.* **89,** 199 (1976).

19

Granulocyte Transfusion in Very Small Newborn Infants with Sepsis

F. LAURENTI,[1] R. FERRO,[1] G. ISACCHI,[2] F. MALAGNINO,[2] M. ROSSINI,[3]
G. MARZETTI,[1] F. MANDELLI,[2] and G. BUCCI[1]

Polymorphonuclear leukocytes (PMNs) are one of the most important factors in host defence against acute bacterial infection. In adults with severe infection the number of circulating PMNs is usually increased and various PMN activities appear to be enhanced, such as chemotaxis, phagocytosis, microbicidal activity, NBT reduction, and hexosomonophosphate shunt, whereas only in few cases with overwhelming infection are such activities depressed.[24, 25, 43, 54] In contrast, several PMN functional activities appear to be depressed in healthy and, more markedly, in septic newborn infants. In healthy newborns, chemotaxis and microbicidal activity were reportedly decreased as compared to adult standards.[11, 13, 28, 29, 39, 40, 55] In septic newborns microbicidal activity was furtherly depressed and phagocytosis was also decreased.[10, 42, 52, 53, 55, 58] As to chemotaxis, in a recent study from our research group on infected preterm neonates chemotactic activity was usually enhanced in the presence of surface colonization (nasal, pharyngeal, conjunctival, umbilical) whereas with septicemia, in contrast to the usual adult response, the chemotactic activity was virtually abolished.[34] Moreover, several studies suggest that various metabolic activities are unstable and easily exhaustible,[6, 13, 42, 47, 55] especially in the course of neonatal sepsis. PMN hexosemonophosphate shunt, normally increased in adult phagocytosing PMNs, drops significantly in infected infants.[4, 55] The degree of positivity of the NBT test, which in healthy infants is similar to adult values or may show a slight spontaneous reduction

---

[1] *Institute of Pediatrics, University of Rome*
[2] *Department of Hematology, University of Rome*
[3] *CNR Centre for Respiratory Viruses*

even in the absence of stimulation,[26, 46] diminishes instead of increasing in neonatal infection.[4, 12, 42] Finally, the PMN chemiluminescence caused by superoxide compounds falls in infected as compared to healthy newborns.[52, 53]

The above findings suggest that in newborn infants with severe infection, even in the absence of neutropenia, PMN defence mechanisms may be markedly impaired and that the transfusion of adult PMNs may be helpful.[32] In recent years in our newborn ICU we have frequently observed severe infection due to Klebsiella, Pseudomonas, or other opportunistic microorganisms, which were usually highly resistant to available antibiotics. Although contamination was widespread among all weight groups, septicemia with a high fatality rate was almost exclusively confined to infants with very low birth weight. We speculated that severe infection due to opportunistic, antibiotic resistant germs in a host with severely impaired PMN defence mechanisms represented an almost ideal indication for PMN administration, and we performed the present clinical trial in a consecutive series of newborn infants weighing 1200 g or less with septicemia.

MATERIALS AND METHODS

All newborns admitted to the ICU with a weight of 1200 g or less were eligible for the study. On admission, nasal, pharyngeal, umbilical, and rectal swabs were taken, and blood culture was performed. Standard treatment included: ampicillin and gentamycin administration, followed by other antibiotics if suggested by sensitivity tests; glucose-saline IV infusion, followed by orojejunal feeding with pasteurized human milk; low-level continuous positive airway pressure by nasal prongs, according to a previously reported protocol.[3] Caffeine was also given after the onset of apneic spells. In the last part of the study, IPPV was given by nasal prongs in the presence of intractable apneic spells.[45]

According to the protocol, PMN transfusion was to be started as soon as clinical and laboratory signs of severe infection were observed, and it was to be repeated daily or at least every other day until recovery. Clinical signs of severe infection included sclerema, abdominal distension, apneic spells, and systemic hypotension. Relevant blood chemistry findings included acidosis and hyperglycemia. Blood picture findings included neutropenia or increased band cells, with toxic granulations and vacuolizations, and megathrombocytes. Blood cultures were taken immediately before initiating PMN treatment, and repeated until recovery or postmortem. In some of the cases the Chemotactic Index (CI) was evaluated before, during, and after PMN therapy according to a previously reported technique.[33]

Packed PMNs were collected by leukofiltration of ABO/Rh compatible blood, according to the methods of Djerassi, et al.[17] and De Fliedner, et al.,[15] partially modified. Briefly, blood is drawn from one antecubital vein at a rate of 40–50 ml/min and flows through tubing and a filter set (Leukopak, Feuwal) returning later to the donor's opposite arm by means of a peristaltic pump. The extracorporeal blood volume is approximately 200 ml and 7 liters of blood are filtered in about 150–180 min. Filters are rinsed with 250 ml of saline in order to displace most of the red cells and to return them to the donor. Elution is done by flushing each filter with 500 ml of isotonic phosphate buffered 0.02% Na_2EDTA ($pH = 7.4$) at a flow rate of 30 ml/min, running the pump in "reverse." The sera of the donors were assayed for syphilis, hepatitis, cytomegalovirus, and toxoplasma antibodes. 20 ml of the cell suspension, containing 0.5–1×10^9 cells, were administered per kg body weight. In this preparation the contaminating lymphocytes did not exceed 5% of the cells.

RESULTS

Only patients with a positive blood culture before the onset of PMNs administration have been included in the present report. The most relevant data in the 13 patients who met this criterion in the study period have been reported in Table I. As to additional data, exchange transfusion (ET) was performed in one survivor because of signs of disseminated intravascular coagulation (DIC). The isolated microorganisms were highly resistant to most antibiotics, a slight sensitivity being found only to cefuroxin in 46%, to gentamycin or to tobramycin in 23%, and to amikacin in 8% of the strains tested. It is also worth reporting that one survivor had Klebsiella meningitis in addition to septicemia.

With respect to the number of PMN transfusions actually given, it must be emphasized that the treatment protocol was actually met only in eight patients, who received from five to 15 transfusions each, whereas in the remaining five patients an insufficient number of transfusions (from one to three for each infant) was given because of difficulties in the supply of the PMN preparation. A comparison between the two groups of patients with or without adequate PMN administration is reported in Table II, showing that the two groups were

TABLE I

Most Relevant Data in the Study Series

No. of cases	13	
Birth weight (g)	1033 ± 114	(820–1200 g)
Gestational age (weeks)	27.1 ± 1.3	(25–29)
Males	61%	
Laboratory studies before treatment		
Blood culture[a]		
Klebsiella, n (%)	11 (84)	
Pseudom. aer., n (%)	3 (23)	
Blood cells count/mm^3	18000 ± 9.56	
Total PMNs	12600 ± 343	(4800–29,000)
Band-cells	2960 ± 1760	(1500–4000)
Age at 1st PMN transfusion (days)	6.23 ± 3.14	(3–14)
PMN transfusions given (n)	6.73 ± 4	(1–15)
Patients given nasal IPPV, n	4[b]	
Deaths, n (%)	6 (46%)	

[a] Both Klebsiella and Pseudom. aer. found in one patient.

[b] Two survivors.

TABLE II

Comparison between Patients in the Study Series with or without Adequate PMN Administration

	PMN Treatment	
	Adequate	Inadequate
No. of cases	8	5
Birthweight (g)	1077 ± 99	962 ± 107
Gestational age (weeks)	27.5 ± 1.5	26.6 ± 0.9
Blood culture		
Klebsiella, n	7	4
Pseudom. aer., n	2	1
Age at 1st PMN transfusion (days)	6 ± 2.1	5.3 ± 3.1
Duration of single infection episode (days)	5.7 ± 1.9	6.6 ± 4.6
PMN transfusions given (n)	10.25 ± 3.4 (5–15)	1.8 ± 0.45 (1–3)
PMN transfusions per symptomatic days	1:1.4	1:6
Patients given nasal IPPV	2	2
Deaths, n (%)[a]	1 (12.5)	5 (100)

[a] $p < 0.005$.

similar with respect to the clinical and bacteriological findings, whereas the mortality rate was significantly lower in the adequately treated group. It is also of interest to report that in the only patient dying after adequate PMN treatment haemoperitoneum with sterile blood cultures were found postmortem, whereas blood cultures were positive for the offending microorganism in all of the five inadequately treated patients. In the latter group postmortem examination revealed brain hemorrhage in three cases (associated in two with necrotizing enterocolitis) and pneumonia in the remaining two patients.

The PMN CI was determined in 11 patients during septicemia, and in some of them also before and after infection. Results are illustrated in Figure 1. In keeping with previous findings[34] the CI was very low (mean 3.1 cells/HPF, range 1–10 cells/HPF) during septicemia, and returned to normal with recovery.

We did not observe any untoward effects of PMN transfusions, such as chills, fever, rash, tachypnea, and cyanosis following the procedure, or possible early and late signs of graft-versus-host disease (GVHD).

DISCUSSION

Although controlled trials would be needed in order to obtain conclusive evidence on the effectiveness of the present approach, several considerations suggest that PMN transfusion was highly effective in the present series of patients. In fact, the mortality rate was remarkably low, when considering the nature of the disease and the degree of prematurity of the patients. The intact survival of the only patient with meningitis was also remarkable. An unplanned control group within the study series was represented by the small group of infants who, by chance and for reasons beyond our control, were not adequately treated with PMN transfusions. In this poorly treated group the mortality rate

CELLS/HPF

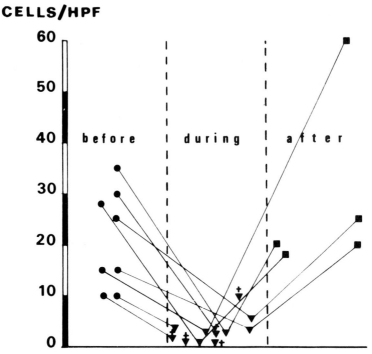

Fig. 1. The Chemotactic Index (cells/HPF) in 11 patients before, during, and after septicemia. The crosses indicate the patients who died. When more than one determination was available in any given period, the average was calculated.

was significantly lower than in adequately treated patients, and it was similar to the one usually observed in our unit before the introduction of PMN therapy.

In order to substantiate the latter statement, we retrospectively evaluated a series of 22 newborn infants with very low birth weight, consecutively admitted in the 2 years preceding the study period. In this series the birth weight (mean 1020 ± 165 g, range 700–1200 g), the gestational age (mean 27.6 ± 1.3 weeks, range 25–30 weeks), and the sex ratio (46% males) were similar to the study series. Blood culture yielded Klebsiella in 59%, Pseudom. aer. in 27%, and Candida albicans in 14% of the cases, with marked antibiotic insensitivity as in the strains found in the study series. In this retrospective series ET was performed in three cases (all died) for signs of DIC. Treatment was in all other respects identical to the study series, with the only exception being that prolonged IPPV ventilation was not used. However, this difference could not markedly influence the results, since only two of the four patients in the study series who received IPPV survived. The mortality rate in these 22 patients was 82%, which was similar to the mortality rate in the poorly treated group in the study series, and significantly ($p < 0.05$) higher than in the entire study series. Interestingly, necrotizing enterocolitis was not seen in the eight adequately treated patients, whereas it was observed in two of the five poorly treated infants and in 31% of the 13 untreated infants in whom postmortem examination was performed.

For all these reasons it seems likely that the PMN transfusion therapy was responsible for the dramatic decrease in the mortality rate in very small septic infants observed in our unit in the study period. Observations on the study cases and on even more septic newborn infants, not included in the present report, suggested that the amount of PMNs given each transfusion was adequate and that in most cases, in order to achieve good results, this amount needed to be repeated from twice a day to once every other day as long as septic signs persisted. It should, however, be emphasized that in the great majority of cases of the present series infection was not fulminating in character. Therefore, in fulminating infection, with severe shock, different results may be expected, and more intensive treatment schedules may be required.

At the beginning of the study period part of the difficulties in the PMN supply were due to the fact that, in view of the previously reported evidence of the functional decay of filtered and stored PMNs,[30, 50, 59] we used only freshly collected preparations. However, recent studies from our research group,[35] in keeping with other reports,[13, 37] failed to show relevant functional changes in PMNs stored for as long as 48 h. Following these observations, we treated the last five patients with PMNs stored up to 48 h: this not only resulted in a greater availability of PMN units, but also enabled us to give to any single patient cells from a more limited number of donors, thereby decreasing the risk of immunization against incompatible PMNs.

Immunological replacement therapy in neonatal infection has so far included fresh frozen plasma, gamma globulins, and exchange transfusion (ET). Fresh frozen plasma has been used in consideration of the multiple deficiencies of humoral factors (mostly IgM, IgA, and complement factors) in the newborn infant,[1, 2, 19, 20, 21, 22, 36] but the limited number of studies available[14, 41] has so far failed to produce convincing evidence on the effectiveness of this treatment. In our opinion the failure of fresh frozen plasma to produce clear-cut benefits in neonatal sepsis is not surprising, since fresh adult plasma may mostly improve the defective opsonization of gram-negative bacteria, which by itself does not result in bacterial killing and may be only helpful if the subsequent steps of cellular immune defences are functioning well. Furthermore, as soon as opsonization is attained, an excess of opsonins is useless. A direct bactericidal effect may be obtained with hyperimmune plasma, but, unfortunately, specific hyperimmune plasma has been thus far prepared and successfully used only for group B streptococcus infection,[51] whereas preparations against other common agents of neonatal sepsis are not available at present. In any case, the association of fresh frozen plasma and PMN transfusion may have some theoretical benefits, and may be worthy of future investigation. ET has been extensively used in several centers, with reportedly good results,[7, 49, 56, 57] but in our opinion the lack of truly controlled trials and the heterogeneity of the clinical material investigated does not allow a full understanding of its role in the treatment of neonatal infection. ET leads mainly to removal of germs, toxins, abnormal split coagulation products, and of other components some-times overproduced in the course of sepsis, such as F_2 prostaglandins.[56] It also provides IgM, IgA, and complement factors, as well as endotoxin serum inhibitors. For these reasons ET seems especially indicated if DIC or shock are present in the course of infection. Another nonimmunological beneficial effect of ET may be related, according to some authors,[44] to the substitution of adult for fetal erythrocytes, thereby shifting the oxygen dissociation curve to the right and increasing the availability of oxygen to tissues.

An effect shared by both the ET and PMN transfusion may be represented by the introduction of white blood cells, mostly PMNs and lymphocytes. The accurate calculation of the number of PMNs and of lymphocytes actually given by ET is almost impossible for several reasons, but it can be roughly assumed that a remarkably smaller amount of PMNs and a moderately greater amount of lymphocytes are added to the patient's WBC pool by a standard ET as compared to the PMN transfusions used in the present study. The introduction of foreign lymphocytes is, of course, undesirable, since GVHD may result if immunocompetence is not yet fully established. However, GVHD has rarely been reported even in extremely premature fetuses transfused *in utero*,[48] and signs of GVHD have not been observed in the present series of patients. This is presumably due to the fact that T-lymphocyte function is usually fully established very early in gestation,[5, 8, 9, 16, 23, 27] as also documented by a normal E-rosette test in three infants in the present series where this test was performed. In any case, we fully agree that the administration of foreign lymphocytes should be avoided as much as possible. In fact, due to recent improvements of the filtration technique the percentage of lymphocytes in our preparation has become as low as 1–2%. In order to completely abolish living lymphocytes, cell irradiation may be considered.

As to the administration of PMNs, this too might produce untoward effects, including early reactions such as chills, fever, rash, tachypnea, and cyanosis or, subsequently, immune neutropenia.[38] These effects might be avoided by thor-ough typing of donors' PMNs, but we did not perform HLA typing in order to avoid additional difficulties in the emergency supply of the PMN preparation, and also in consideration of the fact that other, so far poorly identified antigens, may be as important as HLA in producing immune neutropenia.[31, 38] In any case, untoward effects possibly due to heterologus PMNs were not observed in the present series. Another theoretical untoward effect of transfused PMNs might occur in DIC, where an excess of PMNs could activate the platelet aggregation and clotting sequence through the release of thromboplastin-like precursors.

A final point to be considered when comparing ET and PMN transfusion in the treatment of neonatal infection is that PMN transfusion can easily be repeated at short intervals if necessary, whereas this may be difficult with ET, especially in severely compromised or in very small newborn infants.

From the above considerations, we suggest that ET should be preferred in the presence of DIC or of septic shock, whereas PMN transfusion should be the treatment of choice in uncomplicated septicemia. Both treatments might therefore be required in the same patient at different times. Of course this working hypothesis should be substantiated by well-controlled clinical trials.

ACKNOWLEDGMENT

This study was supported by a grant of the CNR, Project MPP3, No. 79.01022.83.

REFERENCES

1. Adamkin, D., Stitzel, A., Urmson, J., Farnett, M. L., Post, E., and Spitzer, R., Activity of the alternative pathway of complement in the newborn infant. *J. Pediatr.* **93,** 604 (1978).
2. Adinolfi, M., Levels of two components of complement (C_4' and C_3') in human fetal and newborn sera. *Dev. Med. Child. Neruol.* **12,** 306 (1970).
3. Agostino, R., Marzetti, G., Pellegrini-Caliumi, G., Moretti, C., Savignoni, P. G., Nodari, S., Picece-Bucci, S., and Bucci, G., Early Nasal Continuous Positive Pressure (CPAP) Breathing in Newborns Weighing 800–1200 g and without Severe Lung Disease, in *Intensive Care in the Newborn, II*, Stern, Ed. Masson, New York, 1978, p. 63.
4. Anderson, D. C., Pickering, L. K., and Feigin, R. D., Leukocyte function in normal and infected neonates. *J. Pediatr.* **85,** 420 (1974).
5. August, C. S., Berkel, I., Driscoll, S., and Merler, E., Onset of lymphocyte function in the developing human fetus. *Pediatr. Res.* **5,** 539 (1971).
6. Bellanti, J. A., Cantz, B. E., Yang, M. C., von Thadden, H., and Schlegel, R. J., Biochemical Changes in Human Polymorphonuclear Leukocytes during Maturation, in *The Phagocytic Cell in Host Resistance*, Bellanti, J. A., and Dayton, D. H., Eds. Raven Press, New York, 1975, p. 321.
7. Belohradsky, B. H., Klose, H. J., and Marget, W., Results of combined chemotherapy and immunotherapy by exchange transfusion in neonatal septicemia, Abstracted no. 305. Perinat. Med., 6th European Congress, Wien 1978.
8. Campbell, A. C., Waller, C., Wood, J., Aynsley-Green, A., and Yu, V., Lymphocyte populations in the blood of newborn infants. *Clin. Exp. Immunol.* **18,** 469 (1974).
9. Christiansen, J. S., Osther, K., Pietersen, B., *et al.* B, T and null lymphocytes in newborn infants and their mothers. *Acta Paediat. Scand.* **65,** 425 (1976).
10. Ciccimarra, F., Della Pietra, D., Pignata, C., Troncone, R., Risolo, E., and Tancredi, F., Attività fagocitica e battericida in neonati affetti da gravi infezioni batteriche. IV Congr. Soc. Ital. Immun. Immunopat., Bari, 21–23 April 1978.
11. Cocchi, P., and Marianelli, L., Phagocytosis and intracellular killing of Pseudomonas aeruginosa in premature infants. *Helv. Pediatr. Acta* **1,** 110 (1967).
12. Cocchi, P., Mori, S., and Becalturi, A., NBT reduction by neutrophils of newborn infants; in vitro phagocytosis test. *Acta Pediatr. Scand.* **60,** 475 (1971).
13. Coen, R., Grush, O., and Kauder, E., Studies of bactericidal activity and metabolis of the leukocyte in full-term neonates. *J. Pediatr.* **75,** 400 (1969).
14. Davis, A. T., Blum, P. M., and Quic, P. G.: Studies on opsonic activity for E. coli in premature infants after blood transfusion, abstracted. *Proc. Soc. Pediatr. Res.*, 233 (1971).
15. De Fliedner, V., Meuret, G., and Senn, N. I., Leucophérèse par filtration. *Nouv. Rev. Fr. Hematol.* **16,** 98 (1976).
16. De Muralt, G., Maturation of Cellular and Humoral Immunity, in *Perin. Phys.*, Stave, U., Ed. Plenum Publ., New York, 1978, p. 267.
17. Djerassi, I., Kim, J. S., Suvanki, U., Mitrakul, C., and Cieselka, W., Continuous flow filtration leukapheresis. *Transfusion* **12,** 75 (1972).
18. Djerassi, I., and Kim, J. S., Problems and solutions with filtration leukapheresis, in *The Granulocyte: Function and Clinical Utilization*, Greenwalt, T. J., and Jamieson, G. A., Ed. Alan R. Liss, New York, 1977, p. 305.
19. Dosset, J. H., and Quic, P. G., Opsonins and polymorphonuclear leukocytes function in mothers and newborns, abstracted. *Proc. Soc. Pediatr. Res.*, 135 (1968).

20. Dosset, J. H., Williams, R. C., and Quic, P. G., Studies on interaction of bacteria serum factors and PMN leukocytes in mothers and newborns. *Pediatrics* **44**(1) 49 (1969).

21. Feinstein, P. A., and Kplen, S. R., The alternative pathway of complement activation in the neonate. *Pediatr. Res.* **9**, 803 (1975).

22. Fireman, P., Zuchowski, D. A., and Taylor, P. M., Development of human complement system. *J. Immunol.* **103**, 25 (1969).

23. Hayward, A. R., and Ezer, G., Development of lymphocyte population in the human foetal thymus and spleen. *Clin. Exp. Immunol.* **17**, 169 (1974).

24. Hill, H. R., Gerrard, J. M., Hogan, N. A., and Quic, P. G., Hyperactivity of neutrophil leukotactic responses during active bacterical infection. *J. Clin. Invest.* **53**, 996 (1974).

25. Hill, H. R., Warwick, W. J., Dettloff, B. S., and Quic, P. G., Neutrophil granulocyte function in patients with pulmonary infection. *J. Pediatr.* **84**, 55 (1974).

26. Humbert, J. R., Kurtz, M. L., and Hathaway, W. E., Increased reduction of NBT by neutrophils of newborn infants. *Pediatrics* **45**, 125 (1970).

27. Jones, W. R., Fetal and Neonatal Immunology, in *Immunology of Human Reproduction*, Scott, J. S., and Jones, W. R. Eds. Academic Press, Grune-Stratton, New York, 1976.

28. Klein, R. B., Rich, K. C., Biberstein, M., Stiehm, E. R., Defective mononuclear and neutrophilic phagocyte chemotaxis in the newborn. *Clin. Res.* **24**, 180A (1976).

29. Klein, R. B., Fisher, T. J., Gard, S. E., Giberstein, M., Rich, K. C., and Stiehm, E. R., Decreased mononuclear and polymorphonuclear chemotaxis in human newborns, infants and young children. *Pediatrics* **60**, 467 (1977).

30. Klock, J. C., and Bainton, D. F., Degranulation and abnormal bactericidal function of granulocytes procured by reversible adhesion to nylon wool. *Blood* **48**, 149 (1976).

31. Lalezari, P., Neutrophil Antigens: Immunology and Clinica Implication, in *The Granulocyte*: *Function and Clinica Utilization*, Greenwalt, T. J., and Jamieson, G. A., Eds. Alan R. Liss, New York, 1977, p. 209.

32. Laurenti, F., La Greca, G., Ferro, R., and Bucci, G., Transfusion of polymorphonuclear neutrophils in a premature infant with Klebsiella sepsis. *Lancet* **2**, 111 (1978).

33. Laurenti, F., Rossini, M., Balducci, L., and Ferro, R., Descrizione di un apparecchio originale per la determinazione multipma della chemiotassi leucocitaria. *La Clinica Pediatrica* **61**, 78 (1979).

34. Laurenti, F., Ferro, R., Marzetti, G., Rossini, M., and Bucci, G., Neutrophil chemotaxis in preterm infants with infections. *J. Pediatr.* **96**, 468 (1980).

35. Laurenti, F., Balducci, R., Crispino, P., *et al.*, Functional activity of packed polymorphonuclear leukocytes (PMN) obtained by leukofiltration, abstracted. *Eur. Soc. Pediatr. Res.*, Loven, 1979.

36. McCraken, G. H., and Eichenwald, H. F., Leukocyte function and the development of opsonic and complement activity in the neonate. *Am. J. Dis. Child.* **121**, 120 (1971).

37. McCullough, J., Weinblen, B. J., Deinard, A. R., *et al.*, In vitro function and post-transfusion survival of granulocytes collected by continuous-flow centrifugation and by filtration leukopheresis. *Blood* **48**, 315 (1976).

38. McCullough, J., Wood, N. Weinblen, B. J., *et al.*, The Role of Histocompatibility Testing in Granulocyte Transfusion. In *The Granulocyte*: *Function and Clinical Utilization*, Greenwal, T. J., and Jamieson, G. A., Eds. Alan R. Liss, New York, 1977, p. 321.

39. Miller, M. E., Phagocytosis in the newborns infant: humoral and cellular factors. *J. Pediatr.* **74**, 255 (1969).

40. Miller, M. E., Chemotactic function in the human neonate: humoral and cellular aspects. *Pediatr. Res.* **5**, 487 (1971).

41. Miller, M. E., Demonstration and replacement of a functional defect of the fifth component of complement in newborn serum. A major tool in the therapy of neonatal septicemia, abstracted. *Pediatr. Res.* **5**, 379 (1971).

42. Miller, M. E., *Host Defenses in the Human Neonate*, Monographs in Neonatology. Grune and Stratton, New York, 1978.

43. Mowat, A. G., and Baum, J., Polymorphonuclear leukocyte chemotaxis in patients with bacterial infections. *Br. Med. J.* **3**, 617 (1971).

44. Oski, F. A., Fetal hemoglobin, the neonatal red cell, and 2,3-Diphosphoglycerate. *Pediatr. Clin. North Am.* **19,** 907 (1972).

45. Panero, A., Nodari, S., Agostino, R., Moretti, C., Marzetti, G., Mendicini, M., Savignoni, P. G., and Bucci, G., Monitor activated IPPV applied by nasal prongs for the treatment of apnoea of prematurity: a preliminary report, abstracted. Eur. Soc. Pediatr. Res., Turku, 1978.

46. Park, B. H., Holmes, B. M., Rodey, G. E., and Good, R. A., NBT test in children with fetal granulomatous disease and in newborn infants. *Lancet* **1,** 157 (1969).

47. Park, B. H., Holmes, B., and Good, R. A., Metabolic activities in leukocytes of newborn infants. *J. Pediatr.* **76,** 237 (1970).

48. Parkman, R., Mozir, D., Umansky, I., Cochran, W., Carpenter, C. B., and Rosen, F. S., Graft-versus-Host disease after transfusion for hemolysis in newborn. *N. Engl. J. Med.* **290,** 359 (1974).

49. Prod'hom, L. S., Choffat, J. M., Frenck, N., Mazoumi, M., Relier, J. P., and Torrado, A., Care of the seriously ill neonate with hyaline membrane disease and with sepsis (Sclerema Neonatorum). *Pediatrics* **53,** 170 (1974).

50. Roy, A. J., Yankee, R. A., Brivkalns, A., and Fitch, M., Viability of granulocytes obtained by filtration leukapheresis. *Transfusion* **15,** 539 (1975).

51. Shigeoka, A. O., Hall, R. T., and Hill, H. R., Blood transfusion in Group B Streptococcal sepsis. *Lancet* **1,** 636 (1978).

52. Shigeoka, A. O., Allred, C. D., and Hill, H. R., Chemiluminiscence response of neonatal leukocytes, abstracted. *Pediatr. Res.* **12**(4), 486 (1978).

53. Shigeoka, A. O., Santos, J. I., and Hill, H. R., Functional analysis of neutrophil granulocytes from healthy, infected, and stressed neonates. *J. Pediatr.* **95,** 454 (1979).

54. Solberg, C. O., and Hellum, K. B., Neutrophil granulocyte function in bacterial infections. *Lancet* **2,** 727 (1972).

55. Stoerner, J. W., Pickering, L. K., Adcock, E. W., and Morriss, F. H., Polymorphonuclear leukocyte function in newborn infants. *J. Pediatr* **93,** 862 (1978).

56. Töllner, V., Pohlandt, F., Heinze, F., and Henrichs, I., Treatment of septicemia in the newborn infant: choice of initial antimicrobial drugs and the role of exchange transfusion. *Acta Paediatr.* Scand. **66,** 605 (1977).

57. Vain, N. E., Newborld, J. L., Quilligan, J. J., *et al.,* The role of exchange transfusion in the treatment of severe septicemia and sclerema neonatorum, abstracted. *Am. Soc. Pediatr. Res.,* 500 (1978).

58. Wright, W. C., Ank, B. J., Herbert, J., and Stiehm, E. R., Decreased bactericidal activity of leukocytes of stressed newborn infants. *Pediatrics* **56,** 569 (1975).

59. Wright, D. G., Kauffmann, J. C., Chusid, M. J., *et al.,* Functional abnormalities of human neutrophils collected by continuous flow filtration leukapheresis. *Blood* **46,** 901 (1975).

20

Congenital Toxoplasmosis: A 15-Year Prospective Study

JANNA G. KOPPE, H. DE ROEVER-BONNET, and D. H. LOEWER-SIEGER

Toxoplasma gondii, a parasite, was discovered in Algeria by Nicolle and Manceau at the beginning of the century (Fig. 1). The parasite is found in most parts of the world and infects all warm-blood animals, including birds. Infection can occur by eating raw or undercooked meat, especially in Europe where infestation is high (Table I).

In the late 1960s, a new focus of infection was described by Hutchison, *et al.,*[6] who reported that *cats* were a host, not only for the asexual cycle, as for example in human beings and dogs, but for a sexual cycle in the wall of the intestine as well. The cat can excrete oocysts in the faeces which become sporocysts that may infect humans and other species. Thus, vegetarians may become infected in this way.

The first cases of clinical congenital toxoplasmosis were described in 1939 by Wolf, *et al.,*[10] with the well-known "classic triad": hydrocephaly, chorioretinitis, and intracranial calcifications (Figs. 2 and 3).

When clinically overt, a "neurologic form" occurs with chorioretinitis, abnormal spinal fluid, hydrocephalus, microcephaly, microphthalmia, and neurologic abnormalities, and a "generalized form," with hepatosplenomegaly, anemia, thrombocytopenia, and elevated IgM levels.

As a cause of blindness in children a collaborative study in Europe[5] has found between 1.7 and 4.6% due to toxoplasmosis (Table II). In the southern United States Remington and Klein[9] report toxoplasmosis as responsible for 4% of blind students.

The varying manifestations of congenital toxoplasmosis can only be studied

Departments of Neonatology, Parasitology and Ophthalmology, Wilhelmina Gasthuis, University of Amsterdam, The Netherlands

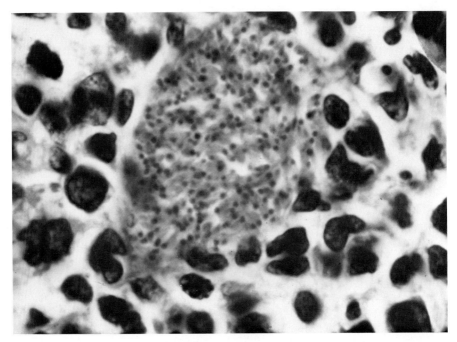

Fig. 1. Toxoplasma cyst.

TABLE I

Isolation of Toxoplasma from Meat

	Netherlands	California, U.S.
Beef loin	30%	0%
Pork loin	65%	32%
Lamb	95%	4%

in a prospective way, as reported in France by Desmonts and Couvreur[4] and in Amsterdam by Koppe, *et al.*[7]

METHODS

In our study, beginning in 1964, 3040 pregnant women were studied with the Sabin Feldman test of which 1821 were studied twice during pregnancy.

Of these 1821 women, about 60% were infected before their pregnancy. 249 mothers and their babies were chosen for follow-up, because they meet one of the following criteria: a change of Sabin-Feldman titre from negative to ≥512, a high titre at first control, a small increase in titre, or a history of toxoplasmosis before pregnancy (Table III). 207 of the babies had passively transferred antibodies. Some babies required more than a year to be free of antibodies. When a baby still had antibodies after 2 years, it was considered to be infected. In all, 12 children were infected; five of them showed signs shortly after birth, and they were treated; the other seven were asymptomatic, and they were not treated (Table IV); the incidence was 6.5‰. In agreement with Desmonts, *et*

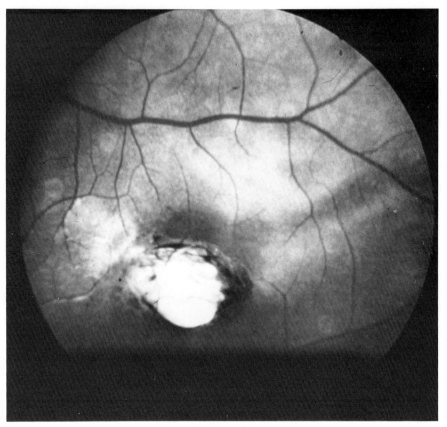

Fig. 2. Chorioretinitis-scar.

al.,[4] 40% of our babies became infected when the mother acquired toxoplasmosis during pregnancy.

The 12 infected children were followed regularly on a yearly basis. Between 5 and 12 years of age, relapses of chorioretinitis in the periphery of the retina were seen in most of the children. The relapses were seen in the treated as well as in the untreated children, without a rise in antibody titre. As an example the follow-up of a treated and a nontreated child is shown in Tables V and VI.

RESULTS

The results of 14 years of follow-up of the 12 infected children are shown in Table VII. Their school performances are normal, and only one had squinting. The other abnormalities in the eyes would not have been found except for this study.

Apart from the 12 infected children there were 10 children who may have been infected. Their Sabin-Feldman titres remained positive for as long as 18 months; although we presumed that they are not infected congenitally, they were included in the follow-up as possible congenital infections. One child, who

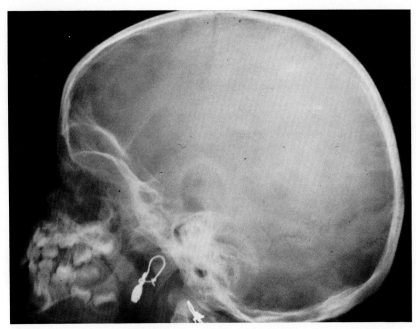

Fig. 3. Intracranial calcifications.

TABLE II

Congenital Toxoplasmosis as Cause of Blindness in Children

Netherlands	4.6%
Belgium	2.8%
Sweden	2.9%
Norway	2.0%
Denmark	1.7%

TABLE III

Categories of Mothers Whose Children Were Followed after Birth

1. Change of dye-test titres from negative or very low to ⩾512	63
2. Dye-test titre ⩾512 at first control	
3. Small increase in dye-test titre	183
4. History of probable infection before pregnancy	3
Total	249

TABLE IV

Clinical Findings at Birth in Five Children out of 12 Infected Children

B 4	scar in left eye
A 7	culture of placenta positive, culture of liquor cerebrospinalis positive, without other signs of disease
A 9	two scars in left eye
A 10	culture of liquor cerebrospinalis positive, scar in left eye
A 11	scar in left eye
7 others	asymptomatic

TABLE V

A 11. Sabin-Feldman Titre and CBR in a Patient with Congenital Toxoplasmosis Treated in the Postneonatal Period

		Sabin-Feldman	CBR
Scar left eye	cord blood	1:1024	1:4
	1 year	1:1024	1:2
	2 years		
	3 years	1:512	
	4 years	1:128	
	5 years	1:64	neg.
	6 years	1:64	1:8
	7 years	1:64	1:2
	8 years	1:64	neg.
	9 years	1:64	neg.
	10 years	1:64	neg.
New scar right eye	12 years	1:16	neg.
	13 years	1:16	neg.

TABLE VI

B 2. Sabin-Feldman Titre and CBR in a Patient with Asymptomatic Congenital Toxoplasmosis *Not* Treated in the Postneonatal Period

		Sabin-Feldman	CBR
	cord blood	1:2048	
	1 year	1:256	1:4
	2 years	1:64	1:4
	3 years		
	4 years		
	5 years	1:4	1:2
	6 years	1:128	1:4
	7 years	1:256	1:2
	8 years	1:256	neg.
	9 years	1:512	1:8
	10 years	1:512	1:2
	11 years		
	12 years	1:256	1:2
New fresh scar in right eye	13 years	1:4	1:2

TABLE VII

After 14 Years of Follow-up

12 infected children "congenital toxoplasmosis"
8 have scars in one or both eyes
4 of 5 treated children have new scars in both eyes
1 of 5 treated children has paroxysmal tachycardia
3 of 7 untreated children have new scars in both eyes

had a negative Sabin-Feldman titre at 18 months and at 3 years, had a sharp rise in Sabin-Feldman titre at 5 years of age, with a fresh scar close to the macula in his right eye, lowering the vision in the eye at 1:10. This appears to be an acquired infection, because after being negative for 3 years, he had such a sharp rise in his Sabin-Feldman titre. Of the other nine questionable cases, one is probably congenitally infected, as his Sabin-Feldman test remained positve at a very low titre (¼) until his 10th year, whereas three acquired a toxoplasmosis infection without clinical signs between 5 and 12 years of age.

The question arose whether or not all relapses in the congenitally infected children were acquired reinfections of toxoplasmosis. To answer this, we checked the other 207 children again, originally selected for follow-up and who were all found to be negative for congenital toxoplasmosis in the postneonatal period, both by eye examinations and measurements of antibody titre.

Until now, we have followed 60 patients out of the above-mentioned 207; 40% have postive Sabin-Feldman titres, due to acquired toxoplasmosis. None of them have chorioretinitis. Keeping cats did not affect the frequency of infection (30% of the infected group and 39% of the noninfected group).

Chorioretinitis due to acquired toxoplasmosis is probably extremely rare and only seen in patients in whom the Sabin-Feldman titre rises sharply, in contrast to the relatively frequent relapses of chorioretinitis due to congenital toxoplasmosis.

Alford, et al.[1] reported that 20% (two out of 10) of congenitally infected infants showed a severe form of the disease, i.e., perinatal death, blindness, or extreme mental retardation. In contrast, the data of Daamen[2] as well as our own study show that the percentage of severe disease in patients with congenital toxoplasmosis is significantly lower in Holland. As summarized in Table VIII only 35 of 1100 infants were severely damaged, a frequency of 3%. Perhaps the difference is due to our prospective study in screening many pregnant mothers with the Sabin-Feldman test, or it may reflect a different definition of the severe form of the disease.

PREVENTION

The problem of prevention is not yet solved. There is no vaccine. From our data noted above, killing all cats is not a rational solution.

Deep-freezing all meat may help kill the parasite. In the U.S., where almost all meat is deep-frozen, the prevalance is lower (1–2/1000)[1] than in Europe (6–7/1000).

TABLE VIII
Congenital Toxoplasmosis in The Netherlands

Total number of births	±170,000/year
Incidence congenital toxoplasmosis	6.5% = ±1100/year
stillborn	4
neonatal deaths	9
dead in first 3 years of life	7
blind	9
severe brain damage	6
chorioretinitis	±400
after 14 years chorioretinitis	±750

Deliberately infecting girls before pregnancy is too dangerous, due to the unknown virulence of the parasite.

Screening pregnant women is possible. When the infection is early in the first trimester an abortion can be done. However, only 15% of the children of mothers with an acquired infection in this stage of pregnancy become infected, so that six abortions would be necessary for one infected fetus.

Desmonts, et al.[4] recommend screening during pregnancy on a regular basis every 4 weeks, and treatment with spiramycine if there is seroconversion. However, no lowering of severe congenital cases occurred, and the only significant reduction was in the mild asymptomatic cases, which originate from acquired infections in the last trimester of pregnancy. Furthermore, it is not clear if spiramycine crosses the placenta-barrier, or if it is effective in an infected baby. To treat a later diagnosed infection is difficult, since the use of sulfa and daraprim is contraindicated in pregnancy. In 60% of the infants treatment of the mother will be unnecessary, as the baby is not infected.

Because of these problems in diagnosis and treatment, we decided in Holland not to screen every pregnancy. Screening babies after birth is useless, as the damage has already occurred. Besides there was no effect on the percentage of relapses of chorioretinitis later on in the treated versus the nontreated group of children with congenital infections.

CONCLUSION

Congenital toxoplasmosis remains an important unsolved problem. The incidence in Europe is high, being about 6/1000 births. Yet, most infections are clinically asymptomatic. Treatment in the neonatal period and the first year of life does not prevent relapses of chorioretinitis later. About 70% of all infants with congenital infections have scars in their eyes by 14 years of age. A peak of relapses occurs between 5 and 12 years. Relapses of chorioretinitis in congenital toxoplasmosis in our experience are not associated with a high level of antibodies, whereas recent acquired infections are. There is no vaccine. Deliberately infecting girls before pregnancy is too dangerous. Screening of pregnant women is possible, but no clear-cut safe therapy is available. Screening the baby after birth is too late.

REFERENCES

1. Alford, C. A., Stagno, S., and Reynolds, D. W. Congenital toxoplasmosis: clinical, laboratory and therapeutic considerations, with special reference to subclinical disease. *Bull. N. Y. Acad. Med.* **50,** 160 (1974).
2. Daamen, C. B. F., Perinatale sterfte in Rotterdam. Thesis, Rotterdam (1966).
3. Desmonts, G., Couvreur, J., and Ben Rachid, M. S., Le toxoplasme, la mère et l'enfant. *Arch. Fr. Pédiatr.* **22,** 1183 (1965).
4. Desmonts, G., and Couvreur, J., Toxoplasmosis in pregnancy and its transmission to the fetus. *Bull. N. Y. Acad. Med. 2nd Ser.* **50,** 146–159 (1974).
5. *Doc. Ophthalmol.* **39**(2), (December 30, 1975).
6. Hutchison, W. M., Dunachie, J. F., Siim, J. C., and Work, K., The life cycle of the coccidian

parasite, Toxoplasma gondii, in the domestic cat. *Trans. Soc. Trop. Med. Hyg.* **65,** 380–399 (1971).

7. Koppe, J. G., Kloosterman, G. J., de Roever-Bonnet, H., Eckert-Stroink, J. A., Loewer-Sieger, D. H., and de Bruijne, J. I., Toxoplasmosis and pregnancy, with a long-term follow-up of the children. *Eur. J. Obstet. Gynecol. Reprod. Biol.* **4,** 101–109 (1974).

8. Nicolle, C., and Manceaux, L., Sur un protozoaire nouveau du gondi. *C. R. Acad. Sci. Paris* **148,** 369–372 (1909).

9. Remington, J. S., Klein, J. O., Eds. *Infectious Diseases of the Fetus and Newborn Infant.* Saunders, Philadelphia-London-Toronto, 1976.

10. Wolf, A., Cowen, D., and Haige, B. H., Human toxoplasmosis. (Occurrence in infants as an encephalomyelitis. Verification by transmission to animals.) Science **89,** 226 (1939).

21

The Volume and Composition of Suckled Breast Milk

J. D. BAUM, M.D., FRCP

Recent evidence strongly supports the belief that human milk is the optimal food for human babies.[1] There are, however, many questions as yet unanswered in relation to the strictly nutritional value of human milk. This applies to any baby feeding at the breast, but particularly babies who are failing to gain weight adequately[2] and to populations of babies in developing countries where there are serious concerns about infant nutrition.[3]

The majority of previous studies on human milk have been based on the biochemical analysis of expressed breast milk[4] together with information on the volume of milk that a baby receives determined by test weighing.[5] However, these data give no information on the composition of the milk that a baby actually receives when sucking at the breast (suckled breast milk), which is known to change in its composition from time to time during a feed and from feed to feed within a day.[6] Furthermore, such information must be looked at together with the total volume of milk transferred from mother to baby during a feed and over a 24-hr period. This is particularly the case in developing countries where test weighing is inappropriate since infants feed on demand and they demand continuously. We therefore set out to develop methods for studying the volume and composition of suckled breast milk to derive an integrated statement of what the breast feeding infant actually receives during a feed and during a day.

THE VOLUME OF SUCKLED BREAST MILK

As an initial step in the investigation of the composition of suckled breast milk the pattern of milk transfer from mothers to babies was measured during

Department of Paediatrics, University of Oxford, John Radcliffe Hospital, Headington, Oxford

normal feeds.[7] This was done by a cross-sectional analysis of 122 mothers and babies breast feeding on the 6th day after birth. Infants were weighed before a feed and after 2, 4, or 7 min or at the end of a feed. Separate data were collected for the first breast and the second breast, and one mother and baby pair gave only one point of information since taking the baby off the breast was considered likely to interfere with the normal physiology of the rest of the feed. The mean interval from the previous feed was 4 hr. Weighings were performed using a Sartorius electronic balance which is accurate to 1 g.

This study showed that the mean total volume of intake on the first breast was 37 ml and that 50% of the milk was obtained by the baby in the first 2 min of the feed and 90% in the first 4 min. The mean total volume intake on the second breast was 29 ml; 50% was obtained by the baby in 2 min and 80% in 4 min (Fig. 1). It thus appears that the milk flow from each breast conforms to a particular pattern when studied on the 6th day after birth. Preliminary studies at 1 month after birth suggest that the pattern of milk transfer conforms to this general picture.

THE COMPOSITION OF SUCKLED BREAST MILK

The method of cross-sectional analysis provides information for a population of mothers and babies about the volume and pattern of milk transfer. The next step in our investigation was to interpose a latex nipple shield (Fig. 2) between a mother and her baby, thus providing a route for sampling milk sequentially during a feed. In this way a picture can be built up of the total composition of the feed based on the mean pattern of milk flow. However, before this can be done with any confidence, it needs to be established that the presence of the latex shield does not in itself interfere with the physiology of lactation.

We have three sets of information to support the fact that the presence of the latex shield interferes minimally with the normal physiology of lactation. First, we have a number of anecdotes in which mothers who have experienced difficulties with lactation, either resulting from sore nipples or flat nipples, have reported that the use of the latex shield has actually facilitated the establishment of lactation.[8] Second, videotape recordings made of babies breast feeding with and without the latex shield in place have shown that the pattern of suckling is very similar both in terms of the intersuck intervals and the duration and distribution of pauses between bouts of suckling.[9, 10] Third, a series of cross-sectional weighing experiments with the latex nipple shield in place show that the total volume and rate of transfer of milk from the mothers to the babies is no different with the shield in place compared to the data collected without the shield[11] (Fig. 3). Given that the presence of the nipple shield does not interfere with the physiology of lactation, we then have available a route for sampling milk during a feed for sequential measurement of its composition.

The most important single variable in the nutritional value of human milk is its fat content which we have measured using the "Creamatocrit."[12] This is

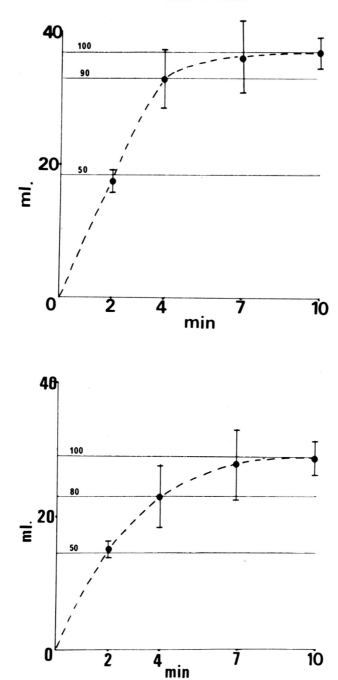

Fig. 1. Pattern of milk intake (mean and SEM) from (above) first breast and (below) the second breast. Horizontal lines represent the percentage of feed taken.

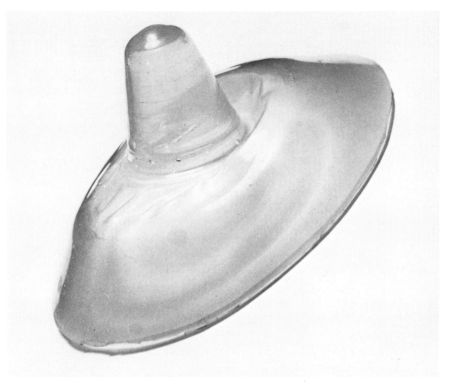

Fig. 2. The latex nipple shield.

a simple micromethod which employs a routine haematocrit centrifuge together with capillary tubes and provides an accurate estimation of the milk fat content on very small milk samples. Using the creamatocrit, small samples were drawn from behind the shield by hand syringe and catheter, at minute intervals during a feed. In this way a profile of the fat composition of milk during a feed can be described (Fig. 4). Using the mean line from the volume of milk transfer data, we can now fit the fat concentration of the milk at minute intervals to this line and thus determine the total composition of the feed for an individual mother and baby provided that the infant is weighed before and after feeding at each breast (Fig. 5).

THE MILK FLOW METER

The method of analysis described above depends upon test weighing and the pattern of volume transfer of milk derived from a population of mothers and babies. This would not provide precise information for studies on an individual mother and baby nor be appropriate for mothers and babies with a pattern of frequent and irregular feeds as in a developing country. In order to describe the situation in an individual mother and baby pair, we have devised a miniaturised ultrasonic flow meter which can be incorporated into the latex

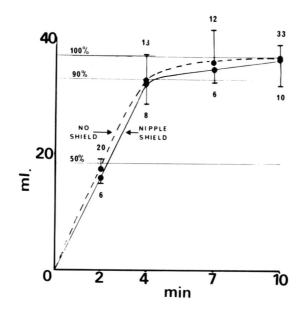

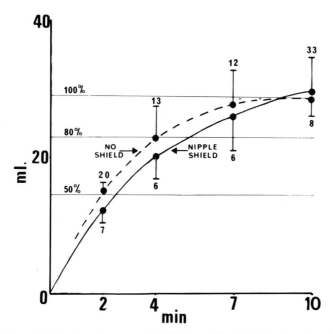

Fig. 3. The pattern of milk intake (mean and SEM) from (above) the first breast and (below) the second breast. The interrupted line represents the data without the nipple shield in place from Figure 1. The continuous line represents the data with the nipple shield in place.

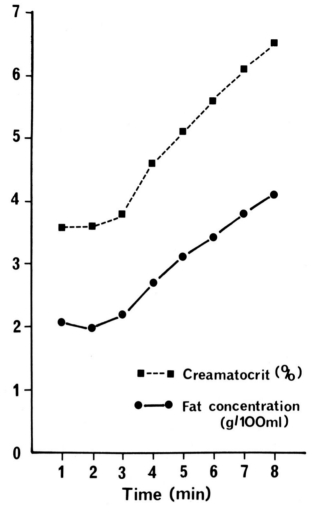

Fig. 4. The changing composition of milk within a feed. The mean of eight studies from the first breast. Milk samples were drawn from behind the nipple shield at minute intervals and the creamatocrit measured and the fat concentration derived from the nomogram.[12]

nipple shield.[13] In this way it is possible to make individual measurements of milk flow throughout a feed and throughout a day whatever the pattern of infant feeding. The flow meter is shown diagramatically in Figure 6 and consists of an ultrasonic transducer, a signal processor, and a recording device. The flow meter is small enough not to interfere with sucking and has a linear response to flow from 0 to 300 ml/min. The signal is unaffected by changes in composition and viscosity of the milk. A critical element in the design of the transducer is the elliptical bell-shaped entrance which converts the turbulent pattern of milk flow into a flat velocity profile within the transducer, thus enabling the doppler method of measurement to be applied.

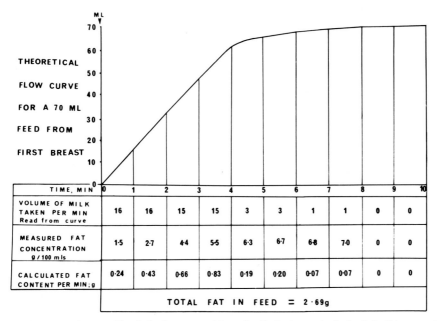

TIME, MIN	0	1	2	3	4	5	6	7	8	9	10
VOLUME OF MILK TAKEN PER MIN Read from curve		16	16	15	15	3	3	1	1	0	0
MEASURED FAT CONCENTRATION g / 100 m ls		1·5	2·7	4·4	5·5	6·3	6·7	6·8	7·0	0	0
CALCULATED FAT CONTENT PER MIN; g		0·24	0·43	0·66	0·83	0·19	0·20	0·07	0·07	0	0
TOTAL FAT IN FEED = 2·69g											

Fig. 5. The complete profile of the fat composition of milk during a single feed. In this example the total volume of the feed was 70 ml. The pattern of volume transfer is derived theoretically from the mean line shown in Figure 1. The fat concentration at minute intervals is derived using the creamatocrit. The fat content/min and the total fat taken during the feed are then calculated from the minute volume and fat concentration.

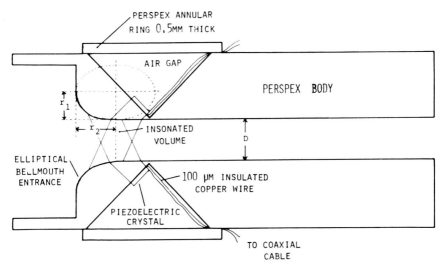

Fig. 6. Longitudinal section of prototype flow transducer 20 mm long by 8.5 mm maximum diameter with internal diameter of 2 mm.

THE INTEGRATED SYSTEM

With the total system incorporating a latex nipple shield, a flow meter, and a sampling line, it is therefore possible to collect real information on the total composition of milk that an individual baby or populations of babies receive when feeding at the breast. Such dynamic information should give us further insight into the actual diet of human infants and infants of other mammalian species.

ACKNOWLEDGMENTS

Much of this work was done as part of the ongoing project to investigate the composition of suckled breast milk with a grant from the International Council of Infant Food Industries (ICIFI).

The following collaborators have been directly involved in this work, the asterisk denoting those whose work has been directly supported as part of the ICIFI grant: Mr. M. Ashmore, Dr. R. F. Drewett, Dr. J. Gibbs, Dr. T. How,* Dr. A. Lucas,* Mrs. P. Lucas,* Dr. P. Rolfe, and Dr. M. Woolridge.*

REFERENCES

1. *Present Day Practice in Infant Feeding*, DHSS Report on Health and Social Subjects No. 9. HMSO, 1974.
2. Davies, D. P., Is inadequate breast feeding an important cause of failure to thrive? *Lancet* **1**, 541 (1979).
3. Coward, W. A., Sawyer, M. B., Whitehead, R. G., Prentice, A. M., and Evans, J., New method for measuring milk intake in breast-fed babies. *Lancet* **2**, 13 (1979).
4. *The Composition of Mature Human Milk*, DHSS Report on Health and Social Subjects No. 12. HMSO, 1977.
5. Waterlow, J. C., and Thomson, A. M., Observations on the adequacy of breast feeding. *Lancet* **2**, 238 (1979).
6. Hytten, F. E., Individual differences in milk composition. *Br. Med. J.* **1**, 253 (1954).
7. Lucas, A., Lucas, P., and Baum, J. D., Pattern of milk flow in breast-fed infants. *Lancet* **2**, 57 (1979).
8. Lucas, P., personal communication.
9. Drewett, R. F., and Woolridge, M., Sucking Patterns of Human Babies on the Breast, in *Early Human Development.* **3**, 315 (1979).
10. Woolridge, M., Baum, J. D., and Drewett, R. F., Effect of a traditional and a new nipple shield on sucking patterns and milk flow. *Early Human Development.* 1980 in press.
11. Lucas, A., Lucas, P., and Baum, J. D., The nipple-shield sampling system: a device for measuring the dietary intake of breast fed infants. *Early Human Development.* 1980 in press.
12. Lucas, A., Gibbs, J. A. H., Lyster, R. L. J., and Baum, J. D., Creamatocrit: sample clinical technique for estimating fat concentration and energy value of human milk. *Br. Med. J.* **1**, 1018 (1978).
13. How, T. V., Ashmore, M. P., Rolfe, P., Lucas A., Lucas P., and Baum, J. D., A Doppler untrasound technique for measuring human milk flow. *J. Med. Eng. Technol.* **3**, 66 (1979).

22

Phagocytes of Human Colostrum and Their Function

M. XANTHOU,[1] M.D., E. MANDYLA-SFAGOU,[2] M.D., C. MARAVELIAS,[3] M.A., J. D. BAUM,[4] M.A., M.Sc., M.D., FRCP, DCH, and N. MATSANIOTIS,[5] M.D.

INTRODUCTION

There is now growing information documenting that human breast milk is superior to cow's milk in minimizing both the morbidity and mortality of infants.[6, 7, 36, 43] This is more obvious in the less affluent and less informed populations of the world[3, 13] and as Mendelsohn (1971)[25] puts it "... if one consciously sets out to kill infants of the poor, he might begin by persuading or forcing their mothers to artificially feed them." Breast-feeding protects infants against a variety of illnesses including intestinal infections,[5, 40] respiratory infections,[10, 36] and necrotizing enterocolitis.[27, 41] The immunological factors in human milk that offer resistance against infection to the neonates are summarized in several review articles.[33, 35, 42]

The white cells of human colostrum, although first observed in 1839 by the biologist-microscopist-photographer Alexander Donné,[9] have only quite recently attracted the attention of immunologists and neonatologists. Thus it was Smith in Goldman's laboratory who rediscovered them in 1966.[38] These cells were found to be present at concentrations of 0.5–10 million cells/ml in colostrum and comprise macrophages 30–85%, polymorphonuclears 1–80%, and

[1] Associate Professor of Paediatrics, Director of the Newborn Intensive Care Unit, First Department of Paediatrics, Athens University
[2] Registrar of the Newborn Intensive Care Unit, First Department of Paediatrics, Athens University
[3] Research Registrar in Physiology, Newborn Instensive Care Unit, First Department of Paediatrics, Athens University
[4] Clinical Reader in Paediatrics, University of Oxford, John Radcliffe Hospital, Oxford
[5] Professor and Chairman of the First Department of Paediatrics, Athens University

T and B lymphocytes 1–15%.[23] The maternal milk contains a much smaller number of milk cells; however, the increasing volume of milk compensates for this change.[23]

Regarding the function of milk white cells largely the lymphocyte population has been studied.[8, 29, 39] The lymphocyte population, though relatively small, appears to the quite significant in function. Thus milk lymphocytes were shown to respond weakly to nonspecific mitogens[8, 29] and to histocompatibility antigens on allogeneic cells.[29] They were also shown to respond quite well to a number of microbial antigens not necessarily the same to which blood lymphocytes from the same person respond.[28, 29] This dichotomy of reactivity appears to reflect the accumulation of particular lymphocyte clones in the breast and the nature of mammary tissue immunity at the T-lymphocyte level.[28]

Macrophages which represent the majority of cells found in human milk have been studied far less. The monocytic phagocytes are lipid laden motile cells which adhere to glass.[38] They have Fc receptors and C_3b receptors and contain intracellular IgA.[32] They are responsible for the synthesis of several host resistance factors of milk, including lysozyme, C_3 and C_4 complement components, and lactoferrin.[16, 32] Two recent studies performed to test the ability of milk phagocytes (macrophages, polymorphonuclear neutrophils) to phagocytose and kill pathogenic organisms have given contradicting results. Robinson, et al. (1978)[37] found macrophages and neutrophils to phagocytose and kill Staph aureus and E. coli in vitro after opsonization by the aqueous phase of milk very efficiently. On the other hand Ho and Lawton (1978)[18] found good phagocytic power of colostral cells but poor killing activity of E. coli.

The aim of the present work was to further study the function of colostral monocytes and polymorphonuclear neutrophils. We tested their ability to elicit antibody-dependent cellular cytotoxicity, i.e., their ability to kill antibody coated target cells in vitro.

MATERIALS AND METHODS

Collection of Colostrum

Colostrum was obtained from 16 women within the first 5 days following delivery. Mothers manually expressed their milk into sterile plastic containers. The samples were brought to the laboratory within 1 hr of collection

Preparation of Colostal Cells

Because of the high fat content of colostrum the usual procedures for identification of the white cells in the peripheral blood could not be applied. Consequently, alternate methods were devised. Samples were centrifuged at 200 g for 25 min. During centrifugation the milk separated into three layers, a cell pellet, a middle layer, and a fat layer. After the middle and fat layers had been removed, the cell pellet was washed twice in Eagle's basal medium (BME) and resuspended in the same tissue culture medium plus 10% foetal calf serum (FCS). The cells were then centrifuged through a Ficoll-Hypaque gradient by the method of Böyum (1968).[2] They were then again washed twice in BME prior to their use in the lytic assay, resuspended in BME + FCS, and counted in a haemocytometer. The viability of cells in suspension was tested after staining the dead cells with trypan blue. Smears were prepared and stained with May-Grünwald-Giemsa.

Preparation of Monocyte-Enriched Colostral Cells

In order to further separate colostral monocytes, equal parts of colostrum and culture medium BME + 10% FCS were incubated for 4 hr in nonsiliconized glass flasks. The cultures were incubated at 37°C in 5% CO_2. Following incubation, the supernatant fluid was removed and the glass adherent cellular layer on the base of the flask was first rinsed with culture medium and then the cells were removed with Trypsin 0.25%. The cells were then washed with BME + 10% FCS and resuspended in the same medium.

Cytochemical Identification of Monocytes and Granulocytes

We used the combined method for nonspecific esterase and chloroacetate esterase in order to demonstrate monocytes and granulocytes simultaneously on the same cytologic preparation.[46] This was done by using α-naphthyl acetate esterase as substrate for staining nonspecific esterase of monocytes and naphthol-AS-D-chloroacetate esterase for staining chloroacetate esterase of granulocytes.

Preparation of Blood Leucocytes

Eight mls of heparinized venous blood was obtained from 11 healthy adult volunteers and 3 ml from 12 healthy premature neonates 3–15 days old. Lymphocyte and monocyte mixtures were isolated on Ficoll-Hypaque gradient by the method of Böyum (1968).[2] They were then washed twice in BME.

Human Immune Anti-A_1 Serum

This was a gift from North West Thames Blood Transfusion Center. It had a heamaglutinic titre of 1:2048 against human A_1 erythrocytes. It was heat inactivated at 56° for 1 hr, and the same batch was used in all experiments.

Target Cells

A_1 erythrocytes were obtained from a constant donor and were washed twice with BME with heparin before they were labeled with radioactive chromium.

Labeling of Target Cells with Cr^{51}

A pellet of approximately 10^8 A_1 erythrocytes was incubated with 100 μCi of [^{51}Cr]chromate (Radio-Chemical Center Amersham, Bucks, specific activity 2–

10 mCi/mM) for 1 hr. They were then washed three times with BME and suspended in BME + FCS at a concentration of 2×10^5/ml.

Haemolytic Assay

The method used was similar to that described by Holm, *et al.* (1974).[20] A varying number of colostral phagocytes (ranging from 0.125×10^6 to 4×10^6) in 0.5 ml of BME + FCS were added to sterile plastic tubes containing 10^5 A$_1$ erythrocytes and antiserum to a total volume of 1.5 ml. The tubes were capped and incubated for 18 hrs at 37°C. After 18 hr the radioactivity of the cell-free supernatant and sediment was determined separately and the percentage of isotope release and the specific cytotoxicity were calculated as described by Brunner, *et al.* (1968).[4] Assays were done in triplicate and the following controls were included in each experiment: target cells only, target and effector cells, target cells and antiserum only.

RESULTS

Cells of Human Colostrum

The colostral cells were mainly mononuclear macrophages, polymorphonuclear neutrophils, and lymphocytes. Morphologically, the polymorphonuclear neutrophils were typical of those seen in peripheral blood except that they contained numerous fat globules (Fig. 1). Monocytes or macrophages were mononuclear cells with abundant cytoplasm containing many fat globules and other granular material (Fig. 2). Lymphocytes were found to be of various sizes similar to those found in the blood (Fig. 2). Because of the fat ingestion it was

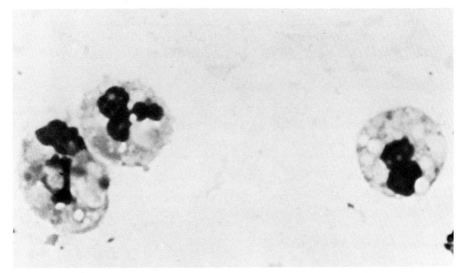

Fig. 1. Colostral neutrophils containing fat vacuoles. (May- Grünwald Giemsa stain).

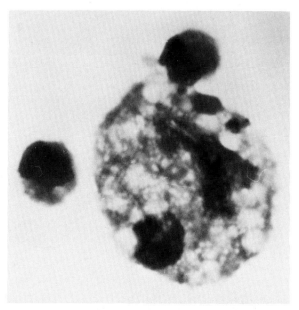

Fig. 2. A macrophage containing fat vacuoles and granular material in the cytoplasm. One of the two lymphocytes around it is shown to have a typical lymphocyte-macrophage interaction. (May-Grünwald-Giemsa stain).

very difficult to differentiate polymorphonuclear neutrophils from monocytes with the usual May-Grünwald-Giemsa stain. We therefore used cytochemical methods for staining nonspecific esterase of monocytes and chloroacetate esterase of granulocytes. With the double staining used, granulocytes showed red granulation while monocytes showed black granulation, and thus we had no difficulty in distinguishing them (Fig. 3). Apart from the cells already described, occasional epithelial cells and epithelial cell fragments were found in colostrum.

After the colostal white cells were separated and passed through Ficoll-Hypaque gradient, they gave a differential count of 50–60% monocytes, 30–40% polymorphonuclear neutrophils, and up to 5% lymphocytes. Our monocyte-enriched colostral white cell preparation gave a monocyte purity of around 90%. It is of interest that after 4 hr incubation these cells had lost most of their fat globules (Fig. 4).

Leucocytes of Adult and Neonatal Peripheral Blood

After passing the cells through Ficoll-Hypaque gradient the differential counts of the white cells obtained consisted of 80–90% lymphocytes, 10–20% monocytes, and 0–2% polymorphonuclear neutrophils.

Antibody-Dependent Cytotoxicity of Colostrum Phagocytes

As shown in Figure 5, colostral monocytes and polymorphonuclear neutrophils have the ability to function quite well in antibody-dependent cell-medi-

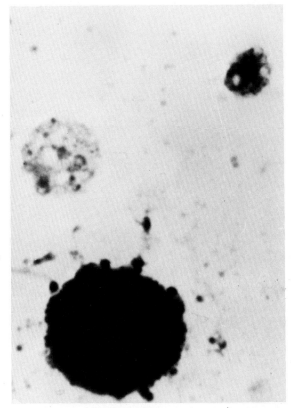

Fig. 3. a. A monocyte stained with an α-naphthyl acetate and showing diffuse black granulation. b. A polymorphonuclear neutrophil stained with naphthol-AS-D chloracetate esterase and showing red granulation. (↓)

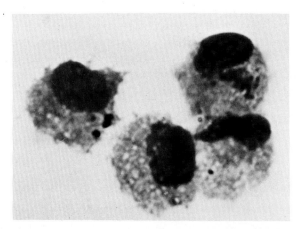

Fig. 4. Colostral monocytes after 4 hr incubation at 37°C.

ated cytotoxicity. The effector/target cell ratios we used were 1:1, 2.5:1, 5:1, 10:1, 20:1, and 40:1. The specific cytotoxicity of colostral phagocytes increased as the effector/target cell ratio rose from 1:1 to 20:1 ($p < 0.001$). Further increase in effector cells (1:40) caused a significant fall in cytotoxicity ($p < 0.05$).

Antibody-Dependent Cytotoxicity of Colostrum and Peripheral Blood Monocytes

There was no difference in the ability of neonatal and adult peripheral blood monocytes to function in antibody-dependent cytotoxicity (Fig. 6). Colostrum monocytes, however, showed a reduced cytotoxic capacity when compared to those of adult ($p < 0.001$) or neonatal blood ($p < 0.001$) at a low effector/target cell ratio (1:1).

DISCUSSION

We studied the colostral-phagocytes function by testing their ability to elicit antibody dependent cellular cytotoxicity (ADCC). This test in peripheral blood monocytes of adults has proved to be a very useful quantitative and qualitative assay of their function.[34] This cytotoxicity involves the specific killing of

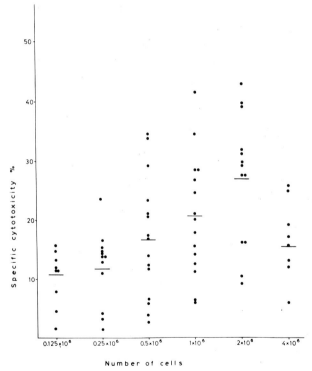

Fig. 5. Antibody-dependent-cytotoxicity of colostral monocytes and polymorphonuclear neutrophils.

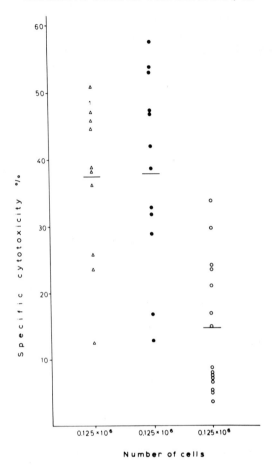

Fig. 6. Antibody-dependent cytotoxicity of colostral and peripheral blood monocytes of adults and neonates. Δ = adult monocytes; ● = neonatal monocytes; ○ = colostral monocytes.

antibody-coated target cells by nonimmune effector cells which have in common the presence of a receptor for the Fc portion of IgG antibody.[30] In man, lymphocytes,[31] null cells or K cells,[44, 45] polymorphonuclear leukocytes,[12] and monocytes and macrophages[19] have all been shown to be capable of mediating ADCC against appropriate target cells. The type of target cell and the source of antibody appear to dictate the nature of the effector cells mediating cytolysis.[24] Lysis of human erythrocytes in the presence of immune isoantibody has been reported to be effected by monocytes and polymorphonuclear leucocytes but not by lymphocytes.[14, 21, 24]

    We have found that colostral monocytes and polymorphonuclear neutrophils have the ability to function in antibody-dependent cellular cytotoxicity. Although there are a few studies on milk colostral phagocytes' ability to ingest and kill pathogenic microorganisms,[18, 37] their ability to elicit ADCC has not been tested as far as we know.

We subsequently tried to compare ADCC of monocytes taken from the peripheral blood of adults or neonates and colostrum.

We found no difference between adult and neonatal peripheral blood monocytes in their ability to elicit ADCC. Two previous studies, using cord blood monocytes as effector cells and human erythrocytes[26] or herpes-simplex-virus-infected Chang liver cells[22] as targets, showed good ADCC. We have found no study about this particular monocyte function during the neonatal period.

We found colostral monocytes to have a reduced cytotoxic capacity when compared with those of adult or neonatal peripheral blood. Gale and Zighelboim (1975)[12] suggested that antibody-dependent lysis by polymorphonuclear neutrophils is an extracellular event whereas the studies of Holm and Hammarström (1973)[21] and Gill, et al. (1977)[14] suggested that phagocytosis is an important component of monocyte mediated lysis. If this is so, the ingestion of lipid by milk monocytes may be the cause of their reduced killing power. It has been suggested that the ingestion of lipid results in disruption of lysosomes and depletion of lysosomal enzymes. Moreover, Holm and Hammarström (1973)[21] have shown that loading of peripheral blood monocytes with heat-killed Candida albicans or carbonyl iron particles suppressed their haemolytic action. However, there are other studies claiming that monocytes are capable of mediating cytolysis through an extracellular lytic process.[17, 46] At the present time, the mechanism by which normal monocytes destroy antibody-coated erythrocytes is not completely understood.

The reduced monocyte cytotoxicity could also be attributed to other colostral factors analogous to those which cause the lymphocytes of the colostrum to show a reduced response to PHA.[8] Finally the fat globules which are attached to the monocyte surface may block the contact of their Fc receptors to the antibody coated erythrocytes.

Although colostral monocytes have a lower cytotoxic ability when compared to that elicited by peripheral blood monocytes, colostral phagocytes show good activity in this type of function particularly at an effector/target cell ratio of 20:1. What is the significance of this colostral leucocyte function *in vivo*? Pitt (1977)[32] in an elegant study demonstrated in a rat model that Klebsiella-induced necrotizing enterocolitis could be prevented by feeding rat colostral macrophages but not by feeding the soluble colostral factors. Similar experiments have not been performed in human neonates, but epidemiological studies have shown that necrotizing enterocolitis is a very infrequent disease of infants fed with untreated breast milk.[27, 41] There is no doubt that there is a definite biological significance in the living functional phagocytes of the human colostrum; however, further studies are needed to clarify it.

SUMMARY

Monocytes and polymorphonuclear neutrophils of human colostrum were identified using cytochemical staining procedures.

The ability of colostral phagocytes to function in antibody-dependent cellular cytotoxicity (ADCC) was found to be satisfactory at a high effector/target cell ratio (20:1).

Colostal monocytes, however, showed a diminished cytotoxicity when compared to monocytes of adult or neonatal peripheral blood at a low effector/target cell ratio (1:1). This could be due to the extensive fat ingestion by these cells.

REFERENCES

1. Beer, A. E., and Billingham, R. E., Immunologic benefits and hazards of milk in maternal-perinatal relationships. *Ann. Int. Med.* **83**, 865 (1975).
2. Böyum, A., Isolation of mononuclear cells and granulocytes from human blood. Isolation of mononuclear cells by one centrifugation and of granulocytes by combined centrifugation and sedimentation at Ig. *Scand. J. Clin. Lab. Invest.* **21** (*Suppl.* 97), 77 (1968).
3. Brown, R. E., Breast feeding in modern times. *Am. J. Clin. Nutr.* **26**, 556 (1973).
4. Brunner, K. T., Manel, J., Cerottini, J. C., and Chapuis, B., Quantitative assay of the lytic action of immune lymphoid cells on Cr^{51} labeled allogeneic target cells in vitro. Inhibition by isoantibody and by drugs. *Immunology* **14**, 181 (1968).
5. Bullen, C. C., and Willis, A. T., Resistance of the breast-fed infant to gastroenteritis. *Br. Med. J.* **3**, 338 (1971).
6. Cunningham, A. S., Morbidity in breast-fed and artificially fed infants. *J. Pediat.* **90**, 726 (1977).
7. Cunningham, A. S., Morbidity in breast-fed and artificially fed infants II. *J. Pediatr.* **95**, 685 (1979).
8. Diaz-Jouanen, E., and Williams, R. C., T and B lymphocytes in human colostrum. *Clin. Immunol. Immunopathol.* **3**, 248 (1974).
9. Donné, A., *Cours de microscopie*, Vol. 1 and Atlas No. 1. Baillière, Paris, 1844–45.
10. Downham, M. A. P. S., Scott, R., Sims, D. G., Webb, J. K. G., and Gardner P. S., Breast-feeding protects against respiratory syncytial virus infections. *Br. Med. J.* **2**, 273 (1976).
11. Gale, P. R., and Zighelboim, J., Polymorphonuclear leucocytes in antibody-dependent cellular cytotoxicity. *J. Immunol.* **114**, 1047 (1975).
12. Gale, P. R., and Zighelboim, J., Modulation of polymorphonuclear leucocyte-mediated antibody-dependent cellular cytotoxicity. *J. Immunol.* **113**, 1973 (1974).
13. Gerrard, J. W., Breast feeding: second thoughts. *Pediatrics* **54**, 757 (1974).
14. Gill, P. G., Waller, C. A., and MacLennan, I. C. M., Relationships between different functional properties of human monocytes. *Immunology* **33**, 873 (1977).
15. Golde, D. W., Territo, M., Finley, T. N., and Cline, M. J., Defective lung macrophages in pulmonary alveolar-proteinosis. *Ann. Intern. Med.* **85**, 304 (1976).
16. Goldman, A. S., and Smith, C. W., Host resistance factors in human milk. *J. Pediatr.* **82**, 1082 (1973).
17. Hibbs, J. B., Heterocytolysis by macrophages activated by Bacillus Calmette-Guerin. Lysosome exocytosis into tumor cells. *Science* **184**, 468 (1974).
18. Ho, P. C., and Lawton, J. W. M., Human colostral cells: Phagocytosis and killing of E. coli and C. albicans. *J. Pediatr.* **93**, 910 (1978).
19. Holm, G., Lysis of antibody-treated human erythrocytes by human leukocytes and macrophages in tissue culture. *Int. Arch. Allergy* **43**, 671 (1972).
20. Holm, G., Engwall, E., Hammarström, S., and Natvig, J. B., Antibody-induced haemolytic activity of human blood monocytes. The role of antibody class and subclass. *Scand. J. Immunol.* **3**, 173 (1974).
21. Holm, G., and Hammarström, S., Haemolytic activity of human blood monocytes. Lysis of human erythrocytes treated with anti-A-serum. *Clin. Exp. Immunol.* **13**, 29 (1973).
22. Kohl, S., Shaban, S. S., Starr, S. E., Wood, P. A., and Nahmias, A. J., Human neonatal and maternal monocyte-macrophage and lymphocyte-mediated antibody-dependent cytotoxicity to cells infected with herpes simplex. *J. Pediatr.* **93**, 206 (1978).
23. Lawton, J. W. M., and Shortridge, K. F., Protective factors in human breast milk and colostrum. *Lancet* **1**, 253 (1977).

24. MacDonald, H. R., Bonnard, G. D., Sordat, B., and Zawodnik, S. A., Antibody-dependent cell-mediated cytotoxicity. Heterogeneity of effector cells in human peripheral blood. *Scand. J. Immunol.* **4**, 487 (1975).

25. Mendelsohn, R. S., In Defence of Laleche, in *Chicago Tribune* June 9, 1971.

26. Milgrom, H., and Shore, S. L., Assessment of monocyte function in the normal newborn infant by antibody-dependent cellular cytotoxicity. *J. Pediatr.* **91**, 612 (1977).

27. Mizzawi, A., Barlow, O., Berdon, W., Blanc, W. A., and Silverman, W. A., Necrotizing enterocolitis in premature infants. *J. Pediatr.* **66**, 697 (1965).

28. Parmely, M. J., and Beer, A. E., Colostral cell-mediated immunity and the concept of a common secretory immune system. *J. Dairy Sci.* **60**, 655 (1976).

29. Parmely, M. J., Beer, A. E., and Billingham, R. E., In vitro studies on the T-lymphocyte population of human milk. *J. Exp. Med.* **144**, 358 (1976).

30. Perlman, P., and Holm, G., Cytotoxic effects of lymphoid cells in vitro. *Adv. Immunol.* **11**, 117 (1969).

31. Perlman, P., Perlman, H., and Wigzell, H., Lymphocyte mediated cytotoxicity in vitro: Induction and inhibition by humoral antibody and nature of effector cells. *Transplant Rev.* **13**, 91 (1972).

32. Pitt, J., The milk mononuclear phagocyte. *Pediatrics Suppl.* **64**, 745 (1979).

33. Pittard, W. B., Breast milk immunology. *Am. J. Dis. Child.* **133**, 83 (1979).

34. Poplack, D. G., Bonnard, G. D., Holiman, B. J., and Blaese, R. M., Monocyte mediated antibody-dependent cellular cytotoxicity: A clinical test of monocyte function. *Blood* **48**, 809 (1976).

35. Relter, B., Review of the progress of Dairy Science: Antimicrobial systems in milk. *J. Dairy Res.* **45**, 131 (1978).

36. Robinson, M., Infant morbidity and mortality. *Lancet* **210**, 788 (1951).

37. Robinson, J. E., Harvey, B. A. M., and Soothill, J. F., Phagocytosis and killing of bacteria and yeast by human milk cells after opsonization in aqueous phase of milk. *Br. Med. J.* **1**, 1443 (1978).

38. Smith, C. W., and Goldman, A. S., The cells of human colostrum. I. In vitro studies of morphology and functions. *Pediatr. Res.* **2**, 103 (1968).

39. Smith, C. W., Goldman, A. S., and Yates, R. D., Interactions of lymphocytes and macrophages from human colostrum. Electron microscopic studies of the interacting lymphocyte. *Exp. Cell. Res.* **69**, 409 (1971).

40. Svirsky-Cross, S., Pathogenic strains of E. coli (0:111) among prematures and the use of human milk in controlling the outbreak of diarrhea. *Ann. Pediatr.* **190**, 109 (1968).

41. Touloukian, R., Berton, W., Amoury, R., and Santulli, T. V., Surgical experience with necrotizing enterocolitis. *J. Pediatr. Surg.* **2**, 389 (1967).

42. Welsh, J. K., and May, J. T., Anti-infective properties of breast milk. *J. Pediatr.* **94**, 1 (1979).

43. Winberg, J., and Wessmer, G., Does breast milk protect against septicaemia in the newborn? *Lancet* **1**, 1091 (1971).

44. Wisløff, F., Frøland, S. S., and Michaelson, T. E., Antibody-dependent cytotoxicity mediated by human Fc-receptor-bearing cells lacking markers for B and T-lymphocytes. *Int. Arch. Allergy Appl. Immunol.* **47**, 139 (1974).

45. Xanthou, M., Mandyla-Sfagou, E., Campbell, A. C., Waller, C. A., Economou-Mavrou, C., and Matsaniotis, N., Lymphocyte Subpopulations and Their Function in the Blood of Neonates, in *Intensive Care in the Newborn. I*, Stern, L., Friis-Hansen, B., and Kildeberg, P., Eds. Masson, New York, 1976.

46. Yam, L. T., Li, C. Y., and Crosby, W. H., Cytochemical identification of monocytes and granulocytes. *Am. J. Clin. Pathol.* **55**, 283 (1971).

23

Withdrawal from Methadone by Breast Feeding

J. STEPHEN ROBINSON, DON H. CATLIN, and CYNTHIA T. BARRETT

Neonatal abstinence syndrome from methadone is generally recognized to be more severe and more prolonged than withdrawal from heroin. In addition, significant symptoms of narcotic withdrawal occur in almost 100% of babies following antenatal exposure to methadone in contrast with approximately 75% of babies with antenatal exposure to heroin.[6] Breast feeding by mothers receiving methadone has not been recommended because this agent passes in high concentration into breast milk.[5] In addition, many people in a methadone maintenance program are frequent or occasional users of other potentially dangerous agents which might also be found in breast milk. We have recently had the opportunity to follow three babies whose methadone abstinence was treated with no drugs other than methadone ingested in breast milk. In one of these we were able to measure methadone in mother's milk and baby's urine during the first 4 weeks after delivery and at 6 weeks in mother's milk, plasma and urine, and in the baby's urine over a 24-hr period.

MATERIALS AND METHODS

The three babies were delivered at term with birth weights ranging from 2800 to 4280 g to mothers receiving 40–75 mg methadone daily. All babies had frequent assessments utilizing a neonatal abstinence score developed by Finnegan.[3] None developed significant signs or symptoms of drug withdrawal during the period that they were receiving their mothers's milk, and their mothers were receiving methadone maintenance therapy. One mother was

Departments of Medicine, Pharmacology and Pediatrtics, UCLA School of Medicine, Los Angeles, California 90024

detoxified during a 1-week period when her baby was 3 weeks old, and the other two mothers weaned their infants between 4 and 6 months of age by gradually replacing breast feedings with bottle feedings during a 6-week period.

One mother and baby, after signing appropriate consent forms approved by the Human Subject Protection Committee, were admitted to the Clinical Research Center at the UCLA Hospital and Clinics 6 weeks after delivery for 24 hr, and measurements of methadone concentration in the mother's urine, plasma, and milk and in the infant's urine and plasma were determined at approximately 4-hr intervals. In addition, random samples of mother's milk and infant's urine were analyzed for methadone concentration during the first 4 weeks of life. The concentration of methadone in body fluids was determined by gas chromatography/mass spectrometry. Results are reported as nM/ml body fluid.

RESULTS

Clinical Outcome

The two children who were withdrawn from breast feedings over a gradual period never had any signs or symptoms of narcotic abstinence. The baby whose mother was removed from methadone maintenance 3 weeks after delivery became hyperirritable and had decreased sleep for 3–4 weeks, but did not require medication other than the diazepam prescribed for her mother which was secreted in the breast milk.

Figure 1 shows methadone concentrations in mother's milk and baby's urine obtained at random times during the first 4 weeks after delivery. The first voided specimen of the baby after delivery contained 3.332 nM/ml methadone. At 12 hr of age the concentration was 0.36 nM/ml or approximately 10% of the initial value, and this gradually fell to a concentration between 0.01 and 0.05 nM/ml by 4 weeks of age. In contrast, colostrum obtained on the day of delivery had a methadone concentration of 0.248 nM/ml and thereafter was in the range of 0.25 to 0.40 nM/ml, showing very little change during this period.

Figure 2 shows serial concentrations of methadone in mother's urine, mother's plasma, mother's milk, and baby's urine during the 24-hr study 6 weeks after delivery. Although samples of baby's plasma were also analyzed, concentrations were at all times below 0.001 nM/ml, the level of detectability. Following the oral administration of methadone (45 mg) at 0815 hours, each of the body fluids showed an increase in the concentration of methadone for approximately 4 hr, followed by a gradual decline during the 20 subsequent hours. On two occasions, 8/1 at 0400 and 0800, samples of milk were obtained at the beginning and end of the feedings to determine if methadone concentration changed during a feeding; on both occasions the concentrations at these times were similar. At 0400 methadone concentration was slightly lower at the beginning of the feeding, and at 0800 it was lower at the end of the feeding. Unfortunately, portions of several of the baby's urine specimens were lost; therefore, the total amount of nonmetabolized methadone excreted by the

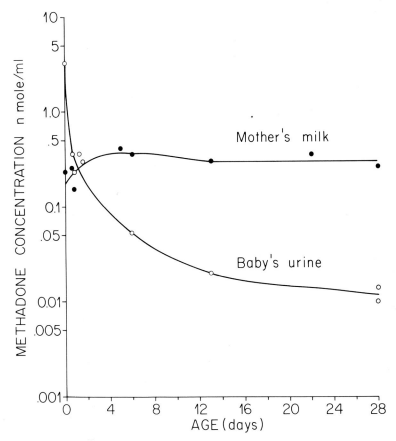

Fig. 1. Concentrations of unchanged methadone (nM/ml) measured in specimens of mother's milk (closed circle) and baby's urine (open circle) are shown during the first 4 weeks after delivery.

baby could not be determined. Similarly, intake could not be precisely quantified. If, however, one assumes that the baby, weighing 5 kg, consumed 700 cc, equally divided among his seven feedings, he would have received approximately 53 μg methadone during the 24-hr period.

DISCUSSION

Many problems exist during the neonatal period for the infant and its mother who are addicted to methadone. The narcotic abstinence syndrome observed with methadone is more severe, may last longer, and have a later onset than that with heroin. Because of the severity of methadone withdrawal, most infants delivered to women in a methadone maintenance program will be admitted to a special care rather than a normal nursery and will remain in the hospital for approximately 2 weeks. In addition, almost all will receive pharmacologic agents to treat the signs and symptoms of their abstinence. Both of these factors may interfere with mother-infant bonding. Our three babies, who

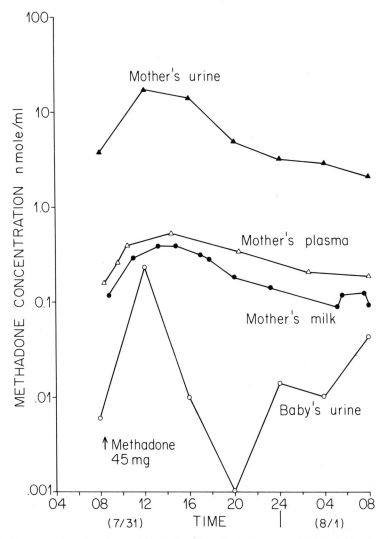

Fig. 2. Concentrations of unchanged methadone (*n* moles/ml) measured in mother's urine (closed triangle), mother's plasma (open triangle), mother's milk (closed circle), and baby's urine (open circle) are shown during a 24-hr period (7/31–8/1). Methadone (45 mg) was administered orally to the mother at 0815, 7/31.

received no pharmacologic agents other than what was present in their mothers' milk, showed no signs or symptoms of methadone withdrawal. They were all cared for in normal nurseries following birth, and all were discharged, asymptomatic, with their mothers at 2–3 days of age.

There are several risks inherent in permitting mothers in a methadone maintenance program to breast feed their babies. Many addicts in methadone maintenance programs use or abuse other legal and illegal substances and thus put a nursing infant at increased risk. In addition, unknown risks may be present in children whose methadone dependence continues into infancy rather than ending with delivery.

The metabolism of methadone in the pregnant woman and her offspring has been studied only sporadically.[1, 2, 4] The agent has been measured in amniotic fluid, cord blood, and neonatal urine. It is extensively metabolized in the liver and excreted in the urine both as unchanged methadone and as metabolites. It is also extensively tissue-bound which tends to prolong its half-life. Thus the newly born infant, with considerable tissue-bound methadone and a decreased capability to metabolize drugs, may have significant amounts of methadone for weeks and thus have a prolonged course or a late onset of symptoms of methadone abstinence. From the concentration-time curve of the baby's urine shown in Figure 1, it is apparent that a steady state was probably not achieved until the fifth week of life.

Although the dose of methadone ingested by the infant in his milk was probably small, 50–100 μg/day, this baby was completely free of symptoms of narcotic abstinence. In addition, he demonstrated none of the behavioral disturbances that have been reported in infants receiving more usual therapeutic regimens of barbiturates, diazepam, or phenothiazine.

CONCLUSIONS

Management of infants delivered to mothers addicted to methadone must include pharmacologic agents to treat symptoms of narcotic abstinence. Breast feeding by mothers receiving methadone is usually not encouraged because of the risk that the mother may also be taking other mood-altering pharmacologic agents which could compromise the well-being of her infant. In addition, potential risks of maintaining an infant on methadone during infancy are unknown. In a selected population, however, that can be followed closely, management of the infant by breast feeding alone can avert symptoms of narcotic withdrawal. It is imperative, however, that the mother not be detoxified over a short period of time and that withdrawal from breast feeding be a very gradual process. We have found that 2–3 weeks seems to be a safe weaning period.

SUMMARY

We have successfully treated infants with antenatal exposure to methadone with methadone administered in breast milk. None had symptoms of narcotic abstinence while on this treatment regimen. One mother and baby studied during the first 6 weeks of life with measurements of methadone in maternal milk and infant's urine demonstrated that a steady state was attained by approximately 4 weeks after delivery. In some instances, breast feeding may be an appropriate way to treat infants with antenatal methadone exposure as it may potentially augment mother-infant bonding and avoid morbidity from the side effects of conventionally administered pharmacologic agents.

REFERENCES

1. Blinick, G., Inturrisi, C. E., Jerez, E., and Wallach, R. C., Amniotic fluid methadone in women maintained on methadone. *Mt. Sinai J. Med.* **41,** 254 (1974).
2. Blinick, G., Inturrisi, C. E., Jerez, E., and Wallach, R. C., Methadone assays in pregnant women and progeny. *Am. J. Obstet. Gynecol.* **121,** 617 (1975).
3. Finnegan, L. P., Connaughton, J. F., Kron, R. E., and Emich, J. P., Neonatal Abstinence Syndrome: Assessment and Management, in *Perinatal Addiction,* Harbison, R. D., Ed. Spectrum Publications, New York, 1975, pp. 141–158.
4. Kreek, M. J., Schecter, A., Gutjahr, C. L., Bowen, D., Field, F., Queenan, J., and Merkatz, I., Analyses of methadone and other drugs in maternal and neonatal body fluids: use in evaluation of symptoms in a neonate of mother maintained on methadone. *Am. J. Drug Alcohol Abuse* **1,** 409 (1974).
5. Rothstein, P., and Gould, J. P., Born with a habit: infants of drug-addicted mothers. *Pediatr. Clin. North Am.* **21,** 307 (1974).
6. Zelson, C., Lee, S. J., and Casalino, M., Neonatal narcotic addiction: comparative effects of maternal intake of heroin and methadone. *N. Engl. J. Med.* **289,** 1216 (1973).

24

Energy Cost of Intravenous Alimentation in the Newborn Infant

TIBOR HEIM, M.D., Ph.D.,[1] GUY PUTET, M.D.,[2]
GASTON VERELLEN, M.D.,[3] PHILIPPE CHESSEX,
M.D.,[4] PAUL R. SWYER, M.A., M.B. (CANTAB)
F.R.C.P.(C),[5] JOHN M. SMITH, PhD., M.A.Sc.,[6] and
ROBERT M. FILLER, M.D.[7]

The nutritional problems of the newborn, especially those of premature infants, differ from those of children and adults for several reasons: (1) all nutrients must provide not only for energy and replacement of tissue but for rapid growth, involving not only the increase in size of all tissues but also substantial qualitative changes in body composition,[11-13, 26, 37, 42, 76, 77] (2) the metabolism of particular nutrients in many organs and tissues of the newborn or premature infant can be limited functionally in comparison with that of the child or adult,[46, 49, 75] and (3) many metabolic activities including heat loss and

[1] Visiting Professor of Pediatrics and Developmental Biology, Research Institute of Hospital for Sick Children, Department of Pediatrics, Medical Faculty, University of Toronto, Toronto, Ontario, Canada

[2] Research Fellow, Neonatal Division, Hospital for Sick Chilren, Department of Pediatrics, Medical Faculty, University of Toronto, Toronto, Ontario, Canada

[3] Research Fellow, Neonatal Division, Hospital for Sick Children, Department of Pediatrics, Medical Faculty, University of Toronto, Toronto, Ontario, Canada

[4] Research Fellow, Neonatal Division, Hospital for Sick Children Department of Pediatrics, Medical Faculty, University of Toronto, Toronto, Ontario, Canada

[5] Professor of Pediatrics, Director, Neonatal Division, Hospital for Sick Children, Department of Pediatrics, Medical Faculty, University of Toronto, Toronto, Ontario, Canada

[6] Director of the Department of Medical Engineering, Hospital for Sick Children, University of Toronto, Toronto, Ontario, Canada

[7] Professor of Surgery, Department of Surgery, Medical Faculty, University of Toronto, Head, Department of Pediatric Surgery, Hospital for Sick Children, Toronto, Ontario, Canada

energy requirements are closely related to body surface area. The ratio of surface area to body weight is exceptionally high in premature and small-for-gestational-age (SGA) newborn infants, thus nutritional requirements need to be adjusted accordingly.[9, 30-34, 38, 43]

For the past 3 years a series of studies has been conducted in newborn infants in which we have investigated the partition of metabolizable energy and nutrient intake for oxidation and deposition.[31, 59-62, 70, 73] Methods of experimental nutrition at the bedside under normal nursing conditions have been applied which permitted an extensive evaluation of different types of oral and intravenous nutritional regimes.[31, 70] The objective of this investigation has been to design a rational nutritional regime for very low birth weight and high-risk infants on total parenteral nutrition (TPN) by (1) estimation of coverage of the energy cost of resting and global metabolism by the three principal nutrients, i.e., carbohydrate, fat, and protein; (2) estimation of the desirable protein and fat deposition for maintenance and growth.

MATERIAL AND METHODS

The majority of subjects were surgical patients on total parenteral nutrition (TPN) (Table I). The study commenced 2 to 3 days postoperatively when the patient's physiological functions became stabilized.

The protocol for investigation of the metabolic effects of TPN was adapted to the actual treatment of the patient (Fig. 1). In *Phase I* the patients were alimented by glucose only or 10% glucose plus 2% amino acid infusion in the form of Amigen®, which is a casein hydrolysate. In order to design rational Intralipid® therapy without undesirable side effects, one day (*Phase II*) was devoted to testing the infant's capability for metabolising fat emulsion. After the Intralipid® utilization test the intravenous alimentation was continued with glucose/amino acid/Intralipid® infusion (*Phase III*).

To achieve these goals the following methods were used: nutrient balance for carbohydrate, protein, and fat; indirect calorimetry using a combination of the high sensitivity Pauling system based on the paramagnetic determination of oxygen concentrations[20, 45, 52] and the infrared carbon dioxide analyser for

TABLE I

Clinical Data of the Infants Subject to the Energy Metabolism Studies[a]

Gest. age (wk) $n = 30$	Birth weight (g) $n = 30$	Postnatal Age (days) (body weight at the time of tests, in g)		
		Phase I (GL or GL/AA) $n = 25$	Phase II (IL tests) $n = 14$	Phase III (GL/AA/IL) $n = 17$
36.3 ± 0.9	2615 ± 166	16.2 ± 3.6	19 ± 3.5	21 ± 4.1
		(2528 ± 170)	(2400 ± 243)	(2640 ± 140)

[a] Values given are $M \pm SE$; n = number of patients. Since not all patients went through each phase of the study, the numbers are different in Phase I, II, and III.

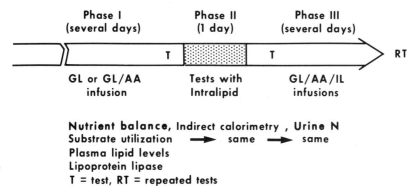

Fig. 1. The protocol for investigation of the metabolic effects of total parenteral nutrition (TPN).

CO_2 measurements; and timed urinary nitrogen output.[31, 70, 71] From these direct measurements substrate utilization could be calculated in each phase of our study.[54, 68, 69, 70] Some indices of lipid metabolism such as plasma lipid levels and lipoprotein lipase activity were assessed as well.[4, 5, 25, 34, 44, 55] The indirect calorimeter (Fig. 2) was built on rollers and could be moved from one ward to another and attached to the incubator in which the infant under study was nursed. The calorimeter used by us is attached to a Hewlett-Packard (Type 9845A desk-top) computer which permits on-line recording of the following data: CO_2 in sample, O_2 sample, CO_2 and O_2 concentration differences, air flow, temperatures from which heat storage can be eventually computed, heart rate, etc. (Fig. 3). Mean and standard deviation can be recalled for any given period of time.

The results can graphically be demonstrated on the TV monitor of the computer and are stored continuously on magnetic tapes or floppy disks. Each segment of the study can be visualized by printing out on the teletype (Fig. 4). A complete neonatal metabolic study thus contains the identification of the patient, anthropometric data, and substrate utilization for each minute or the whole day or whatever period of time the investigator happened to be interested in, computed on the chart (Fig. 5).

Finally, when laboratory results of the nutrient balance (intake–output) are ready and fed into the appropriate place of our computer programme, oxidation and tissue deposition for all three principal nutrients were calculated (Table II). When the intake from a particular nutrient was less than that of the oxidized portion, obviously the balance was derived from endogenous sources. In this case the lipids were being mobilized from adipose tissue.

RESULTS AND COMMENTS

In the next few figures selected examples will be presented on how nutritional adequacy can be measured by this technology in the very-low-birth-weight (VLBW) premature infant and how these results facilitate the design of suitable dietary regimes for infants fed intravenously.

One of the characteristic features of substrate utilization during Phase I, i.e.,

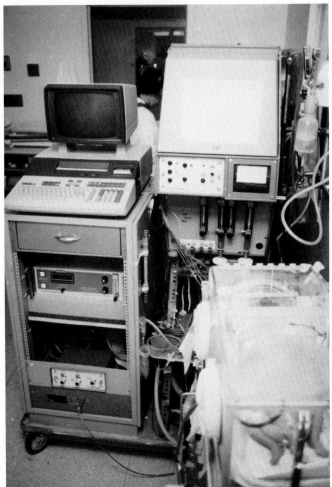

Fig. 2. Computerized indirect calorimeter assembled and programmed in the Department of Medical Engineering at the Hospital for Sick Children. The principal parts of the equipment: Taylor-Servomex (OA 184) dual channel paramagnetic oxygen analyser, Beckman LB_2 infrared carbon dioxide analyser, Fleisch pneumotachometer with Validyne transducer, and Hewlett-Packard (Type 9845 A) desk-top computer.

glucose (GL) or glucose/amino acid (GL/AA) infusion, is demonstrated in Figure 6. Caloric intake is plotted against the percentage of calories produced by oxidation of endogenous fat. A highly significant inverse relationship was found between caloric intake and endogenous fat oxidation with a correlation coefficient of 0.91.

Phase II of our protocol was devoted to test the capacity of the infant to oxidize exogenous lipids. The test was composed of three periods (Fig. 7). Prior to and during the first period lasting 3–4 hr, the infant received the GL/AA infusion at a steady caloric intake for at least 24 hr (2.4–3.9 kcal/kg/hr). Then the GL/AA infusion was replaced by an isocaloric and isovolumetric infusion

DATA SUMMARY FOR PERIOD ENDING   280 MINUTES

VARIABLE	MEAN	STAND. DEV
CO2 Sample	.5770	.0040
O2 Ref	20.8700	0.0000
O2 Sample	20.3150	.0027
O2 Diff	.5782	.0018
Flow (STP)	2628.9300	7.7712
T-Front	36.6171	.0008
T-Abdomen	36.9100	.0036
T-Upper Arm	36.2013	.0040
T-Thigh	36.2880	.0310
T-Hand	36.3379	.0166
T-Foot	35.3013	.0055
T-Core	37.0496	.0079
T-Hood	31.8940	.2707
T-Isolette	32.4733	.0022
T-Room	27.5104	.0032
Baro. Pressure	746.0000	
RH-Isolette	44.0000	
Heart Rate	166.0000	
CO2 Ref	.0450	
CO2 Diff	.5320	
RQ	.9010	
O2 Flow	6.7491	
CO2 Flow	6.0812	
T-Mean Skin	36.5126	
RH-Room	57.5697	

Fig. 3. Data actually measured by the indirect calorimeter and computed in every 20 sec by the on-line computer during the energy metabolism studies.

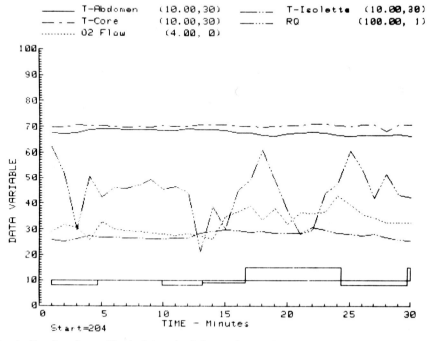

Fig. 4. Results of any 30-min interval of the study can be selected and visualized on the computer's screen.

```
Protday                  .753370786517
                    NEONATAL METABOLIC STUDY


    1.Date...........   2/2/79        2.Expt. No.......    14
    3.Name...........   Cooper        4.Chart No.......    1124850
    5.Sex............   f             6.Birthdate......    24/1/79
    7.Birth Wt. Kg...   3.5           8.Expt. Wt. Kg...    2.67
    9.Expt. Age......   9            10.Length cm......    47
   11.B.S.P..........   .189         12.Baro. Press....   750
   13.Rel. Humid. %..   61           14.CO2 Ref........   .056


              SUBSTRATE UTILISATION


       Parameters       Units/min      Units/day


       grams N2/kg        .0001           .1205
       Global VO2        6.8726         9896.60
       Global VCO2       5.5421         7980.61
       Global PO          .8064
       Grams CHO/kg       .0031           4.40
       Grams fat/kg       .0022           3.15
       Grams prot/kg      .0005           .75
       Met rate kcal/kg   .0330          47.59
       Met rate kcal/M2   .4669         672.28
       Heat prod kcal     .0882         127.06
       Time period                                    111.0
       Fract CHO                                         .34
       Fract fat                                         .66
```

Fig. 5. Chart of a complete energy metabolism study by computerized indirect calorimetry.

of Intralipid (IL) for 3–4 hr (2.1–3.5 ml/kg/hr). Finally, the same GL/AA infusion as in the first period was reinstated. $\dot{V}O_2$, $\dot{V}CO_2$, and deep colonic and mean skin temperatures were continuously measured and the infant's activity according to the Brück scale (−4 to +4) was recorded.[9, 70] The respiratory quotient was 0.91 during the GL/AA infusion, dropped quickly to 0.72 during Intralipid infusion, and increased slowly to the original level when the GL/AA infusion was reinstated. $\dot{V}O_2$ was 6.3 ml/kg/min on GL/AA, rose to 7.3 ml/kg/min during IL (15% increase), and returned to the initial level after reinstating GL/AA.

A thermic effect of lipid with rises in colonic and mean skin temperatures was usually present, resulting in a considerable heat storage 2.7 kcal/kg bwt (Fig. 8).

By determining the timed urinary nitrogen output and protein-free respiratory quotient the partition of utilization of the infused substrates could be calculated (Fig. 9). Although each test lasted 4–6 hr, the results are expressed in g/day/kg body weight for purposes of comparison and clarity. During the first period of GL/AA infusion approximately one-third of AA (0.9 of 2.7) and approximately three-fourths (10 of 13 g) of carbohydrate intake were oxidized, while 1 g of fat burned from endogenous sources. During the IL infusion some AA were oxidized (0.8 g) from the endogenous pool. The 2.3 g carbohydrate oxidized during IL Infusion was derived partially from the glycerol component of the infusion (1.4 g) and partially from endogenous sources (0.9 g). Two-

TABLE II

Partition of the Gross Energy Intake for Oxidation and Tissue Deposition of Carbohydrate, Fat, and Protein During Total Parenteral Nutrition in an Infant Receiving IV Alimentation by Glucose (10%) Plus Amino Acid (2%) Plus Intralipid (10%)[a]

Nutrient	Intake	Oxidized	Lost in Urine	Stored in Tissues
Calories (kcal/kg/day)[b]	77.33	47.85	0.83	28.65
Carbohydrate (g/kg/day)				
glucose	12.10	4.40	0.22	8.04
glycerol	0.56			
Amino acid (g/kg/day)	2.40	0.75	—	1.65
Fat (g/kg/day)	2.25	3.15	—	—

[a] The study period (as determined by the timed urinary nitrogen output) lasted 120 min, thus timed urinary nitrogen and glucose output could be determined. The urine collection and indirect calorimetry measurements were continued and each period of the study is computed in similar fashion. If the oxidized portion is greater than the intake, the balance is derived from endogenous sources, e.g.: in this study 0.9 g endogenous fat was oxidized which resulted in 8.1 Kcal energy loss from adinose tissue.

[b] Calorie equivalents of one gram of: Carbohydrate 3.75 (hydrous glucose); Amino Acid 4; Fat 9.

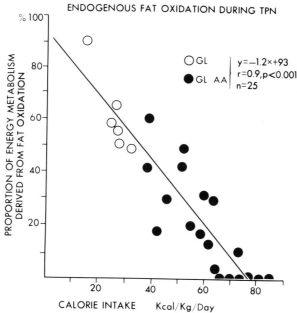

Fig. 6. Correlation between calorie intake and the percentage contribution of endogenous fat oxidation to the global energy metabolism of newborn infants ($n = 25$) on fat-free TPN: ○, glucose infusion ($n = 6$) ●, Glucose plus amino acid infusion ($n = 19$).

thirds of the infused IL was oxidized. It is equivalent to 4.2 g/kg/day fat oxidation. After return to the GL/AA infusion the intake, oxidation and storage were roughly the same as during the initial period.

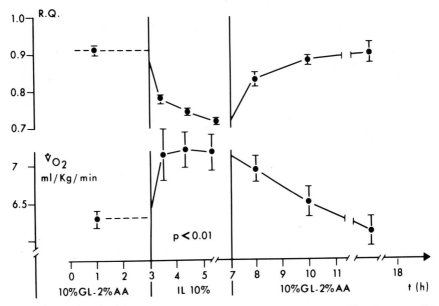

Fig. 7. Test designed for determination of the capacity of the patient to oxidize exogenous fatty acids. Two periods of amino acid (2%) plus glucose (10%) infusion (5–8 ml/kg/hr) was interrupted by a single 3–4 hr period of isocaloric (2.4–3.9 kcal/kg/hr) and isovolemic infusion of fat emulsion (10% Intralipid® 2.1–3.5 ml/kg/hr). To achieve isovolemia (5–8 ml/kg/hr) the Intralipid was diluted with physiologic saline. Oxygen consumption at STPD ($\dot{V}O_2$), and CO_2 production ml/kg/min and respiratory quotient (RQ) were calculated from those quiet periods when the Brück activity scale was −2 to −4.[9]

The relative distribution of nutrients oxidized during isocaloric infusion of AA/GL and IL is illustrated in Figure 10. During GL/AA 70% of the caloric production was derived from oxidation of carbohydrate, 22% from fat, and 8% from AA. During IL infusion there was a completely reversed situation: 75% of calories were produced by oxidation of fat, 18% by carbohydrate, and 7% by AA. During the repeated GL/AA infusion the results were similar to that of the initial GL/AA phase.

Whether the contribution of the particular nutrient to the energy metabolism is dependent on the calorie intake was analysed in Figure 11. The patients were divided into two groups: one was receiving less than 70 kcal/kg/day, the other more than 70 kcal/kg/day during isocaloric TPN with GL/AA, then with IL alone, and with GL/AA again. In infants receiving less than 70 kcal/kg/day as GL/AA, 30% of the energy metabolism was provided by endogenous fat oxidation. If the intake was increased to >70 kcal/kg/day with GL/AA infusion almost the total energy metabolism was maintained by glucose oxidation. In contrast, nearly equal proportions of fat were oxidized in the low (<70 kcal/kg/day) and the higher (>70 kcal/kg/day) caloric intake group.

When good endogenous and exogenous (above 60% of intake) fat oxidation was demonstrated during Phase I and Phase II, TPN with GL/AA/IL was recommended. Our measurements were also continued as Phase III. The

**CHANGE IN CORE AND MEAN SKIN TEMPERATURES
DURING ISOCALORIC INFUSION OF GLUCOSE AND
AMINO ACID OR INTRALIPID (n=12;M ± SE)**

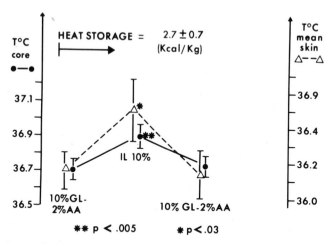

Fig. 8. Thermic effect of Intralipid® (10%) infusion for 3–4 hr at a rate 5–8 ml/kg body wt/hr. Changes in core, mean skin temperature, and heat storage are indicated.

INTAKE OXID. STORAGE OF IV NUTRIENTS (n=12)

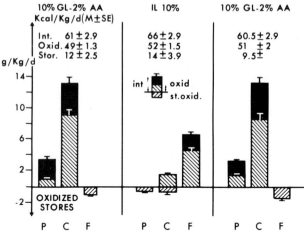

Fig. 9. Partition of utilization of the principal nutrients (P = protein, C = carbohydrate, F = fat) during the three periods of IV alimentation with glucose (10%) plus amino acid (Amigen® 2%), Intralipid® (10%), and glucose (10%) plus amino acid (Amigen 2%) again. The whole column represents the intake in grams, the shaded part (▨) indicates the oxidized portion of the nutrient, the solid part (▬) that of the stored. When there was no intake of a specific nutrient, the oxidation from endogenous sources is represented below the base line.

results are demonstrated in Figure 12. The proportion of energy metabolism covered by exogenous fat oxidation is demonstrated on the right side of the figure. Although the number of cases are not large for final statistical evaluation, it appears that over a caloric intake of 70–80 kcal/kg/day the contribution

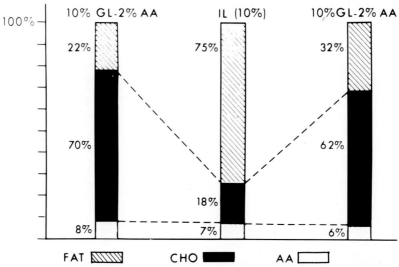

Fig. 10. Relative distribution of principal nutrients (fat ▨, carbohydrate ■, amino acid ▢) oxidized during isocaloric and isovolumetric infusion of glucose (10%) plus amino acid (Amigen 2%), Intralipid® (10%), and glucose (10%) plus amino acid (Amigen 2%) again. The global energy metabolism is represented by the whole column (100%).

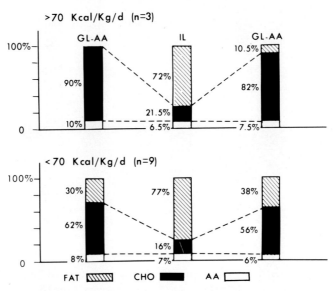

Fig. 11. Contribution of the three principal nutrients to the global energy metabolism (100%) at a gross calorie intake of less than 70 kcal/kg/day and more than 70 kcal/kg/day. (Abbreviations are the same as in Fig. 10.)

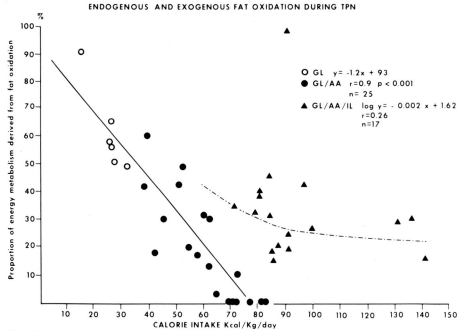

Fig. 12. Proportion of global energy metabolism from fat oxidation during fat-free IV alimentation by glucose (○, GL) and glucose plus amino acid (●, GL + AA), or by complete total parenteral nutrition by glucose/amino acid/Intralipid® (▲, GL/AA/IL) is plotted against the gross caloric intake (kcal/kg/day). Number of patients, regression equations, and correlation coefficients are indicated.

of fat oxidation to total energy metabolism decreases slightly from 35% at 70–80 kcal/kg/day intake to 22% at an intake of 130–140 kcal/kg/day.

Nitrogen balance and protein sparing during total parenteral nutrition (TPN) by either glucose (GL), glucose + amino acid (GL/AA), or glucose + amino acid + Intralipid (GL/AA/IL) at variable protein intake are demonstrated in Figure 13. The latter two infusates differed only in their caloric content. During hypocaloric infusion by glucose the nitrogen balance is negative (average −70 mg/kg/day). Glucose + amino acid infusion resulted in a positive nitrogen balance and correlated significantly with the daily protein intake which varied between 0.5 and 3.5 g/kg/day. By addition of Intralipid, i.e., by increasing the caloric intake at a fixed protein intake, the nitrogen retention becomes substantially higher (by 51 mg/kg/day), resulting in approximately 0.3 g/kg/day extra protein deposition.

DISCUSSION AND CONCLUSIONS

With improved respiratory care, infants of very low birth weight are surviving in increasing numbers. Postnatal nutrition has become a major item of concern for these infants, since there is suspicion that some neuropsychiatric disorders encountered at follow-up may occur as a result of nutritional imbalances in

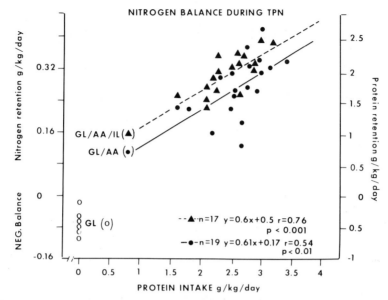

Fig. 13. Nitrogen balance and tissue deposition of protein is plotted against protein intake during IV alimentation by either glucose (○, GL) or glucose plus amino acid (--●---●--, GL/AA) or glucose/amino acid/Intralipid® (--▲--▲--, GL/AA/IL). The intrauterine rate of nitrogen deposition (325 mg/kg/day) was attained at a protein intake of 3.25 g/kg/day provided by glucose plus amino acid mixture and at an intake of 2.75 g/kg/day when the infusate was enriched by Intralipid (GL/AA/IL). Number of patients, regression equations, and correlation coefficients are indicated.

early life.[17, 18, 65] There is no consensus on what diet is optimal.[26] The role of parenteral nutrition in the preterm and postoperative newborn infant is well defined.[1, 2, 6–8, 10, 14–16, 19, 21–24, 29, 35–37, 47, 53, 64, 67, 79, 80] It is part of the supportive management in case of gastrointestinal immaturity and life-saving therapy in patients undergoing extensive gastrointestinal surgery. Parenteral feeding carefully and sensibly employed can improve the outlook for unhandicapped survival in this small and vulnerable patient population.[14, 79]

The usual policy is to start total parenteral nutrition with glucose then continue with glucose/amino acid solution (Phase I of our study), and finally when all contraindications such as hyperbilirubinaemia, infection, respiratory distress, and hypoxia are excluded,[10, 63, 66] fat emulsion (Intralipid) is employed (Phase II and Phase III). Since IV alimentation with GL/AA may be prolonged, the fat-free feeding may cover basal energy metabolism but cannot sustain weight gain comparable to normal growth and development. We have therefore devoted special attention to the role of endogenous fat (Phase I = GL and GL/AA) and exogenous fat (Phase II and III = IL and GL/AA/IL) as a rich energy source.

By analysing the characteristic features of energy metabolism and substrate utilisation during Phase I of our studies (Fig. 6) it became obvious that the newborn infant relies on the oxidation of endogenous fatty acids during hypocaloric fat-free TPN. For instance at 30 kcal/kg/day intake more than

60% of the metabolic energy is derived from endogenous fat. With increasing caloric intake fat oxidation is gradually diminished and above 70–80 kcal/kg/day intake no endogenous fat was oxidized.

Classically, increased fat oxidation is associated with starvation and weight loss or at least failure to thrive. Our results imply that a 70 kcal/kg/day IV caloric intake is the level of energy equilibrium, where endogenous fat oxidation is no longer necessary to support resting metabolism. How does this finding fit into the current concepts of infant's nutrition? This point is analysed in Figure 14. Our results are depicted in the histogram on the right side and compared with Sinclair's data on the left.[68] He calculated that 120 kcal/kg is the minimal daily caloric requirement for a growing infant fed orally: 55 kcal/kg/day can cover the basal energy metabolism; 15 kcal are oxidized during muscular activity, 29 kcal are required for growth, laying down proteins (17 kcal) and lipid (12 kcal); 11 kcal are lost by stool; and 10 calories are used up for chemical thermogenesis. According to our data "high risk" infants nursed in incubators in a thermoneutral environment[9, 38, 68, 70] and receiving TPN have practically no fecal caloric loss and do not use calories for thermoregulatory heat production. In fact a 70 kcal/kg/day intake satisfies the resting metabolic requirement as well the energy requirements for muscular activity. Growth, however, cannot be expected. According to our findings a 70 kcal/kg/day IV caloric intake is

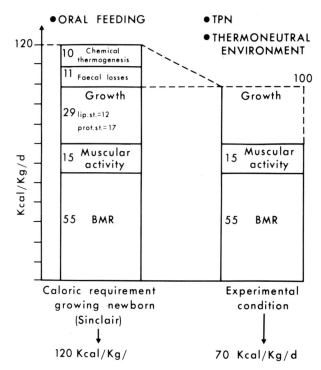

Fig. 14. Partition of the gross caloric intake in orally fed healthy infants[68] and in those intravenously alimented at a thermoneutral environment.

the turning point when endogenous fat oxidation concludes (Fig. 6), thus the infant is in energy equilibrium.

To achieve growth we obviously should enrich the infusate with caloric dense material, i.e., fat emulsion. Can we do this undisturbed or should we be influenced by the bad publicity of dietary fat with respect to its relation to arteriosclerosis and obesity.[39, 50] We challenged this general attitude which greatly influences the judgment of many physicians, and hypothesized that until the fat emulsion is oxidized, i.e., expired as CO_2 and excreted as H_2O, there should be no fear from undesirable side effects.[3, 10, 24, 48, 56, 63, 72, 80] To decide this point, the capacity of the patient to oxidize fatty acids was tested in Phase II of our protocol (Figs. 7–11). The results implied: (1) a quick and good adaptation to the available energy substrate; (2) during fat-free intravenous alimentation by (GL/AA) a fair amount of endogenous fat is oxidized; and (3) oxidation of amino acids is low and fairly constant in spite of the variable intake, they cover only 6–8% of global energy metabolism.

The next question to be answered was: is fat preferentially used for calorigenesis and eliminated as harmless end products such as CO_2 and H_2O even if the caloric intake is increased above the level of the maintenance requirement, i.e., 70 kcal/kg/day? Results depicted in Fig. 11 serve to answer this question. On fat-free TPN with glucose and amino acid the bulk of the energy metabolism can in fact be covered by glucose oxidation. However, this method of increasing caloric intake is neither desirable nor practical because excessive glucose intake leads to an undesirable osmotic load and an increase in amino acid intake might result in high circulating levels of phenylalanine and tyrosine with possible deleterious consequences on brain development.[57] Moreover, in the newborn infant excessive parenteral protein and glucose administration have been reported to be associated with an earlier onset, increased magnitude, and frequency of cholestatic jaundice.[74] According to our results, the oxidation rate of lipids was equally high at intakes of less or more than the 70 kcal/kg/day maintenance level, indicating that the infants preferentially use fat oxidation for covering energy requirements at low and higher caloric intake alike. As a consequence glucose and amino acid can be spared for synthetic processes, required for growth and development of the newborn.

The high rate of fat oxidation during Intralipid infusion was always accompanied by increased heat production and heat conservation (Figs. 7 and 8). The possible reasons for this thermic effect are: (1) the uncoupling effect of fatty acids on oxidative phosphorylation in the mitochondrial electron transfer chain;[51, 58] (2) stimulated recycling of nonesterified fatty acids in the fat cells, thus stimulating the triglyceride hydrolysis reesterification cycle;[30–32, 34, 58] or (3) the stimulation of protein synthesis by energy liberated from the oxidation of fatty acids, such synthesis being costly in kilocalories and therefore leading to the production of heat.[34] Indirect evidence suggests that both the uncoupling effect of increased free fatty acids and the protein sparing effect of Intralipid (Fig. 13) may play a role in the calorigenic effect of fat emulsion.[1, 2, 34, 42, 62, 63, 73]

In the light of the results presented can we attempt to answer the next question: "What is the rational use of Intralipid?" According to our concept it should be tested in each "high risk" case and depending on the result of the test the patient can receive even a high rate of Intralipid if it is preferentially oxidized and not deposited. Figure 12 shows our relevant preliminary observation. During complete IV alimentation by GL + AA + IL the contribution of fat oxidation to the energy metabolism has been measured, and using those values one can compute that at a daily intake of 70–80 kcal/kg by intravenous alimentation and 55 kcal/kg/day resting metabolism the infant is likely to oxidize a minimum of 19 kcal energy as fat, i.e., 2.1 g/kg/day [(55 × 35)/100 = 19/9 = 2.1, where 35 is the percentage contribution of fat oxidation to the resting metabolism as derived from Fig. 13 and 9 is the metabolic value of 1 g lipid oxidized]. The same infant at 130–140 kcal/kg/day total intake and 55 kcal/kg/day resting metabolism will oxidize a minimum of 12 kcal equivalent of fat, i.e., 1.4 g/kg/day [(55 × 22)/100] = 12; 12/9 = 1.4). Keeping in mind these proportions, excessive lipid levels and undesirable side effects may be avoided, and fat accumulation similar to the rate of intrauterine deposition (4–7 g/kg/day)[26, 76, 77] as well as an adequate supply of essential fatty acids[27, 28, 40, 41, 78] can be provided for.

Finally, there is a long-term advantage of well-designed intravenous alimentation with fat emulsion to normal growth inherent in a satisfactory rate of protein synthesis. Results presented in Figures 7–12 demonstrated that exogenous fat emulsion was oxidized, thus yielding considerable energy for protein synthesis (Fig. 13). These findings *strongly suggest* that the salutary effects of protein sparing may be attributable to the utilization of fat.

In summary, Phase I of our study demonstrated that during IV alimentation by glucose and glucose/amino acid solution, i.e., fat-free TPN, endogenous fat up to 4.5 g/kg/day was oxidized in proportion to the kcal deficit until the metabolism of 70 kcal/kg/day was derived from exogenous sources.

Phase II, i.e., the Intralipid (IL), tests allowed us to conclude that (1) neonates show metabolic flexibility for diverse substrates; (2) the proportion of protein oxidized is independent of calorie intake; and (3) fat emulsion is used preferentially as an energy substrate with more than 60–70% oxidation and less than 30–40% deposition.

From Phase III, i.e., Intravenous, therapy with glucose/amino acid/Intralipid we have learned that (1) the proportion of energy metabolism covered by exogenous fat oxidation decreases slightly as caloric intake is increased; (2) over 70 kcal/kg/day intake, 22–35% of the basal energy metabolism is covered by fat oxidation, i.e., 1.4–2.1 g/kg/day fat is oxidized; (3) favorable nitrogen balance during TPN can be achieved if a high rate of lipid oxidation is maintained simultaneously; and (4) "Rational Intralipid Therapy" can only be based on appropriate measurements.

This paper is not intended to be a comprehensive review, therefore many aspects of the intravenous nutrition in the neonate have been omitted or barely touched upon. The aim has been to demonstrate that the tools of experimental nutrition can be applied at the bedside in the form of a sophisticated noninvasive method, and the information gained expands not only our theoretical knowledge about infant nutrition but also provides valuable information for the everyday management of the premature and high risk infant.

ACKNOWLEDGMENTS

Thanks are due to Mrs. S. Chandramowli and Mrs. O. Stubna for technical assistance and Mrs. Lina Gerebizza for preparation of the manuscript. The project was supported by grants from National Health and Welfare of Canada No. 606-1482 and the Medical Research Council of Canada No. MA-7277. Dr. Guy Putet was a fellow of the National Research Council of Canada (Franco-Canadian Cultural Exchange). Dr. Gaston Verellen held a NATO Fellowship and Dr. Philippe Chessex an MRC Fellowship.

REFERENCES

1. Andrew, G., Chan, G., and Schiff, D., Lipid metabolism in the neonate: I. The effect of Intralipid infusion on plasma triglyceride and free fatty acid concentrations in the neonate. *J. Pediat.* **88,** 273 (1976).

2. Andrew, G., Chan, G., and Schiff, D., Lipid metabolism in the neonate: II. The effect of Intralipid on bilirubin binding *in vitro* and *in vivo. J. Pediat.* **88,** 279 (1976).

3. Barson, A. G., Chiswick, M. L., and Doig, C. M., Fat embolism in infancy after intravenous fat infusions. *Arch. Dis. Child.* **53,** 218 (1978).

4. Boberg, J., and Carlson, L. A., Determination of heparin-induced lipoprotein lipase activity in human plasma. *Clin. Chim. Acta.* **10,** 420 (1964).

5. Boberg, J., Quantitative determination of heparin released lipoprotein lipase activity in human plasma. *Lipids* **5,** 452 (1970).

6. Bode, H. H., History of parenteral alimentation, In *Parenteral Nutrition in Infancy and Childhood.* H. H. Bode and J. B. Warshaw (eds.), Plenum Press, New York, 1974, Vol. 46, p. 1.

7. Borresen, H., Bjordal, R., and Knutrud, O., Postoperative parenteral feeding of neonates: Peripheral vein infusion technique, fat administration and metabolic studies. In *Parenteral Nutrition in Infancy and Childhood.* H. H. Bode and J. B. Warshaw (eds.), Plenum Press, New York, 1974, Vol. 46, p. 165.

8. Borresen, H. C., and Knutrud, O., Intravenous feeding of low birth weight infants. *Nutr. Metab. (Suppl. 1)* **20,** 88 (1976).

9. Brück, K., Parmelee, A. H., Jr., and Brück, M., Neutral temperature range and range of "thermal comfort" in premature infants. *Biol. Neonate* **4,** 32 (1962).

10. Bryan, H., Shennan, A., Griffin, E., and Angel, A., Intralipid—Its rational use in parenteral nutrition of the newborn. *Pediatrics* **58,** 787 (1976).

11. Clandinin, M. T., Chapell, J. E., and Heim, T., Intrauterine fatty acid accretion in human brain. *Fed. Proc.* **39,** 440 (1980).

12. Clandinin, M. T., Chapell, J. E., Leong, S., Heim, T., Swyer, P. R., and Chance, G. W., Extrauterine fatty acid accretion in infant brain: implications for fatty acid requirements. *Early Human Development* **4/2,** 121 (1980).

13. Clandinin, M. T., Chapell, J. E., Leong, S., Heim, T., Swyer, P. R., and Chance, G. W., Intrauterine fatty acid accretion rates in human brain: implications for fatty acid requirements. *Early Human Development* **4/12,** 131 (1980).

14. Cockburn, F., The place of parenteral nuitrition in the pre-term infant. *Curr. Med. Res. Opin. Suppl. 1* **4,** 90 (1976).

15. Cockburn, F., Intravenous feeding of the newborn. *Clin. Endocrinol. Metabol.* **5,** 191 (1976).

16. Coran, A., The intravenous use of fat for the total parenteral nutrition of the infant. *Lipids* **7,** 455 (1972).

17. Davies, P. A., and Steward, A. L., Low birthweight infants: Neurological sequelae and later intelligence. *Br. Med. Bull.* **31,** 85 (1975).

18. Davies, P. A., and Davies, J. P., Very low birthweight and subsequent head growth. *Lancet* **2,** 1216 (1970).

19. Dudrick, S. J., Wilmore, D. W., Vars, H. M., and Rhoads, J. E., Can intravenous feeding as the sole means of nutrition support growth in the child and restore weight loss in an adult? *Ann. Surg.* **169,** 974 (1969).

20. Ellis, F. R., and Nunn, J. F., The measurement of gaseous oxygen tension utilizing paramagnetism, an evaluation of the "Servomex" OA 150 analyser. *Br. J. Anaesth.* **50,** 569 (1968).

21. Filler, R. M., Eraklis, A. G., Rubin, V. G., and Das, J. B., Long-term parenteral nutrition in infants. *New Engl. J. Med.* **281,** 589 (1969).

22. Filler, R. M., Experience with total parenteral feeding of infants. *Pediatrician* **3,** 220 (1974).

23. Filler, R. M., and Eraklis, A. J., Care of the critically ill child: intravenous alimentation. *Pediatrics* **46,** 456 (1970).

24. Filler, R. M., Takada, Y., Carreras, T., and Heim, T., Serum Intralipid levels in neonates during parenteral nutrition: the relation to gestational age. *J. Pediat. Surg.* **15/4,** (1980) in press.

25. Folch, J., Lees, M., and Sloane-Stanley, G. A., A simple method for the isolation and purification of total lipids from animal tissues. *J. Biol. Chem.* **226,** 497 (1957).

26. Fomon, S. J., *Infant Nutrition*, 2nd ed., W. B. Saunders, Philadelphia, 1974.

27. Friedman, Z., Danon, M. D., Stahlman, M. T., and Oates, J. A., Rapid onset of essential fatty acid deficiency in the newborn. *Pediatrics* **58,** 640 (1976).

28. Friedman, Z., Marks, K. H., Maisels, J. M., Thorson, R., and Naeye, R., Effect of parenteral fat emulsion on the pulmonary and reticuloendothelial systems in the newborn infant. *Pediatrics* **61,** 694 (1978).

29. Ghadimi, H., Arulanatham, K., and Rathi, M., Evaluation of nutritional management of the low birth weight newborn. *Amer. J. Clin. Nutr.* **26,** 473 (1973).

30. Heim, T., Thermogenesis in the newborn infant. *Clin. Obstet. Gynecol. N.Y.* **14,** 790 (1971).

31. Heim, T., Cser, Á., Jászai, V., Donhoffer, H., Varga, F., Swyer, P., Putet, G., and Smith, J. M., Energy metabolism and thermal homeostasis in the newborn infant. In *Intensive Care in the Newborn, II.* L. Stern, W. Oh, B. Friis-Hansen (eds.), Masson Publishing USA, Inc., New York, 1978, pp. 275–305.

32. Heim, T., Fetal and neonatal metabolism. In *Perinatal Medicine.* E. Kerpel-Fronius, P. Véghelyi, J. Rosta (eds.), Hungarian Academy Sciences Publishing House, Budapest, 1978, pp. 873–902.

33. Heim, T., Energy Balance of the preterm baby. In *Perinatal Medicine.* E. Kerpel-Fronius, P. Véghelyi, J. Rosta (eds.), Hungarian Academy of Sciences Publishing House, Budapest, 1978, pp. 575–577.

34. Heim, T., Homeothermy and its metabolic cost. In *Scientific Foundations of Paediatrics.* J. A. Davis and G. Dobbing (eds), William Heinemann Medical Books Ltd., London, 1980.

35. Heird, W., Dirscoll, J., and Winters, R., Total intravenous alimentation in low birth weight premature infants In *Parentral Nutrition in Infancy and Childhood*, H. H. Bode and J. B. Warshaw (eds.), Plenum Press, New York, 1974, Vol. 46, p. 199.

36. Heird, W., Winters, R., and Dudrick, S., Metabolic complications of total parenteral nutrition. In *Parenteral Nutrition in Infancy and Childhood,* H. H. Bode and J. B. Warshaw (eds.), Plenum Press, New York, Vol. 46, p. 256.

37. Heird, W. C., and Anderson, T. L., Nutritional requirements and methods of feeding low birthweight infants. *Curr. Probl. Pediatr.* **7,** 2 (1977).

38. Hey, E., Thermal neutrality. *Br. Med. Bull.* **31,** 69 (1975).

39. Holman, R. T., Atherosclerosis—a pediatric nutrition problem. *Amer. J. Clin. Nutr.* **9,** 565 (1961).

40. Holman, R. T., Essential fatty acid deficiency. In *Progress in Chemistry of Fat and Other Lipids,* Pergamon Press Inc., Elmsford, N.Y., 1968, p. 279.

41. Holman, R. T., Essential fatty acid deficiency in human. In *Dietary Lipids and Postnatal Development.* C. Galli, C. Jacini, A. Pecile (eds.), Raven Press, New York, 1973, p. 127.

42. Hommes, F. A., Drost, Y. M., Geraets, W. X. M., and Reijenga, M. A. A., The energy requirement for growth: An application of Atkinson's metabolic price system. *Pediatr. Res.* **9**, 51 (1975).

43. Kajtár, P., Jecquier, E., and Prodhom, L. S., Heat losses in newborn infants of different body size measured by direct calorimetry in a thermoneutral and a cold environment. *Biol. Neonate* **30**, 55 (1976).

44. Kaplan, A., and Lee, V. F., A micromethod for determination of serum triglyceride. *Proc. Soc. Exp. Biol. Med.* **118**, 296 (1965).

45. Kappagoda, C. T., and Linden, R. J., A critical assessment of an open circuit technique for measuring oxygen consumption. *Cardiovasc. Res.* **6**, 589 (1974).

46. Katz, L., and Hamilton, J. R., Fat absorption in infants of birthweight less than 1,300 gm. *J. Pediatr.* **85**, 608 (1974).

47. Kerner, J. A., and Sunshine, P., Parenteral alimentation. *Semin. Perinatol.* **3**, 417 (1979).

48. Koga, Y., Swanson, V., and Hays, D., Hepatic "Intravenous Fat Pigment" in infants and children receiving lipid emulsion. *J. Ped. Surg.* **10**, 641 (1975).

49. Kretchmer, N., Levine, S. A., and McNamara, H., The *in vitro* metabolism of tyrosine and its intermediates in the liver of the premature infants. *Am. J. Dis. Child.* **93**, 19 (1957).

50. Kwitterovich, P. O., Jr., Neonatal screening for hyperlipidemia. *Pediatrics* **53**, 455 (1974).

51. Lindberg, O., *Brown Adipose Tissue*, Elsevier, New York, 1970.

52. Lister, G., Hoffman, J. I. E., and Rudolph, A. M., Oxygen uptake in infants and children: a simple method of measurement. *Pediatrics* **53**, 656 (1974).

53. Mestyán, J., Energy metabolism and substrate utilization in the newborn. In *Temperature Regulation and Energy Balance in the Newborn*. J. C. Sinclair (Ed.), Grune and Stratton, New York, 1978, pp. 39–74.

54. Nelson, N., A photometric adaptation of the Somogyi method for the determination of glucose. *J. Biol. Chem.* **153**, 375 (1944).

55. Novák, M., Colorimetric ultramicro method for the determination of free fatty acids. *J. Lipid Res.* **6**, 431 (1965).

56. Olegard, R., Gustafson, A., Kjellmer, I., and Victorin, L. H., Nutrition in low birth weight infants. III. Lipolysis and free fatty acid elimination after intravenous administration of fat emulsion. *Acta Pediat. Scand.* **64**, 745 (1975).

57. Peng, Y., Gubin, J., Harper, A. E., Vavich, M. G., and Kemmerer, A. R., Food intake regulation: amino acid toxicity and changes in rat brain and plasma amino acids. *J. Nutr.* **103**, 608 (1973).

58. Prusiner, S. B., Eisenhart, R. E., Rylander, E., and Lindberg, O., The regulation of oxidative metabolism of isolated brown fat cells. *Biochem. Biophys. Res. Comm.* **30**, 508 (1968).

59. Putet, G., Heim, T., Smith, J., and Swyer, P., Substrate utilization during isocaloric, isovolaemic parenteral nutrition (TPN) with glucose/amino-acid (GL/AA) and fat emulsions (IL). *Pediatr. Res.* **12**, 440 (1978).

60. Putet, G., Verellen, G. J. E., Heim, T., Swyer, P. R., and Smith, J. M., Evaluation of energy requirements by indirect calorimetry (IC) during total intravenous alimentation (TIA) of the "high risk" new born infant. *J. Nutr.* **6**, XXI (1979).

61. Putet, G., Verellen, G., Heim, T., and Swyer, P., Effect of calorie intake on the utilization of cárbohydrate (C), protein (P), and fat (F) as energy substrate in the ill newborn infant on total parenteral nutrition (TPN). *Pediatr. Res.* **13**, 72 (1979).

62. Putet, G. Verellen, G., Heim T., Swyer, P., and Smith, J., The protein sparing of exogenous lipid during i.v. alimentation. *Pediatr. Res.* **14**: 175 (1980).

63. Schiff, D., Andrew, G., and Chan, G., Metabolism of intravenously administered lipid in the newborn. In *Intensive Care in the Newborn, II*, L. Stern, W. Oh, B. Friis-Hansen, (eds.), Masson Publishing USA, Inc., New York, 1978, pp. 267–273.

64. Shaw, J. C. L., Parenteral nutrition in the management of sick low birthweight infants. *Pediatr. Clin. North. Am.* **20**, 333 (1973).

65. Shaw, J. C. L., Malnutrition in very low birthweight preterm infants. *Proc. Nutr. Soc.* **33**, 103 (1974).

66. Shennan, A. T., Cherian, A. G., Angel, A., and Bryan, M. H., The effect of Intralipid on the

estimation of serum bilirubin in the newborn infant. *J. Pediat.* **88,** 285 (1976).

67. Sinclair, J. C. Driscoll, J. M. Heird, W. C., and Winters, R. W., Supportive management of the sick neonate. Parenteral calories, water and electrolytes. *Ped. Clin. N. Amer.* **17,** 863 (1970).

68. Sinclair, J. C., Energy balance of the newborn. In *Temperature Regulation and Energy Balance in the Newborn*, J. C. Sinclair (ed.), Grune and Stratton, New York, 1978, pp. 187–203.

69. Somogyi, M., Notes of sugar determination. *J. Biol. Chem.* **195,** 19 (1952).

70. Swyer, P., Putet, G., Smith, J. M., and Heim, T., Energy metabolism and substrate utilization during total parenteral nutrition in the newborn. In *Intensive Care in the Newborn. II*, L. Stern, W. Oh, B. Friis-Hansen (eds.), Masson Publishing USA, Inc., New York, 1978, pp. 307–316.

71. Ta, R. S., and Zuazaga, G., Micro-Kjeldahl determination of nitrogen. A new indicator and an improved rapid method. *Ind. Eng. Chem. Anal.* **14,** 280 (1942).

72. Thompson, S. W., Thomassen, R. W., and Host, D. H., A study on pigment deposition by intravenous fat emulsion. *J. Nutr.* **71,** 37 (1960).

73. Verellen, G., Putet, G., Heim, T., Swyer, P., and Smith, J., Utilization of endogenous and exogenous lipids during total parenteral nutrition (TPN). *Clin. Res.* **26,** 867A (1978).

74. Vileisis, R. A., Inwood, R. J., and Hunt, C. E., Prospective controlled study of parenteral nutrition associated cholestatic jaundice: effect of protein intake. *Pediatr. Res.* **14,** 512 (1980).

75. Warshaw, J. B., Fatty acid oxidation during development. In *Parenteral Nutrition in Infancy and Childhood*. H. H. Bode, J. B. Warshaw (eds.), Plenum Press, New York, 1974 Vol. 46, p. 88.

76. Widdowson, E. M., Nutrition. In *Scientific Foundations of Pediatrics*, 1st ed., J. A. Davis and J. Dobbing (eds.), William Heinemann Medical Books Ltd., London, 1974, pp. 44–55.

77. Widdowson, E. M., Changes in body proportions and composition during growth, In *Scientific Foundations of Paediatrics*, 1st ed., J. A. Davis and J. Dobbing (eds.), William Heinemann Medical Books Ltd, London, 1974, pp. 153–163.

78. Wiese, H. F., Hansen, A. E., and Adam, D. G. D., Essential fatty acids in infant nutrition. I. Linoleic acid requirement in terms of serum di-, tri- and tetraenic acid levels. *J. Nutr.* **66,** 345 (1958).

79. Winters, R. W., and Hasselmayer, E., *Intravenous Nutrition in the High Risk Infant*, W. R. Winters and H. Hasselmayer (eds.) Wiley, New York, 1975.

80. Wretlind, A., Complete intravenous nutrition. Theoretical and experimental background. *Nutr. Metab. Suppl. 1* **14,** (1972).

25

Delayed Intracranial Hypertension in the Premature Neonate, Following Chronic Fetal Distress

C. AMIEL-TISON, R. KOROBKIN, H. HORNYCH, and C. DALISSON

Increased intracranial pressure (ICP) is a common problem in premature infants; it is usually due to obstruction to cerebrospinal fluid (CSF) outflow following intraventricular hemorrhage (IVH). We have seen four small for gestational age (SGA) premature infants in whom there developed evidence of medically reversible intracranial hypertension, without a history of IVH or subarachnoid hemorrhage (SAH). The increased ICP became evident weeks to months after birth, generally at a time when the babies were approaching term gestational age and were no longer suffering the systemic consequences of their prematurity. All of these infants had normal CSF at the time of diagnosis of intracranial hypertension; none had dilated cerebral ventricles. The symptoms were relieved by lumbar puncture and acetazolamide. In this report we will present the cases, discuss the diagnosis, management, and outcome, and speculate on pathophysiology.

CASE 1 (FIG. 1)

This boy was a 34-week gestational age, 1180-g second-born twin. There was meconium staining of the amniotic fluid, but Apgar scores were 5 at 1 min and 10 at 5 min. There had been several maternal complications of pregnancy. The mother took clomid to stimulate ovulation and then had several episodes of threatened abortion, starting with bleeding in the third month of pregnancy. At the end of the fourth month, a cervical cerclage

Port-Royal Maternity Hospital, 123 Boulevard de Port Royal 75014 Paris Cedex, France

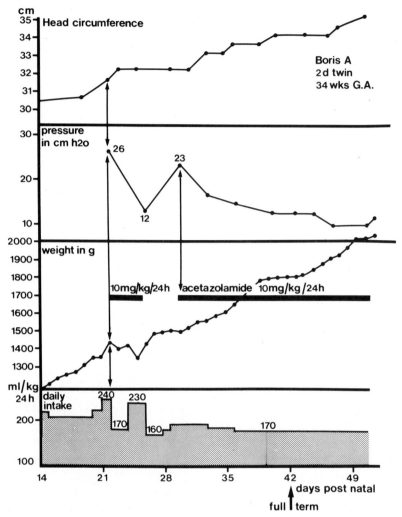

Fig. 1. Case 1: Head circumference, fontanelle pressure, body weight, and total daily fluid volume intake, from 14 to 49 days of age.

procedure was performed. The problem persisted, however, and she was treated with beta stimulants and indomethacin. Other maternal complications included cholestasis and anemia.

The baby did well for the first 2 weeks of life and regained his birthweight by day 14. The neurological examination was consistent with gestational age, but there were very large anterior and posterior fontanelles and disjunction of the sutures without other clinical signs. In the third week of life, he continued to gain weight, taking 240 ml/kg/24 hr formula. He gained as much as 90 g in 1 day and had further disjunction of the sutures. At that time, the anterior fontanelle pressure (measured by applanation pressure transducer) was 26 cm water and the infant was agitated with irregular respirations. There was peripheral edema and he had occasional opisthotonic posturing. The fluids were reduced to 170 ml/kg/24 hr and he was treated with acetazolamide 10 mg/kg/24 hr. Over the ensuing 3 days, he improved and the anterior fontanelle pressure decreased to 12 cm water. The head circumference was 31.5 cm and weight was 1450 g. He then developed abdominal distension and was transferred to a different unit where the acetazolamide was discontinued and high volume fluids (230 ml/kg/24 hr, partly intravenously, partly oral formula) were reinstituted. Within 3 days, the anterior fontanelle pressure again increased to 23 cm water. At that time fluids were reduced to 160 ml/kg/24 hr and the acetazolamide was reinstituted. Three days later the anterior fontanelle pressure had dropped to 14 cm water. A computerized tomographic (CT) brain scan was normal as was an EEG. Acetazolamide was continued for 3 weeks and the anterior fontanelle pressure continued to fall to 8 cm water. The head circumference stabilized and the sutures closed. He is now 10 months old and had normal development.

CASE 2 (FIG. 2)

This girl was a 32-week gestational age, 1000-g infant born to a mother with toxemia of pregnancy. There was poor prenatal care and the baby was born at

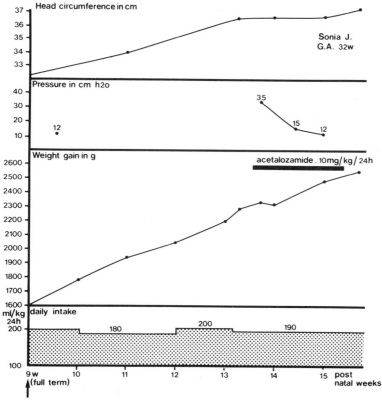

Fig. 2. Case 2: Head circumference, fontanelle pressure, body weight, and total daily fluid volume intake, from 9 to 15 weeks of age.

home. Presentation was breech. Soon after birth, the infant was transported to the hospital where she was cyanotic and bradycardic on arrival. After intubation, she was quickly resuscitated. Body temperature was 31° and the pH was 7.12. She was extubated after the acidosis and hypothermia were corrected. She did well clinically and neurologically over the next few weeks. At 36 weeks corrected age, she had neck extensor hypertonia on neurological examination. This sign persisted, and she developed occasional spontaneous opisthotonic posturing and lid retraction. Head circumference grew at a normal rate, and the infant remained alert and vigilant and followed well with her eyes. Fundoscopy was normal, and transillumination of the cranium was negative. Anterior fontanelle pressure was 12 cm water. At 13 weeks of age, 1 month corrected age, she suddenly developed permanent opisthotonus and a sunset sign. The fontanelle was bulging and she had apnea after crying. The head circumference increased 2.5 cm in 1 week. Anterior fontanelle pressure was between 30 and 40 cm water. She was started on acetazolamide 10 mg/kg/24 hr and within a week she was calmer, she stopped having apnea, the opisthotonus diminished, the eye signs disappeared, and the head circumference stopped expanding rapidly (it did not grow at all in the first week following institution of acetazolamide). Five days after starting acetazolamide, the anterior fontanelle pressure was 12–15 cm water. The CT brain scan was normal. Fifteen days after starting acetazolamide, the fontanelle was normal, the infant was alert and vigilant, and there were minimal signs of neck extensor hypertonia. Acetazolamide was discontinued, and she was discharged home. At 5 months corrected age, the neurological examination and the head circumference were normal. She is now lost to follow-up.

CASE 3 (FIG. 3)

This 1350-g 32-week gestational age second-born twin was the product of an otherwise uncomplicated pregnancy. The twins were biovulate and there was no discordance in weight. There was a complicated breech delivery with forceps extraction. Apgar scores were 4 at 1 min and 6 at 5 min. There was no respiratory distress, and she did well except for two brief episodes of hypoxia associated with aspiration on the fifth and sixth days of life. Fontanelle and sutures were normal and head circumference followed a normal growth curve. At 2½ months of age, that is, 2 weeks corrected age, she appeared irritable and had hypertonia of the neck extensors, a full fontanelle, and edema of the lower extremities. One week previously, the examination had been entirely normal. Diuresis with lasix produced only 130 ml of urine in 24 hr and slight amelioration of the irritability. She had persistent hypertonia of neck extensors over the next several weeks, with opisthotonus provoked by crying or examination, and general irritability, but no peripheral edema or excessive weight gain. Lumbar puncture at 3 months of age, 3 weeks corrected age, produced CSF which seemed under pressure and had a protein content of 45 mg/100 ml. Within hours after this procedure, she was much less irritable and had less marked axial extensor hypertonia; this improvement lasted several days. One

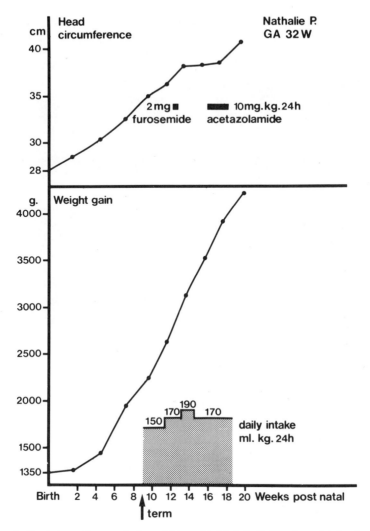

Fig. 3. Case 3: Head circumference, body weight, and total daily fluid volume intake, from birth to 20 weeks of age.

week later, isotope cisternography with ^{111}In DTPA introduced at the lumbar subarachnoid space showed persistence of isotope over the cortical subarachnoid space, especially the Sylvian Fissure (Figs. 4A and 5A). We then began therapy with acetazolamide 10 mg/kg/24 hr and repeated the cisternography 7 days later, (Figs. 4B and 5B). It showed a dramatic improvement in flow, paralleling a remarkable improvement in the clinical course. One week after starting acetazolamide, the neurological examination was normal except for excessive passive hyperextension of the trunk. Acetazolamide was discontinued after 2 weeks of treatment, and the infant remained well. At 3 years of age, she had normal behavior and development except for a delay in speech.

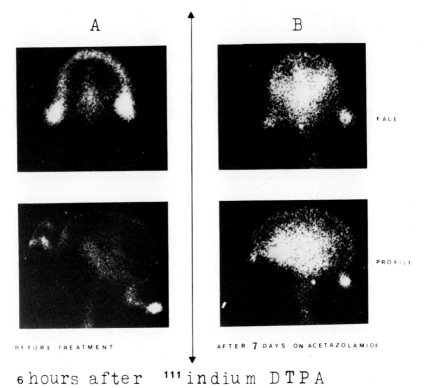

6 hours after ¹¹¹indium DTPA

Fig. 4. Isotope cisternography in Case 3: Brain scan 6 hr after lumbar subarachnoid injection of 111-Indium DTPA. (A) Before therapy; (B) after 7 days therapy with acetazolamide.

CASE 4

This 880-g, 30-week gestational age infant was born to a gravida-1 mother with preeclampsia. Delivery was normal, and Apgar scores were 6 at 1 min and 8 at 5 min. Although he appeared hypotrophic, his examination was otherwise normal for gestational age at birth. He did well clinically, requiring no more than 40% oxygen. Because of hyperbilirubinemia at 4 days of age, an exchange transfusion was performed. He had several brief episodes of apnea in the first weeks of life, but no major problems. At 6 weeks of age, general physical and neurological examinations were normal. One week later, at 7 weeks (corrected age 37 weeks gestation), he was tremulous and had hypertonia of the neck extensors. Serum electrolytes, glucose, and calcium were normal. CSF was normal with protein of 101 mg/100 ml. Weight gain was within normal limits. The infant improved after lumbar puncture and seemed neurologically normal until 2 months later (corrected age 1½ months) when he again had hypertonia of neck extensors, this time associated with disjunction of the sutures. Over the ensuing weeks, several lumbar punctures relieved symptoms transiently, but at the time of discharge 3 weeks later, he was still irritable and had neck extensor hypertonia. At 4 years of age he showed global intellectual retardation

A   B

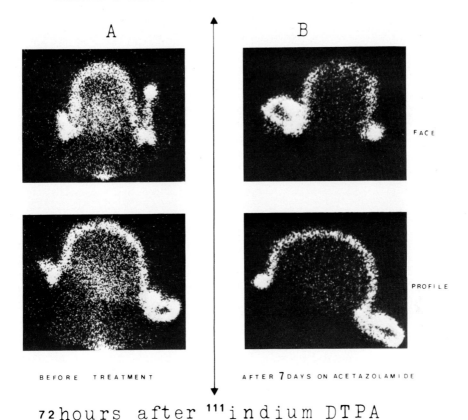

72 hours after ^{111}indium DTPA

Fig. 5. Isotope cisternography in Case 3: 72 hr after lumbar subarachnoid injection of 111-Indium DTPA. (A) Before therapy; (B) after 7 days therapy with acetazolamide.

and had febrile convulsions. After that, he had slow language development, and remained an irritable and hyperactive child. At 9 years of age, his behavior had improved; however, he had difficulty reading and writing and poor fine motor coordination. He had no seizures, did not take medication, and had a normal EEG.

CLINICAL FINDINGS (TABLE I)

The clinical findings are summarized in Table I. Although the four cases belong to a high-risk group of neonates, SGA premature newborns (multiple pregnancy in cases 1 and 3, vascular complications in cases 2 and 4), status at birth was good, and the neonatal course was uncomplicated. Only case 2 required assisted ventilation for a few hours because of hypothermia and acidosis. The first postnatal weeks were without problems; there were no signs of infection or hemorrhage. Thus, in the four cases, the symptom-free interval after birth and the delayed appearances of neurological signs after 3–13 postnatal weeks is a common feature. The conceptional age at the beginning of symptoms was from 37 to 45 weeks. Therefore, this syndrome appears

TABLE I

Gestational and Neonatal History[a]

	BW (g)	GA (weeks)	Toxemia	Multiple Pregnancy	IUGR	Status at Birth	Neonatal Course	Beginning of ICH (weeks)
Case 1	1180	34	−	+ 2nd twin discordant weight	++ <10%	Good	No problems	34 + 3 = 37
Case 2	1000	32	+	−	++ <10%	Acidosis hypothermia	Rapid recovery	32 + 13 = 45
Case 3	1350	32	−	+ 2nd twin	+ <25%	Good	No problems	32 + 11 = 43
Case 4	880	30	++ Preeclampsia	−	++ <10%	Good	No problems	30 + 7 = 37

[a] Abbreviations used are: BW, birth weight; GA, gestational age; IUGR, intrauterine growth retardation; ICH, intracranial hypertension.

Note: Percentile based on Lubchenco intrauterine growth chart (Lubchenco, et al., 1963).

clearly distinct from the early increase of intracranial pressure, probably related to post natal hypoxia.[5, 20, 26] All four infants had clinical signs of increased ICP, as previously described.[1] Irritability and neck extensor hypertonia were the early signs; later on, permanent opisthotonic posturing occurred. A rapid enlargement of head circumference was observed, more striking in cases 1 and 3. Disjunction of cranial sutures, including the squamosal, was constant finding, with bulging fontanelle more marked in case 2. However, these findings are late signs of increased ICP, as demonstrated in obstructive hydrocephalus.[15]

Our patients had no history of perinatal asphyxia, meningitis, or intracranial hemorrhage. It is likely that their neck extensor hypertonia represents slight cerebellar herniation or pressure on the brainstem secondary to increased intracranial pressure. One of our patients had irregular respirations (case 1) and one had apnea (case 2) associated with the clinical syndrome, suggesting some brainstem compromise. The temporary relief of signs and symptoms immediately following lumbar puncture suggests that they were caused by increased intracranial pressure. In all four cases, the CSF was under pressure, with a clear perception of a tense dura during the puncture. The CSF composition was normal; blood electrolytes were normal.

DIAGNOSTIC PROCEDURES

Diagnostic procedures are summarized in Table II.

1. Noninvasive measurement of intracranial pressure was achieved in two patients (cases 1 and 2). Several methods have been recently devised and tested.[9, 21, 22, 25, 27]

TABLE II

Diagnostic Procedures, Treatment, and Outcome[a]

	IC Pressure cm Water	CT Brain Scan	Isotope Cistern-ography	Treatment	Outcome
Case 1	26 Normalized after 3 days of treatment	Normal	Not performed	Acetazolamide	Good at 10 months
Case 2	35 Normalized after 5 days of treatment	Normal	Not performed	Acetazolamide	Good at 5 months
Case 3	Not measured	Not per-formed	Abnormal, nor-malization after 7 days of treatment	Acetazolamide	Good at 3 years
Case 4	Not measured	Not per-formed	Not performed	Repeated LP during 3 weeks	M.B.D. at 9 years

[a] Abbreviations used are: IC, intracranial; CT, computerized tomographic; LP, lumbar puncture; MBD, minimal brain dysfunction.

The applanation pressure transducer (Model HP-APT 16, Hewlett Packard) was used in our patients. *This method permits the measurement of pressure through the intact anterior fontanelle. It is based on the principle that if a plane surface is placed against a membrane distended by internal pressure, the membrane will bulge through any hole in the surface, and the force which must be applied to applanate it must be equal to the internal pressure. The plane reference surface is a plastic plate 27 mm in diameter with a central hole of 6.4 mm diameter in which is placed a spring loaded plunger. The membrane bulges through the hole in the baseplate until the force exerted by the spring is equal to the internal pressure. The movement of the plunger is measured by a differential transformer technique and recorded as pressure. The transducer is first calibrated using a rubber balloon filled with fluid. The intracranial pressure is then expressed in centimeters of water.*

With this simple and reliable measurement, it appears possible to detect the preclinical stage of increased ICP in high risk newborns, 15 cm water being considered as the upper limit in a quiet infant and 20 cm water a definite sign of intracranial hypertension.

2. The CT brain scan was normal when performed, in cases 1 and 2, with normal size of ventricles and normal density of parenchyma.

3. Isotope cisternography was performed in case 3; the half-life was delayed with accumulation of fluid in the Sylvian Fissure (Figs. 4 and 5).

TREATMENT

The remarkable effect of acetazolamide does not help in the pathophysiologic understanding of the syndrome, as it may act on both CSF production and total blood volume as well. Acetazolamide is a carbonic anhydrase inhibitor and, in addition to its well-known diuretic effect, it reduces the formation of CSF.[4, 8, 16] When used in the management of experimental cerebral edema, it may be more effective than corticosteroids, osmotically active agents, or other diuretics.[16] Its mode of action on CSF formation is still not well established. It may act on choroid plexus cells as on renal tubular cells. In the presence of a carbonic anhydrase inhibitor, less hydrogen ions are available for exchange with sodium which is coupled with the passive diffusion of water. Alkaline diuresis at the kidney, and diminution of CSF formation at the choroid plexus are the results.[8, 18]

A side effect of acetazolamide is metabolic acidosis associated with hypokalemia. Acid-base status and electrolytes must be monitored. In our experience, the slight hypokalemia was easily corrected by orally administered potassium chloride. Acidosis was not a problem. The diuretic effect of acetazolamide was moderate and induced slight initial weight loss, but this was not persistent.

OUTCOME

The four patients we described have not had major handicaps, despite the fact that they were small for gestational age prematures. None developed hydrocephalus. Two are normal at 10 and 5 months (corrected age) (cases 1 and 2). One had minor speech delay at 3 years of age (case 3), and one has poor fine motor coordination with some difficulty in reading and writing at 9 years of age (case 4). The 9 year old was treated with lumbar punctures only. The other three infants received acetazolamide after the initial lumbar puncture.

SPECULATIONS ON PATHOPHYSIOLOGY

Increased intracranial pressure presupposes an excess of tissue, blood or CSF within the rigid confines of the cranium. Thus, excessive CSF production or decreased absorption enlarging the CSF compartment, excessive total blood volume or cerebral blood flow enlarging the vascular compartment, an intracranial mass lesion or cell swelling enlarging the tissue compartment can all give signs of increased intracranial pressure. In our four cases, the signs were rapidly reversible, and there was no evidence of an intracranial mass lesion. Two of the infants had normal CT brain scans (cases 1 and 2). Thus, it is likely that the symptoms represent a dynamic problem.

1. *An increase in CSF volume* can be caused by increased CSF production or faulty CSF absorption without any obstruction. In our cases, the absorption of CSF could not keep up with production; this is suggested by isotope cisternography in case 3. The first study, while the infant had significant signs and symptoms of intracranial hypertension, showed delayed absorption of isotope over the hemispheres. One week later, when she had become asymptomatic following therapy with acetazolamide, a second study was normal.

All of the infants had transient relief of signs and symptoms following lumbar puncture. Three of them (cases 1, 2, and 3) had a dramatic improvement within 48 hr of acetazolamide therapy. This effect was well documented by measurements of intracranial pressure in cases 1 and 2. In case 1, an interruption of treatment was followed by a recurrence of intracranial hypertension, only to be relieved again by reinstitution of therapy. This reduction of the CSF compartment relieved symptoms in all cases.

An additional argument for faulty CSF absorption are the soft cranial bones in these SGA premature newborns.[19] This was particularly striking in case 1, the discordant twin having a very soft skull and very wide fontanelles. It has been shown that the intracranial pressure is partly determined by intracranial volume and partly by mechanical force generated by the overlying cranium.[3, 6, 7] Thus poor ossification may be an additional factor compromising CSF absorption.

One cannot ascertain whether the problem is faulty CSF absorption, excessive CSF production, or a combination of the two. There is clearly no permanent obstruction to CSF absorption. The exquisite sensitivity of these infants to fluid overload and their dramatic response to an inhibitor of CSF production leads to the speculation that they are unable to regulate CSF production at this vulnerable age. Extracellular fluid space measured by the inulin space in two groups of prematures was found to be very enlarged in a high volume fluid intake group (170 ml/kg/24 hr) compared to a low volume fluid intake group (120 ml/kg/24 hr).[23] CSF being part of intracranial, extracellular water, these results seem to be in favor of an excessive production of CSF related to an excessive total intake of fluid.

The delayed appearance of the intracranial hypertension could be related to renal maturation. In the premature newborn less than 34 weeks gestational age (our cases are 30–34 weeks) the sodium balance is negative for the first 2–3 weeks of life and later becomes positive.[2] Therefore, a formula containing 10–12 mEq of sodium as occurs with the modified cow's milk in use in our unit often provides too little sodium in the first 2 weeks and too much sodium after 3 weeks of age when the balance becomes positive.[10, 24]

2. *An increase in blood volume* should also be considered. We initially thought that a significant increase in blood volume or cerebral blood flow was unlikely since the infants had no signs of congestive heart failure (hepatic enlargement and only mild peripheral edema in case 1 and 3). However, an increased total blood volume, or an excessive cerebral blood flow cannot be ruled out.

A comparison can be suggested between pseudotumor cerebri and this syndrome of reversible intracranial hypertension in the neonatal period. The pattern of normal ventricular size and delayed resorption of CSF shown by isotope cisternography in pseudotumor is the same as described by case 3;[13, 28] acetazolamide is a satisfactory treatment in both situations. Whatever the mechanism could be, the end result of high intracranial pressure would be cerebral ischemia, when ICP reaches or exceeds arterial perfusion pressure.[11, 12, 14] Early treatment seems therefore advisable.

CONCLUSION

In conclusion, we suggest the following approach to diagnosis and treatment. When previously premature infants develop symptoms of increased intracranial pressure in the first months of life in the absence of infection or known predisposing causes, or when the ICP rises in the high-risk neonate, we recommend the following procedure:

1. Lumbar puncture to look for signs of hemorrhage or infection and as a therapeutic test
2. CT brain scan to eliminate obstructive hydrocephalus, subdural hematoma, or a mass lesion
3. If the infant shows improvement in the hours following lumbar puncture, institute acetazolamide 10 mg/kg/24 hr for about 14 days
4. Adjust total fluid intake to less than 160 ml/kg/24 hr. In the same way that a ductal murmur may lead one to restrict fluids, rising intracranial pressure should be such an indication, as suggested in Figure 6.

The incidence of this syndrome in the high-risk population of SGA prema-

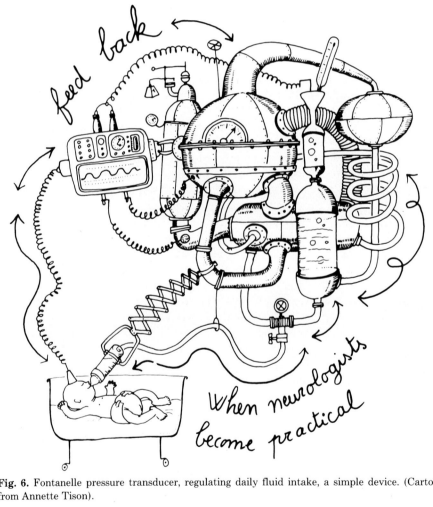

Fig. 6. Fontanelle pressure transducer, regulating daily fluid intake, a simple device. (Cartoon from Annette Tison).

ture newborns cannot be evaluated. In addition to these four severe cases observed within the last 9 years in the Port Royal Maternity Hospital, many mild cases have been observed. A reduction of fluid intake is all that is required for rapid reversal of the problem.

SUMMARY

We define a new syndrome of delayed intracranial hypertension in the neonatal period following chronic fetal distress. The essential features common to our four patients are as follows: premature small for gestational age infants without neurological abnormality who develop signs and symptoms of increased intracranial pressure when they are otherwise clinically stable. There is mild or no peripheral edema, no congestive heart failure, or other sign of fluid overload. Symptoms are relieved by lumbar puncture and/or treatment with acetazolamide. The syndrome is transient; there is no permanent hydrocephalus. The outcome is generally good. We speculate that this syndrome is related to restricted CSF absorption compared to production.

REFERENCES

1. Amiel-Tison, C., Korobkin, R., and Esque-Vaucouloux, M. T., Neck extensors hypertonia: a clinical sign of insult of the Central nervous system of the newborn. *Early Hum. Dev.* 1(2), 181 (1977).
2. Aperia, A., Broberger, O., Herin, P., and Zetterström, R., Renal Tubular Transport Systems as Markers of Cellular Maturation in Newborn Infants, in *Intensive Care in the Newborn*, III Stern *et al.*, Eds. Masson, New York, 1980, p. 000.
3. Bell, W. E., and McCormick, W. F., increased Intracranial Pressure in Children, in *Major Problems in Clinical Pediatrics*, Vol. VIII. W. B. Saunders, Philadelphia. 1978, pp. 193.
4. Domer, F. R., Effects of Diuretics on Cerebrospinal Fluid Formation and Potassium Exchange, in *Renal Pharmacology*, Fisher, J. W., Ed. Butterworths, London, 1971, p. 121.
5. Donn, S. M., and Philip, A. G. S., Early increase in intracranial pressure in preterm infants. *Pediatrics* 61, 904 (1978).
6. Epstein, F. J., Hochwald, G. M., and Ransohoff, J., Neonatal hydrocephalus treated by compressive head wrapping. *Lancet* 1, 634 (1973).
7. Epstein, F. J., Hochwald, G. M., Wald, A., and Ransohoff, J., Avoidance of shunt dependency in hydrocephalus. *Dev. Med. Child. Neurol.* 17 (*Suppl. 35*), 71 (1975).
8. Fishmann, R. A., Current Modes of Therapy of Brain Edema, in *Dynamics of Brain Edema*, Pappius, H. M., and Feindel, W., Eds. Springer-Verlag, New York, 1976, p. 362.
9. Hirsch, J. F., Lacombe, J., Pierre-Kahn, A., and Renier, D., Mesure de la pression intra cranienne par palpeur de fontanelle. *Neurochirurgie* 24, 89 (1978).
10. Hornych, H., and Amiel-Tison, C., Retention hydrosaline chez les enfants de faible poids de naissance. *Arch. Fr. Pediatr.* 34, 206 (1977).
11. Johnston, I. H., Rowan, J. O., Harper, A. M., and Jennett, W. B., Raised intracranial pressure and cerebral blood flow. I. Cisterna magna infusion in primates. *J. Neurol. Neurosurg. Psychiat.* 35, 285 (1972).
12. Johnston, I. H., Rowan, J. O., Harper, A. M., and Jennett, W. B., Raised intracranial pressure and cerebral blood flow. Part 2: Supratentorial and infratentorial mass lesions in primates. *J. Neurol. Neurosurg. Psychiatr.* 36, 161 (1973).
13. Johnston, I. H., and Patterson, A., Benign intracranial hypertension II. Pressure and circulation. *Brain* 97, 301 (1974).
14. Johnston, I. H., Rowan, J. O., Park, D. M., and Rennie, M. J., Raised intracranial pressure and

cerebral blood flow. Part 5: Effects of episodic intracranial pressure waves in primates. *J. Neurol. Neurosurg. Psychiatr.* **38,** 1076 (1975).

15. Korobkin, R., The relationship between head circumference and development of communicating hydrocephalus following intraventricular hemorrhage. *Pediatrics* **56,** 74 (1975).
16. Long, D. M., Maxwell, R., and Choi, K. S., A New Therapy Regimen for Brain Edema, in *Dynamics of Brain Edema*, Pappius, H. M., and Feindel, W., Eds. Springer-Verlag, New York, 1976, p. 293.
17. Lubchenco, L. O., Hansman, C., Dressler, M., *et al.*, Intrauterine growth as estimated from live born birth weight data at 24 to 42 weeks of gestation. *Pediatrics* **32,** 793 (1963).
18. Maren, T. H., Carbonic anhydrase: chemistry, physiology and inhibition. *Physiol. Rev.* **47,** 595 (1967).
19. Philip, A. G. S., Fontanel size and epiphyseal ossification in neonates with intrauterine growth retardation. *J. Pediatr.* **84,** 204 (1974).
20. Philip, A. G. S., Noninvasive monitoring of intracranial pressure. *Clin. Perinatol.* **6,** 123 (1979).
21. Robinson, R. O., Rolfe, P., and Sutton, P., Noninvasive method for measuring intracranial pressure in normal newborn infants. *Dev. Med. Child. Neurol.* **19,** 305 (1977).
22. Salmon, J. H., Hajjar, W., and Bada, H. S., The fontogram: A noninvasive intracranial pressure monitor. *Pediatrics* **60,** 721 (1977).
23. Stonestreet, B., Bell, E., Warburton, D., and Oh, W., The effects of fluid and sodium intake and renal compensation on the postnatal changes of extracellular fluid in low birth weight infants. *Pediatr. Res.* **13,** 521 (1979).
24. Sulyok, E., Nemeth, M., Tenyl, I., Csaba, I., Gyory, E., Ertl, T., and Varga, F., Postnatal development of renin angiotensin-aldosterone system, in relation to electrolyte balance in premature infants. *Pediatr. Res.* **13,** 817 (1979).
25. Vidyasagar, D., and Raju, T. N. K., A simple noninvasive technique of measuring intracranial pressure in the newborn. *Pediatrics* **59,** 957 (1977).
26. Vidyasagar, D., Raju, T. N. K., and Chiang, J., clinical significance of monitoring anterior fontanel pressure in sick neonates and infants. *Pediatrics* **62,** 996 (1978).
27. Wealthall, S. R., and Smallwood, R., Methods of measuring intracranial pressure via the fontanel without puncture. *J. Neurol. Neurosurg. Psychiatr.* **37,** 88 (1974).
28. Weisberg, L. A., and Chutorian, A. M., Pseudotumor cerebri of childhood. *Am. J. Dis. Child.* **131,** 1243 (1977).

26

The Pathogenesis of Cerebral Hypoxic Lesions and Intraventricular Hemorrhage in the Newborn Preterm Infant

BENT FRIIS-HANSEN, M.D. Ph.D.,[1] HANS C. LOU, M.D., Ph.D.,[2] NIELS A. LASSEN, M.D., Ph.D.,[3] and PETER D. WIMBERLEY, M.B., M.R.C.P.[4]

Intracranial hemorrhage is the major cause of perinatal death and of permanent brain damage in surviving preterm infants. Intracranial hemorrhage may be divided into two groups (Fig. 1): extracerebral and intracerebral hemorrhages.

"Extracerebral" bleeding is mainly subdural. It is of traumatic origin and is usually seen in full-term infants. This group includes hemorrhages caused by rupture of the falx, the tentorium, the sagittal sinus, or the veins entering the sagittal sinus.

"Intracerebral" hemorrhages are by far the most common type and account for about 90% of all intracranial hemorrhages in the perinatal period, occuring especially in premature infants. They include both hemorrhages and necrosis and, most commonly, a combination of both (Fig. 1).

It is now generally accepted that in most cases the hemorrhages start as capillary bleeding in subependymal layers of the germinal matrix as shown by Hambleton and Wigglesworth.[12, 22] This richly vascular structure overlying the caudate nucleus is most developed in the fetus from 6 to 8 months of age. It consists of spongioblasts which migrate out to the surface of the brain, where

[1] Rigshospitalet, Department of Neonatology, DK-2100 Ø, Copenhagen, Denmark
[2] Roskilde Hospital, Department of Neurology, DK-4000 Roskilde, Denmark
[3] Bispebjerg Hospital, Department of Clinical Physiology, DK-2400 NV, Copenhagen, Denmark
[4] Rigshospitalet, Department of Neonatology, DK-2100 Ø, Copenhagen, Denmark

INTRACRANIAL HEMORRHAGE IN NEWBORN INFANTS

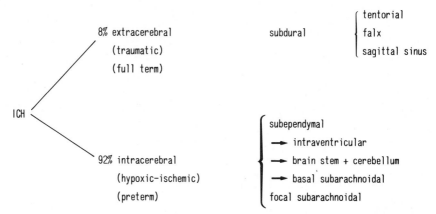

Fig. 1. A simple division of intracranial hemorrhage (ICH) into "extracerebral" and "intracerebral" bleedings.

they given rise to formation of the cerebral cortex. As a rule, bleeding will rupture through the ependymal lining into the ventricular system, but large bleeds may also extend into the parenchymal tissue. It is therefore easily understood why any damage to this highly important tissue will have a serious impact on later development of the infant.

From the lateral ventricles the bleeding expands into the fourth ventricle, through the foraminae, and out onto the surface of the brain, around the brain stem and cerebellum where it enters the subarachnoid space. Rarely, however, there will be only small, focal subarachnoid bleeds seen over the hemispheres.

Since intraventricular hemorrhage (IVH) is the most common type, we shall use this term to describe the entire group of intracerebral hemorrhages. It is seen in about 50% of all small premature infants dying during the first week of life, the incidence increasing with the degree of prematurity. Furthermore, it is found in almost all premature infants who have died from RDS—but on the other hand not all infants with IVH have suffered from RDS.

Recent studies by computerised tomography[23] have demonstrated IVH in 40% of all premature infants with a birth weight less than 1500 g. Among the surviving infants in this group one-quarter had IVH, of which several cases had not had any clinical symptoms suggestive of IVH.

PREVIOUSLY PROPOSED ETIOLOGIC FACTORS FOR IVH

Apart from immaturity and asphyxia, a diversity of explanations have been put forward including structural vulnerability of the germinal matrix (Ruchensteiner and Zollner, 1929[24]), maternal toxemia (Craig, 1938[3]), hypoxic venous congestion and capillary damage (Gruenwald, 1951[11]), venestasis and infarction (Larroche, 1964[15]), coagulation disorders (Gray, et al. 1968[10]), severe hypoxia (Harrison, et al., 1968[13]), hypoxia with circulatory failure and infarction and thrombosis of the vessels on the venous side of capillaries (Towbin, 1969[26]), the "no-reflow" phenomenon (Ames, et al., 1968[1]), increased venous pressure due to the use of continuous positive airway pressure (Vert, et al., 1973[28]), and venous hypertension secondary to hypoxic heart failure (Cole, et al. 1974[4]).

The liberal use of hypertonic bicarbonate solutions with leakage of protein into the cerebrospinal fluid (Simmons, et al., 1974[25]) has also been postulated.

Other theories which have been put forward include a combination of hypoxia, stasis, and rupture of the thin-walled veins poorly supported in the germinal matrix with abnormal coagulation (Leech and Kohnen, 1974[16]), cerebral oedema (Brann and Meyers, 1975[2]), increased capillary and arterial pressure (Hambleton and Wigglesworth, 1976[12]), an endotoxin (Gilles, et al., 1976[8]), the "luxury perfusion" syndrome (Liu, 1977[17]), and hypercarbia (Kenny, et al., 1978[14]).

It would be difficult to add much to this profuse number of ideas and therefore what we propose is more an overall working hypothesis which includes many of the already mentioned factors and which, hopefully, can offer suggestions for prophylactic treatment.

TIMING OF IVH

Most cases of IVH take place after birth and only about 5% of all cases are found in stillborn infants. Mildred Stahlman and her co-workers[27] were able to demonstrate that the majority of hemorrhages occurred 2–3 days after delivery with a mean of 38 hr. They used an elegant technique of injecting nonradioactive chromium tagged erythrocytes which later were activated when a post mortem clot was found.

Similar results were obtained by Tizard and his group,[5] who measured the timing of IVH by analysing the clot for the concentration of fetal hemoglobin (HbF) and comparing this to the concentration HbF in the circulating blood, which, after repeated small transfusions, was gradually declining during the first days of life. They found that the earliest bleeding took place 3–6 hr postpartum and the latest 3–4 days after delivery. Similar results have also been obtained by Leech in 1974[16] in a pathoanatomical study.

ASPHYXIA AND THE BLOOD BRAIN BARRIER (BBR)

The fact that IVH is rarely seen during or immediately after delivery indicates that the major cause of bleeding is unlikely to be found among the events taking place before delivery and that the many changes taking place during delivery hydrostatic and circulatory changes are presumably of the greatest importance.

During fetal life the arterial oxygen tension is only 3–4 kPa (20–30 mmHg) but a high cerebral blood flow presumably compensates for this low value— even lower values may occur during intrauterine asphyxia. Such low values are very rarely found after birth since the introduction of effective resuscitation and modern means of ventilatory support. This indicates that low oxygen tension in the perinatal period is not an immediate cause of IVH, but, combined with a postnatal diversion of blood flow from the brain to other tissues such as the respiratory muscles, may well be of great importance.

Even short periods of asphyxia are followed by a breakdown of the blood-brain barrier with leakage of albumin into the extracellular space of the brain. This has been illustrated clearly in newborn lambs, where Evans-blue was injected intravenously after delivery. In normal lambs no trace of the dye was found outside the blood vessels, but in asphyxiated lambs, where the dye was injected after recovery, the whole brain was coloured blue due to the albumin-bound dye spreading diffusely throughout the brain (Lou, *et al.*, 1979[19]).

CHANGES IN THE HYDROSTATIC PRESSURE

The skull of a newborn full-term infant is quite rigid and gives firm support to the brain, which is thereby protected against pressure changes occurring

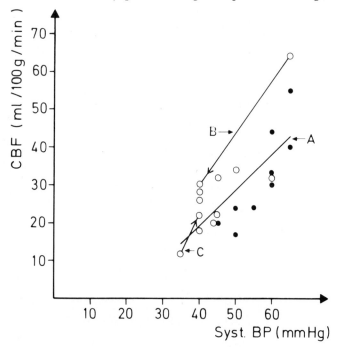

● : Newborns with birth weight ≥ 2000 g

O : Newborns with birth weight < 2000 g

A : Regression line : y = 0.96x − 18.6   r = 0.75

B : Repeated CBF measurements in an infants with spontaneous drops in syst BP

C : Repeated CBF measurements in an infants with spontaneous increase in syst BP

Fig. 2. The relation between CBF and the systolic blood pressure in 19 distressed newborn infants.[6] A is the line of correlation showing a pressure passive CBF. B and C show repeated measurements at a short time interval in two patients.

both inside and outside. In contrast, the skull of a preterm baby is very much softer and thereby less able to protect the brain. During fetal life the hydrostatic pressure of the amniotic fluid is about 15 mmHg, but this pressure surrounds the fetus and is therefore of no importance. After rupture of the membranes and during delivery this pressure disappears. However, with uterine contractions the pressure around the body of the fetus increases by 40–60 mmHg, and when the head is in the birth canal the blood pressure inside the capillaries will be increased by a similar value. This could well cause initial damage, which later might precipitate a rupture of the capillary wall.

AUTOREGULATION OF THE CEREBRAL BLOOD FLOW

In normal children as in adults the cerebral blood flow (CBF) is practically constant within a wide range of variations in the arterial pressure. This mechanism is called "autoregulation" and protects the brain from hypertension as well as hypotension.

Our studies of cerebral blood flow in asphyxiated premature newborn infants has shown that CBF is "pressure-passive" as illustrated in Figure 2, where

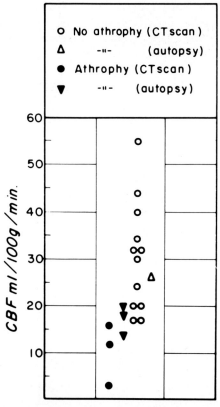

Fig. 3. A diagram showing the central role played by impaired autoregulation of CBF in the development of cerebral necrosis and IVH in perinatal hypoxic-ischemia brain injury.

CBF is found to decrease with decreasing blood pressure and to increase with hypertension.[18]

We have measured CBF in 19 asphyxiated infants and found variations from normal or slightly elevated values of 55 ml/100 g/min to low values of 3–20 ml/100 g/min. Seven of these babies died and the rest were reexamined clinically 1 year later. It is interesting that cerebral atrophy was demonstrated, by autopsy or by CT scan at follow-up, only in the infants with a CBF of 20 ml/100 g/min or less (Fig. 3). Since our method of measuring CBF includes the injection of a small amount of radioactive xenon through a temporarily placed catheter in the aortic arch, they cannot be repeated many times in the same babies. Therefore it remains to be shown whether autoregulation is also impaired after a "normal delivery," and if normal autoregulation is restored after the first few days of life. The latter would explain the observation that IVH rarely takes place after this period.

From our studies we believe that impaired autoregulation of CBF has a central role in the events leading to IVH. This is illustrated in Figure 4.

Perinatal asphyxia of the brain may be caused either by a decrease in arterial oxygen tension, hemoglobin concentration, CBF, or by a combination of all three factors. This causes a breakdown of the blood-brain barrier and the development of brain oedema. This oedema is both extracellular and intracellular including endothelial cells (blebs) as well as neurones and glial cells. Finally the autoregulation of CBF becomes impaired with a maximal dilatation of the arterioles, capillaries, and small thin-walled veins. Thereby CBF becomes

PATHOGENESIS OF PERINATAL HYPOXIC–ISCHEMIC BRAIN INJURY

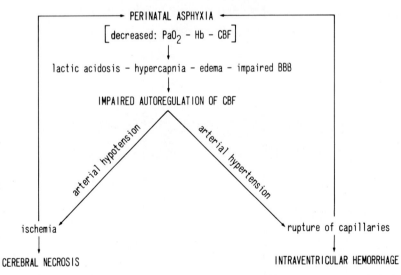

Fig. 4. Cerebral atrophy as verified either by autopsy or by CT scan was found only in infants with a low CBF of 20 ml/100 g/min or less, as compared to a value of 60–70 ml/100 g/min seen in healthy infants.

pressure-passive and in this situation any increase in blood pressure will be transmitted directly to the capillaries which in the premature brain have poor glial support, and bleeding takes place.

On the other hand a fall in the arterial blood pressure will be followed by a decreased CBF which will aggravate any coexisting ischemia and cause necrosis.

It is well known that during asphyxia of the newborn the blood pressure increases, but this is often followed by a period of hypotension, which may be equally harmful to the infant.

That hypotension is an important factor has recently also been demonstrated by Tizard and collaborators[7] in a study of clinical events leading to IVH.

Furthermore, our studies have demonstrated that large changes in blood pressure frequently occur in newborn premature infants, often precipitated by spontaneous motor activity, by routine handling, or during seizures.[21]

That increased blood pressure is of primary importance for the development of IVH has been demonstrated in recent animal experiments. Newborn beagles have a germinal matrix similar to that of the human, and it has been shown

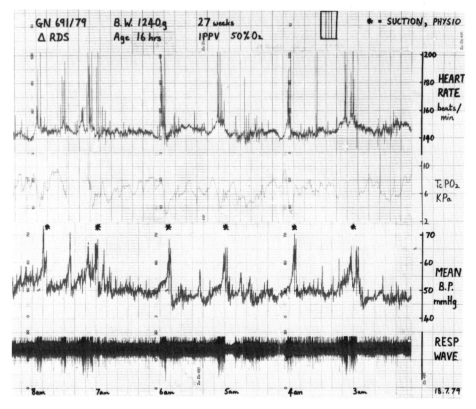

Fig. 5. Each time physiotherapy and suction was carried out acute increases were seen in heart rate, mean arterial blood pressure, and motor activity as reflected by the respiratory wave or transthoracic impedance. At the same time TcpO₂ decreased. Curve to be read from right to left.

that they will develop IVH if the blood pressure is increased without any changes in blood gases and acid-base balance.[9]

In order to demonstrate to what extent newborn infants are exposed to hypertension, we have studied a number of infants by continuous recording of the mean arterial blood pressure (MPB), systolic and diastolic blood pressure, heart rate, transcutaneous oxygen tension ($TcpO_2$), and respiratory rate by transthoracic impedance—which also indicates motor activity.

These recordings have demonstrated that young sick (RDS) premature infants often react to routine handling, such as feeding, suction, etc. with acute increases in MBP from around 50–60 to 80–90 mmHg. At the same time the systolic blood pressure often jumps above 100 mm for periods of a quarter to half an hour or more (Fig. 5). Furthermore we have noticed that the $TcpO_2$ during the first couple of days often decreases during these periods of hypertension, which will aggravate any threatening ischemia of the brain. When, after a couple of days the infant is recovering, the $TcpO_2$ tends to increase with increases in MBP (Fig. 6).

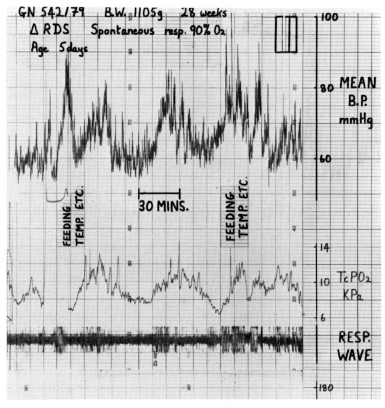

Fig. 6. In connection with temperature taking and feeding, acute increases in mean arterial blood pressure and motor activity (respiratory wave) were seen, but in this infant 5 days of age $TcpO_2$ increased at the same time. Curve to be read from right to left.

SUMMARY

A short account is given of the many factors which have been put forward to explain the development of IVH, and an overall model is proposed which is centered around "impaired autoregulation of CBF" in asphyxiated newborn infants. This explains how both arterial hypotension and hypertension can cause or aggravate ischemia as well as rupture of the capillaries in the subependymal layers of the highly vascular germinal matrix in the premature brain.

Prophylactic measures might therefore include avoidance of asphyxia and pressure damage during delivery, which in the small high risk infants should possibly be by Caesarean section. After delivery large variations in the blood pressure should be counteracted.

REFERENCES

1. Ames, A., Wright, L., Kowada, M., Thurston, J. M., and Majno, G., Cerebral ischemia II. The no-reflow phenomenon. *Am. J. Pathol.* **52,** 437 (1968).
2. Brann, A. W., Jr., and Meyers, R. E., Central nervous system findings in the newborn monkey following severe in utero partial asphyxia. *Neurology* **25,** 327 (1975).
3. Craig, W. S., Intracranial hemorrhage in the newborn. A study of diagnosis and differential diagnosis based upon pathological and clinical findings in 126 cases. *Arch. Dis. Child.* **13,** 89 (1938).
4. Cole, V. A., Durbin, G. M., Olafsson, A., Reynolds, E. O. R., Rivers, R. P. A., and Smith, J. F., Pathogenesis of intraventricular hemorrhage in newborn infants. *Arch. Dis. Child.* **49,** 722 (1974).
5. Emerson, P., Fujimura, M., Howat, P., Howes, D., Keeling, J., Robinson, R. O., Salisbury, D., and Tizard, J. P. M., Timing of intraventricular hemorrhage. *Arch. Dis. Child.* **52,** 183 (1977).
6. Friis-Hansen, B., Lou, H., and Lassen, N., Cerebral blood flow in distressed infants. *Intensive Care in the Newborn II*, Stern, L., Ed. Masson, New York, 1979, p. 119.
7. Fujimura, M., Salisbury, D. M., Robinson, R. O., Howat, P., Emerson, P. M., Keeling, J. W., and Tizard, J. P. M., Clinical events relating to intraventricular hemorrhage in the newborn. *Arch. Dis. Child.* **54,** 409 (1979).
8. Gilles, F. H., Leviton, A., and Kerr, C. S., Endotoxin leucoencephalopathy in the telencephalon of the newborn kitten. *J. Neurol. Sci.* **27,** 183 (1976).
9. Goddard, J., Lewis, R. M., Armstrong, D. L., et al., Intraventricular hemorrhage—an animal model. *Biol. Neonate* **37,** 39 (1980).
10. Gray, O. P., Ackerman, A., and Fraser, A. J., Intracranial hemorrhage and clotting defects in low birth weight infants. *Lancet* **1,** 545 (1968).
11. Gruenwald, P., Subependymal cerebral hemorrhage in premature infants and its relation to various injurious influences at birth. *Am. J. Obstet. Gynecol.* **61,** 1285 (1951).
12. Hambleton, G., and Wigglesworth, J. S., Origin of intraventricular hemorrhage in the pre-term infant. *Arch. Dis. Child.* **51,** 651 (1976).
13. Harrison, V. C., Heese, H. de V., and Klein, M., Intracranial hemorrhage associated with hyaline membrane disease. *Arch. Dis. Child.* **43,** 116 (1968).
14. Kenny, J. D., Garcia-Prats, J. A., Hilliard, J. L., Corbet, A. J. S., and Rudolph, A. J., Hypercarbia at birth: A possible role in the pathogenesis of intraventricular hemorrhage. *Pediatrics* **62,** 465 (1978).
15. Larroche, J. C., Hémorrhagies cérébrales intraventriculaires chez la prématuré. I. Anatomie et pathophysiologie. *Biol. Neonat.* **7,** 26 (1964).
16. Leech, R. W., and Kohnen, P., Subependymal and intraventricular hemorrhages in the newborn. *Am. J. Pathol.* **77,** 465 (1974).

17. Liu, H. M., A new look at an old problem: Intraventricular hemorrhage in the newborn. *Am. J. Pathol.* **86**, 850 (1977).

18. Lou, H., Lassen, N., and Friis-Hansen, B., Low cerebral blood flow in hypotensive perinatal distress. *Acta Neurol. Scand.* **56**, 343 (1977).

19. Lou, H., Lassen, N., Tweed, W. A., Johnson, G., Jones, M., and Palahnuik, R. J., Pressure passive cerebral blood flow and breakdown of the blood-brain barrier in experimental fetal asphyxia. *Acta Paediatr. Scand.* **68**, 57 (1979).

20. Lou, H., Lassen, N., and Friis-Hansen, B., Impaired autoregulation of cerebral blood flow in the distressed newborn infant. *J. Pediatr.* **94**, 118 (1979).

21. Lou, H. C., and Friis-Hansen, B., Elevations in arterial blood pressure during motor activity and epileptic seizures in the newborn. *Acta Pediatr. Scand* **68**, 803 (1979).

22. Pape, K. E., and Wigglesworth, J. S., Hemorrhage, Ischemia and the Perinatal Brain, in *Clinics in Developmental Medicine, Nos. 69/70.* Heineman, London, 1979.

23. Papile, L. A., Burstein, J., Burstein, R., and Koffler, H., Incidence and evolution of subependymal and intraventricular hemorrhage: A study of infants with birth weights less than 1500 g. *J. Pediatr.* **92**, 529 (1978).

24. Ruchensteiner, E., and Zollner, F., Über die Blutungen im Gebiete der Vena terminalis bei Neugeborenen. *Frankf. Z. Pathol.* **37**, 568 (1929) [cited by Fujimura, M., *et al.*, *Arch. Dis. Child.* **54**, 409 (1979)]

25. Simmons, M. A., Adcock, E. W., and Battaglia, F. C., Hypernatremia and intracranial hemorrhage in neonates. *N. Engl. J. Med.* **291**, 6 (1974).

26. Towbin, A., Cerebral hypoxic damage in fetus and newborn. *Arch. Neurol.* **20**, 35 (1969).

27. Tsiantos, A., Victorin, L., Relier, J. P., Dyer, N., Sundell, H., Brill, A. B., and Stahlman, M., Intracranial hemorrhage in the prematurely born infant. *J. Pediatr.* **85**, 854 (1974).

28. Vert, P., André, M., and Sibout, M., Increased venous pressure due to use of continous positive airway pressure. *Lancet* **2**, 319 (1973).

27

Respiratory Muscle Fatigue in Newborn Infants

NESTOR L. MULLER, M.D., A. CHARLES BRYAN, M.D. and
M. HEATHER BRYAN, M.D.

The ventilatory muscles just like any other skeletal muscle can fatigue; that is, they begin to fail as force generators. When this occurs, alveolar ventilation must fall, CO_2 must rise, and by definition the patient is in respiratory failure. This failure is ventilatory muscle failure and the purpose of this paper is to show that ventilatory muscle failure is common in sick newborn infants. In lung disease the work of breathing can become very high, and the newborn infant is particularly susceptible to fatigue at these high work loads. Keens, *et al.*[1] have shown that the oxidative capacity of the preterm infant diaphragm is extremely low. Substrate available for muscle contraction is tenuous as both glycogen and lipid stores are scanty in the preterm infant. In addition respiratory rates are high in newborn infants, and it is a general principle of muscle physiology that the higher the contraction repetition rate, the shorter is the endurance.[2]

Kadefors, *et al.*[3] showed that muscle fatigue could be diagnosed by spectral frequency analysis of the EMG, that is, the distribution of power as a function of frequency. They showed that muscles during nonfatiguing loads had a characteristic frequency spectrum. When subjected to a fatiguing load, there was a characteristic change in the power spectrum, with a fall in the high frequency power and a substantial increase in the low frequency power (Fig. 1). There is controversy as to the cause of this spectral frequency shift, but it is probably the result of a decrease in the velocity of the action potentials within the muscle,[4] secondary to metabolic changes in the muscle.[5]

A major problem in applying this analysis to the newborn infant is that the

The Research Institute, The Hospital for Sick Children
Toronto, Ontario, Canada

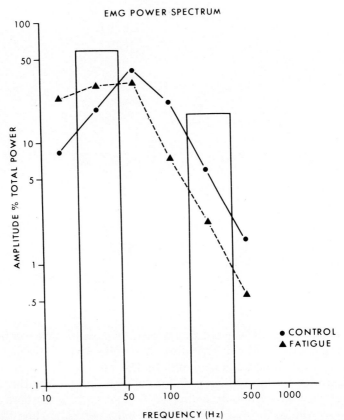

Fig. 1. The diaphragmatic EMG power spectrum plotted with the amplitude (percent of total power) as a function of frequency (Hz). Both scales are logarithmic. The solid lines shows the normal frequency spectrum obtained from the diaphragmatic EMG, while the dotted line indicates the shift in the frequency spectrum which accompanies diaphragmatic fatigue. The upright bars are the two band frequencies (20–40 Hz and 150–350 Hz) where the major power shifts occur and which can be expressed as a ratio. A fall in the high/low frequency ratio denotes muscle fatigue.

diaphragmatic EMG is contaminated by the EKG signal, most of which largely occurs below 100 Hz. We used the R wave of the EKG signal to trigger a digital computer to ignore the next 50 msec, and then to sample the following 200 msec stopping well before the next EKG complex.[6, 7] The pure EMG sample was then analyzed by Fourier transform analysis to yield the power spectrum.

Initially we analyzed the EMG signal in normal newborn infants obtained by surface electrodes,[8] gated out the EKG,[6, 7] and showed that the frequency spectrum was identical to that of any adult skeletal muscle.[9] We also found that when the chest wall of newborn infants was distorting during REM sleep, there was a characteristic change of muscle fatigue, that is, a fall in the high frequency power spectrum with a simultaneous increase in the low frequency power (Fig. 1).

We saw this fatigue pattern, an indicator of failure of the diaphragm as a force generator, in normal infants during REM sleep. They adapted by either changing sleep state, or by a short apneic pause. We also observed that diaphragmatic muscle fatigue played a major role in the response of infants with lung disease (RDS) who were on mechanical ventilators.

As Fourier transform analysis requires elaborate computer based technology, it was impractical as a simple clinical monitoring device. Using the same basic principles, we achieved the same results using a simple "on line" monitoring device. After exclusion or gating of the EKG signal, we used two filter bands, a high frequency band between 150–350 Hz and a low frequency band of 20–40 Hz (Fig. 1), and displayed the ratio of the power in the two bands. With muscle fatigue, the high frequency power falls while the low frequency power rises, and therefore the ratio of the high to low frequencies decreases and this ratio is continuously recorded on a pen recorder.

A typical example is shown in Figure 2 of an infant who had just been weaned from intermittent positive pressure ventilation to CPAP alone. The

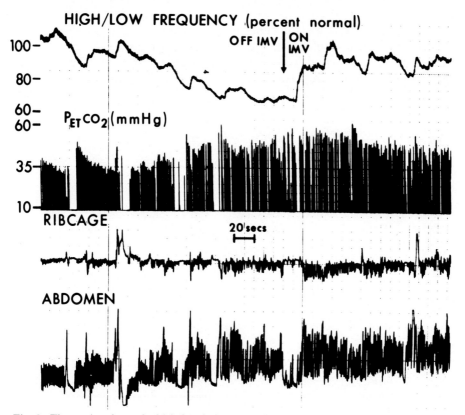

Fig. 2. The tracing shows the high/low frequency ratio monitored from an infant diaphragmatic EMG, end tidal PCO_2, rib cage and abdominal movement. There is a progressive fall in the high/low ratio and steady rise in the PCO_2 following weaning from IMV to CPAP alone. The respiratory failure due to diaphragmatic muscle fatigue is reversed with the restarting of IMV as indicated by the rapid rise and recovery of the high/low ratio and slower return towards normal of the end tidal PCO_2.

high/low frequency ratio progressively falls and end tidal PCO_2 rises. The clinical condition required reinstitution of mechanical ventilation with a prompt rise in the high/low ratio and a slower return of the end tidal PCO_2 towards normal. In another example (Fig. 3) the high/low frequency ratio is shown in an infant weaned from intermittent mandatory ventilation (IMV) to CPAP alone. The high/low ratio shows a marked fall after 10 min, indicating diaphragmatic fatigue. Clinical deterioration, however, as evidenced by cyanosis and apnea was not apparent until 30 min of CPAP alone. There was a prompt recovery in the high/low ratio with the resumption of IMV.

Using this monitoring device, we followed 10 infants during weaning either to a lower ventilator frequency or to CPAP alone. The diaphragmatic EMG was monitored with subcostal surface electrodes. We also recorded end tidal or arterial PCO_2. This information was withheld from the clinician. Because muscle fatigue can occur during hypoxia,[10] we monitored oxygen with a transcutaneous PO_2 electrode (radiometer) keeping the skin PO_2 nearly constant by altering the FIO_2.

In six infants we had a significant fall in the high/low frequency ratio (20% or more below the control ratio), indicating diaphragmatic muscle fatigue. The transcutaneous PO_2 values were relatively constant, while in every case the end tidal PCO_2 rose significantly (Fig. 4). The weaning step had failed, and

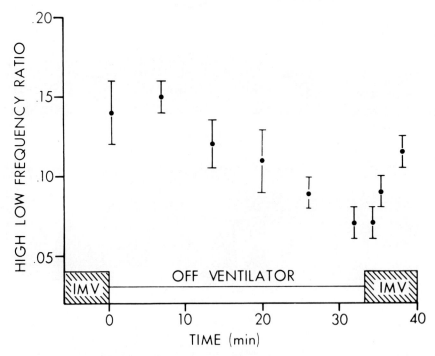

Fig. 3. The high/low frequency ratio progressively falls in this infant when weaned from the ventilator to CPAP alone. IMV was restarted on clinical indications after 30 min although the characteristics of diaphragmatic muscle fatigue are present earlier.

DIAPHRAGMATIC FATIGUE

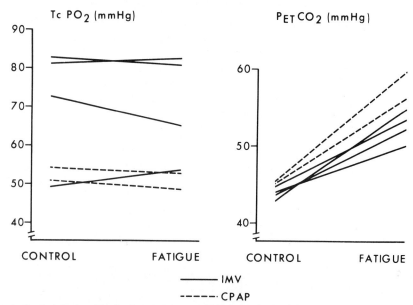

Fig. 4. In six infants with diaphragmatic muscle fatigue obtained from EMG spectral frequency analysis the end tidal PCO_2 rose significantly, indicating respiratory failure. The transcutaneous PO_2 was held relatively constant by altering the inspired oxygen.

NO DIAPHRAGMATIC FATIGUE

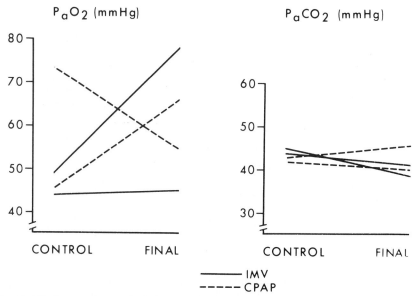

Fig. 5. Diaphragmatic muscle fatigue was not present in these four infants monitored with diaphragmatic EMGs. The arterial PCO_2's did not alter in the absence of diaphragmatic fatigue.

respiratory failure was evident. The clinician reinstituted mechanical ventilation because of the deteriorating clinical condition. In four infants studied there was no significant fall in the diaphragmatic high/low frequency ratio (Fig. 5). Carbon dioxide retention was not seen, and these weaning steps were successful for a period of 12 hr or more.

The monitoring of the high/low frequency ratio derived from the diaphragmatic EMG directed and assisted the weaning of newborn infants from mechanical ventilators. We have observed in several instances that at high mechanical ventilator respiratory rates the EMG signal ceased, indicating no diaphragmatic activity. While one can regard this as a resting period for the diaphragm, we believe that disuse may be the harbinger of atrophy. Successful weaning requires that the diaphragm works hard, but just short of fatigue. An example of one infant is shown in Figure 6. The baby on assisted ventilation of

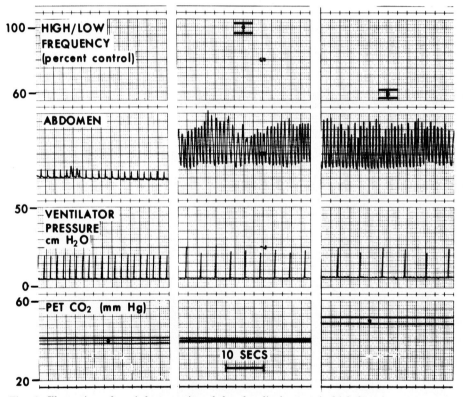

Fig. 6. Illustration of an infant monitored for the diaphragmatic high/low frequency ratio, abdominal movement measured with magnetometers, ventilator pressure and rate, and end tidal PCO_2. At a ventilator rate of 30 breaths/min there is little abdominal movement, an absent high/low ratio indicating no diaphragmatic EMG activity, and a normal end tidal PCO_2. At a ventilator rate of 15 breaths/min there is active diaphragmatic muscle activity indicated by the high/low ratio, good abdominal movement, and a normal end tidal PCO_2. With a ventilator rate of 10 breaths/min the high/low ratio is now showing diaphragmatic muscle fatigue and an increase in PCO_2.

30 breaths/min has a normal end tidal PCO_2 and small abdominal movements in phase with the ventilator. No diaphragmatic EMG activity was present. At a ventilator rate of 15 breaths/min, end tidal PCO_2 was normal and there was an active diaphragm with a normal high/low frequency ratio. At a ventilator rate of 10 breaths/min, however, the diaphragm is active but the high/low ratio has fallen, indicating diaphragmatic fatigue, and the end tidal CO_2 has increased indicating ventilatory failure.

Mechanical ventilators are initially life-saving in babies with RDS, but they are dangerous substitutes for respiratory muscles. Indeed the incidence of bronchopulmonary dysplasia may be aggravated by inappropriate maintenance of ventilator therapy leading to disuse atrophy of the respiratory muscles. Respiratory failure in newborn infants may be peripheral, rather than central, in origin. Respiratory muscle failure plays a major role in newborn lung disease.

REFERENCES

1. Keens, T. G., Bryan, A. C., Levison, H., and Ianuzzo, C. D., Developmental pattern of muscle fiber types in human ventilatory muscles. *J. Appl. Physiol. Respirat. Environ. Exercise Physiol.* **44,** 909 (1978).

2. Molbech, S., Average Percentage Force at Repeated Maximal Isometric Muscle Contractions at Different Frequencies, in *Communications from the Testing and Observations Institute of Danish National Association for Infantile Paralysis, No. 16,* 1963.

3. Kadefors, R., Kaiser, E., and Petersen, I., Dynamic spectrum analysis of myopotentials with special reference to muscle fatigue. *Electromyography* **8,** 39 (1968).

4. Lindstrom, L., Magnusson, R., and Petersen, I., Muscle fatigue and action potential conduction velocity changes studied with frequency analysis of EMG signals. *Electromyogr. Clin. Neurophysiol.* **10,** 341 (1970).

5. Mortimer, J. T., Magnusson, R., and Petersen, I., Conduction velocity in ischemic muscle: effect on EMG frequency spectrum. *Am. J. Physiol.* **219,** 1324 (1970).

6. Prechtl, H. F. R., Van Eykern, L. A., and O'Brien, M. J., Respiratory muscle EMG in newborns: a non-intrusive method. *Early Hum. Dev.* **1,** 265 (1977).

7. Muller, N., Volgyesi, G., Becker, L., Bryan, M. H., and Bryan, A. C., Diaphragmatic muscle tone. *J. Appl. Physiol. Respirat. Environ. Exercise Physiol.* **42,** 279 (1979).

8. Gross, D., Grassino, A., Ross, W. D., and Macklem, P. T., Electromyogram pattern of diaphragmatic fatigue. *J. Appl. Physiol. Respirat. Environ. Exercise Physiol.* **46,** 1 (1979).

9. Muller, N., Gulston, G., Cade, D., Whitton, J., Froese, A. B., Bryan, M. H., and Bryan, A. C., Diaphragmatic muscle fatigue in the newborn. *J. Appl. Physiol. Respirat. Environ. Exercise Physiol.* **46,** 688 (1979).

10. Roussos, C. S., and Macklem, P. T., Diaphragmatic fatigue in man. *J. Appl. Physiol. Respirat. Environ. Exercise Physiol.* **43,** 189 (1977).

28

Ventilation by High Frequency Oscillation (A Preliminary Report)

ALISON B. FROESE and A. CHARLES BRYAN

In the lung gas transport is achieved both by convection and diffusion.[1] The relative magnitude of these two processes can be estimated by the Peclet number, which is the ratio of the velocity times the diameter to the molecular diffusivity. The Peclet number in the trachea is normally in the order of 1000, indicating a dominance of convective transport. But with succeeding generations and decreasing diameter and velocity, the Peclet number falls. A "critical zone" is reached in the terminal bronchioles where the Peclet number is equal to 1 and convective motion is equal to the rate of diffusion, which is exceedingly slow. Gas transport from the critical zone to the alveoli is, however, considerably enhanced by the mechanical action of the heart. The efficacy of cardiogenic mixing suggested that further "stirring" of the air column at the mouth might facilitate gas transport.

In some preliminary experiments pigs were anaesthetised, intubated, and the endotracheal tube attached to a loudspeaker. The animals were then paralysed and the end tidal CO_2 fell to zero. The loudspeaker was then driven at 5 Hz (which gave an air displacement of approximately 25 ml) and CO_2 was very rapidly "shaken" out of the lung.

In dogs we subsequently reported that excellent gas exchange could be maintained during complete paralysis by high frequency oscillation.[2] Oscillation was achieved using a small piston pump. The physiological dead space of these dogs was a mean of 56 ml, and the displacement of the pump was set at 15 ml. The optimum frequency for gas exchange was found to be 15 Hz. These dogs accumulated hundreds of hours of oscillation with no apparent damage to the lungs.

Hospital for Sick Children, Toronto

271

Oscillation in human volunteers has two problems: the soft palate oscillates and this is quite disconcerting; further, the glottis tends to close. We therefore performed awake nasotracheal intubation on four normal volunteers.[3] Oscillations were applied to the endotracheal tube with a volume of 80 ml at 15 Hz. The sensation is quite soothing, but chest wall proprioception is impaired. Breath-holding up to 7 min, with normal $PaCO_2$ at breakpoint, was achieved, but prolonged apnea was not induced. To circumvent the cortical input to breathing, a sleep dose of pentobarbital was given, during oscillation. This produced complete apnea for up to 13 min with normal blood gases throughout.

Before use in patients a safe circuit had to be devised. The requirement was for an exit port for the fresh gas flow to carry away the CO_2 and a pathway to allow spontaneous breathing. The problem is that any exit allows the escape of oscillatory volume. This was partially solved by making the exit an 8-ft-long, 0.5-in. diameter tube with a large gas inertia. As impedance at high frequency is largely inertial, this tube offers a high impedance to high frequency oscillation, but low impedance to the fresh gas flow and normal breathing—it is a fluidic low pass filter. It is still not ideal as its efficiency varies with the relative impedance of the filter and the lung. In a normal subject only about one-half to one-third of the oscillatory volume reaches the lung; in abnormal lungs it is even less efficient. Thus quoted volume displacements and pressure amplitudes have no real meaning. The strategy is to increase the volume displacement until there are "satisfactory" oscillations of the chest wall. The equivalent of continuous positive airway pressure is maintained by varying the rate of fresh gas flow.

Using this system, we have oscillated, for 1-hr periods, 12 patients requiring mechanical ventilation for a variety of reasons. They range in weight from 2.5 kg to 100 kg. Most of the patients were heavily sedated and paralysed. Two were unsedated and not paralysed, one with RDS and the other with chronic obstructive pulmonary disease (COPD). In all patients CO_2 elimination during oscillation was normal, and oxygenation well maintained. Cardiac output was unchanged. The most instructive case was the patient with COPD, who was on a ventilator with an $F_IO_2 = 0.36$, just about to be weaned. Two minutes after starting the oscillator, he stopped breathing. Despite this his CO_2 remained normal and his PaO_2 climbed gradually by 40 mm on the same F_IO_2. The P_aO_2 fell again when he was returned to standard mechanical ventilation.

We have now oscillated four infants with RDS. In one case the infant was very restless throughout and we had to desist because of severe right to left shunting. Results were good in the three other infants. One stopped breathing for a long period. In the other two good oxygenation was maintained with lower inspired oxygen concentrations than were required on the ventilator.

The oscillator is clearly not achieving gas exchange by convective flow as the "tidal volume" is less than dead space volume. Gas exchange therefore appears to be achieved by facilitated diffusion. The velocities are substantially higher than during normal breathing and the increase in the Peclet number moves the "critical zone" closer to the alveoli. Scherer, et al.[4] showed in a five branched lung model that effective diffusivity (D_{eff}) could be very substantially higher than molecular diffusivity (D_{mol}). The magnitude followed the general equation for Taylor dispersion in turbulent flow[5]:

$$D_{eff} = D_{mol} + kud,$$

where k is a constant close to unity, u is the velocity, and d is the diameter. At velocities of 100 cm/sec they showed a 4000-fold increase in effective diffusivity over molecular diffusivity, and our velocities are substantially higher than this.

There are several potential advantages to high frequency oscillation. As the volume displacement is very small, the risk of pulmonary barotrauma is substantially reduced. Further diffusive transport is less dependent on regional time constants than is convective flow.

However, as a "practical" device this requires a great deal of further investigation and considerable work on circuit design, optimum frequencies, and amplitudes, etc.

REFERENCES

1. Engle, L. A., and Macklem, P. T., Gas Mixing and Distribution in the Lung, in *Respiratory Physiology II, International Review of Physiology, Vol 14*, Widdicombe, J. G., Ed. University Park Press, Baltimore, 1977.
2. Bohn, D. J., Miyasaka, K., Marchak, B. E., Thompson, W. K., Froese, A. B., and Bryan, A. C., Ventilation by high frequency oscillation. *J. Appl. Physiol. Respirat. Environ. Exercise Physiol.* **48**(4), 710 (1980).
3. Butler, W. J., Bohn, D. J., Bryan, A. C., and Froese, A. B., Ventilation by high frequency oscillation in humans. *Anesthesia and Analgesia* **59**(8), 577 (1980).
4. Scherer, P. W., Shendalman, L. H., Greene, N. M., and Bouhuys, A., Measurement of axial diffusivity in a model of the bronchial airways. *J. Appl. Physiol.* **38**, 719 (1975).
5. Taylor, G. I., The dispersion of matter in tubulent flow through a pipe. *Proc. R. Soc. Lond. Ser. A* **223**, 446 (1954).

29

Histochemical Identification of Chloride-Secreting Cells in the Fetal Respiratory Tract

ELIZABETH PERKETT, M.D.,* MARY E. GRAY, Ph.D., and MILDRED STAHL-MAN, M.D.

The production of fluid by the mammalian fetal lung appears to be an active process, probably under neural or humoral control.[1] The composition of its ions support this view, in that chloride ions are moved from fetal blood into lung fluid against a concentration and electrical gradient. The theories of chloride cotransport[2] and of standing gradients[3] in the intracellular spaces, along with the proposed presence of Na-K ATP'ases on the basolateral surfaces of epithelial lining cells[4] have been suggested as mechanisms consistent with existing data from other epithelial cell types involved in similar transport. However, the specific cellular type involved in the production of fetal lung fluid has not been identified.

In an attempt to identify the morphology of homologous cell types, gills of the Teleost fish, Poecilia sphenops, have been examined by light and electron microscopy, both before and after exposure to the halide-silver staining that has been described by Philpott.[5] Fish were taken from fresh water adaptation serially to a salt water environment over 72 hr and four concentration changes. Gills were examined following sacrifice after 24 hr at each concentration. On light microscopy, gill plates showed typical large rounded cells with characteristic pits at their lumenal edge situated at the base of respiratory leaflets. With the silver halide stain, silver grains were concentrated around the edge of these pits.

Departments of Pediatrics and Pathology, Newborn Lung Center, Vanderbilt University School of Medicine, Nashville, Tennessee 37232
Supported by Grant # HL 14214-08
* Trainee under Grant # HL 07256

On electron microscopy, these cells were crowded with many sausage-shaped mitochondria, and precipitate was seen in intracellular spaces and in some intercellular spaces, but was most concentrated around the edge of the pits (Fig. 1). More silver-halide-stained cells (presumably silver chloride) were seen in sea water than in fresh water adapted fish, and silver staining was heavier.

Thus far, one fetal lamb killed at birth at 117 days gestation (term = 147 days) and one human fetus of 22 weeks gestation have been similarly studied.

The trachea of the lamb showed heavy silver staining in a number of the ciliated cells, with no appreciable staining of the nonciliated secretory cells (Goblet cells). On electron microscopy, precipitate was concentrated in the

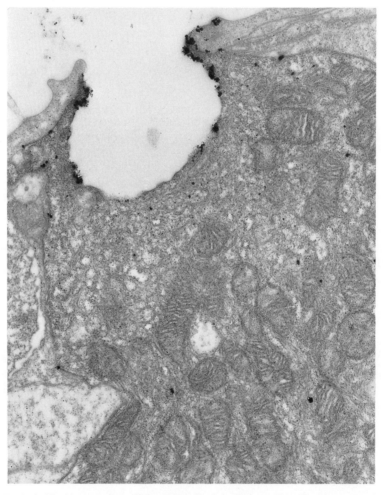

Fig. 1. Typical chloride-secreting cell from the gill of the Teleost, Poecilia sphenops, adapted to sea water. Heaviest silver halide accumulation is seen lining the exposed apical cavity and in scattered accumulations along intercellular borders. Additional finely dispersed silver halide granules are found throughout the cell. (Philpott stain; × 17,125).

intracellular spaces, in scattered intercellular spaces, but was heaviest at the lumenal edge around the cilia (Fig. 2).

In the 22-week human fetus, ciliated cells of the intrapulmonary conducting airways were most heavily stained, in locations similar to those of lamb tracheal ciliated cells, but also heavy accumulation spots were localized on the baso-lateral membranes (Fig. 3).

These preliminary findings suggest that some of the ciliated cells of the fetal tracheobronchial tree are the site of chloride transfer from pulmonary intra-vascular to intralumenal compartments, and that fluid transfer occurs at the same sites.

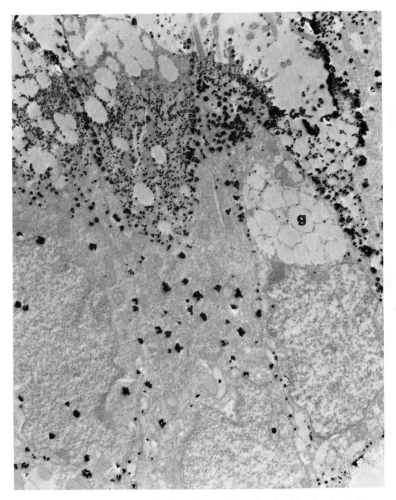

Fig. 2. Ciliated columnar epithelial cells from the trachea of a fetal lamb of 117 days gestation which was killed at birth. Silver halide accumulation is heaviest along the lumenal border of the ciliated cells and in the intercellular spaces. Scattered large accumulations of silver halide appear to be associated with intracellular spaces. Goblet cell (g) is unstained. (Philpott stain; × 8,000).

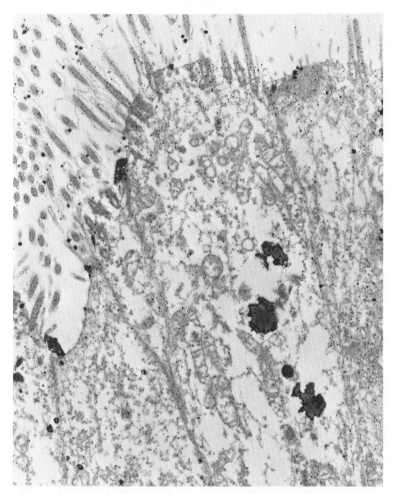

Fig. 3. Ciliated columnar epithelial cells from a small intrapulmonary bronchus of a human fetus of 22 weeks gestation. Silver halide accumulation is heaviest along the lumenal border and around intracellular droplets of lipid. Finely dispersed silver halide appears intracellularly. Silver grains can be seen incorporated into membranes of the cilia. (Philpott stain; × 11,200).

REFERENCES

1. Olver, R. E., Fetal lung liquids. *Fed. Proc.* **36,** 2269 (1977).
2. Frizzel, R. A., Field, M., and Schultz, S. G., Sodium coupled chloride transport by epithelial tissues. *Am. J. Physiol.* **236,** 1 (1979).
3. Diamond, J. M., and Bossert, W. A., Standing-gradient osmotic flow: A mechanism for coupling of water and solute transport in epithelia. *J. Gen. Physiol.* **50,** 2061 (1967).
4. Katz, A. I., and Epstein, F. H. Physiologic role of sodium-potassium-activated adenosive triphosphatase in the transport of cations across biologic membranes. *N. Eng. J. Med.* **278,** 253 (1968).
5. Philpott, C. W., Halide localization in the teleost chloride cell and its identification by selected area electron diffraction. *Protoplasma* **60,** 7–23 (1965).

30

Effects of Vitamin E on Lung Response to Hyperoxic Insult in the Newborn Rabbit

JOSEPH B. WARSHAW, M.D., and DAVID F. WENDER, M.D.

Tissue injury is a recognized effect of prolonged exposure to hyperoxia. The lung is particularly vulnerable to the toxic effects of oxygen because the pulmonary epithelium comes in direct contact with high concentrations of inspired oxygen.[1] Premature infants are often exposed to increased concentrations of oxygen for treatment of hyaline membrane disease (HMD). In infants requiring prolonged therapy for HMD, recovery may be complicated by bronchopulmonary dysplasia (BPD). While the etiology of BPD is most likely multifactorial and relates to endotracheal intubation and positive pressure ventilation[2,3] and lung water content,[4] direct tissue injury by oxygen is postulated to be a major etiologic factor.

The basis for tissue injury by oxygen is damage to cells by free radicals formed in the course of oxygen metabolism. Among such radicals are the superoxide anion (O_2^-), the perhydroxide anion (HOO^-), and the hydroxide anion (OH^-). All react rapidly with membrane components and other cell constituents, resulting, as oxygen exposure continues, in extensive tissue injury. A number of important mechanisms have evolved to protect tissues from oxidant-induced injury. These mechanisms include the enzyme superoxide dismutase, which participates in the dismutation of O_2^- to H_2O, and the glutathione system, which helps maintain membranes and cell proteins in a reduced state.

Previous work from our group suggested that vitamin E ameliorated the course of bronchopulmonary dysplasia in infants.[5] The basis for a protective

Division of Perinatal Medicine, Departments of Pediatrics and, Obstetrics and Gynecology, Yale University School of Medicine, New Haven, Connecticut

influence of vitamin E may be its property as a biological antioxidant capable of scavenging oxygen-free radicals before they can oxidize membrane lipids and cause tissue injury.

METHODS

Using the newborn rabbit as an animal model, we have studied the effects of vitamin E on the response to hyperoxic insult. Rabbit pups were randomized at birth into three groups. Group I was maintained in room air, Group II was maintained in 100% oxygen, and Group III was maintained in 100% oxygen and treated with daily injections of vitamin E, 2 mg/100 g. In studies of lung histology, the vitamin E dose for Group III was increased to 6 mg/100 g/day. During the course of each experiment, pups were gavage fed a modification of the artificial diet described by Aprille.[6] Pups were sacrificed at birth and at 24, 48, and 72 hr. Plasma vitamin E concentrations[7] and *in vitro* erythrocyte sensitivity to hydrogen peroxide (H_2O_2) hemolysis[8] were determined. Biochemical analysis of lung tissue included determinations of vitamin E content,[9] *in vitro* lipid peroxide formation,[10] protein concentration,[11] and the activities of superoxide dismutase,[12] glutathione peroxidase,[13] and glutathione reductase.[14] Histologic specimens were examined by light microscopy, and a morphometric quantitation of the extent of histologic injury was performed.[15] Serum and lung tissue vitamin E data were analyzed statistically by analysis of variance. All other data were analyzed by an analysis of covariance using the plasma vitamin E level as the covariate.

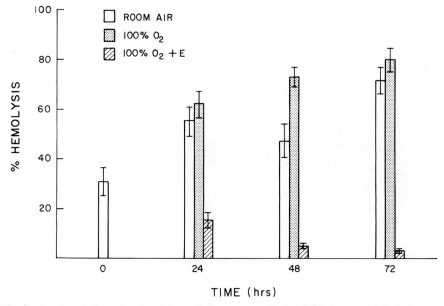

Fig. 1. *In vitro* erythrocyte sensitivity to hydrogen peroxide (H_2O_2) induced hemolysis (mean ± SEM). A marked resistance to hemolysis developed in animals treated with daily injections of vitamin E ($p < 0.01$).

RESULTS

Plasma vitamin E concentrations averaged less than 0.4 mg/dl at birth and increased by about twofold over 72 hr in both the room air and 100% oxygen groups. Plasma vitamin E levels at 72 hr were four times higher at a dose of 2 mg/100 g/day and 12 times higher at a dose of 6 mg/100 g/day than corresponding levels for animals in the room air or 100% oxygen groups. Lung tissue vitamin E concentrations paralleled the increases in plasma concentrations observed with vitamin E treatment.

Results for the red blood cell hydrogen peroxide (H_2O_2) hemolysis test are presented in Figure 1. For both the room air and 100% oxygen groups, percent red cell hemolysis increased during the course of the experiment, a pattern similar to that seen with clinical vitamin E deficiency states in humans. However, for the oxygen-exposed group treated with vitamin E, a marked resistance to H_2O_2-induced hemolysis developed with cumulative vitamin E treatment.

In vitro lung tissue lipid peroxide formation was assessed of animals maintained in 100% oxygen with or without vitamin E treatment. As shown in Figure 2, 72 hr of oxygen exposure resulted in increased lipid peroxide formation

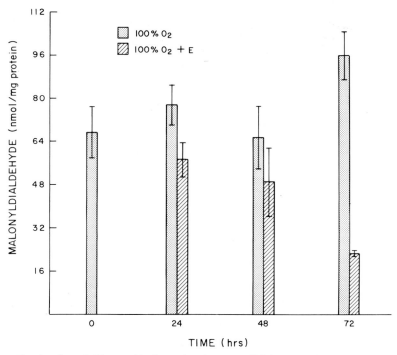

Fig. 2. *In vitro* lung lipid peroxide formation (mean ± SEM). Lung lipid peroxide formation increased with continuous 100% oxygen exposure in animals not treated with vitamin E. In vitamin-E-treated animals, lipid peroxide formation decreased with cumulative vitamin E treatment. By 72 hr, lipid peroxide formation was inhibited by approximately 80% in these animals ($p < 0.01$).

in animals not treated with E. However, in vitamin E treated animals, lipid peroxide formation decreased with cumulative vitamin E treatment so that, by 72 hr, lipid peroxide formation had been inhibited by approximately 80%.

Results for lung superoxide dismutase are presented in Figure 3. For animals in 100% oxygen without vitamin E treatment, superoxide dismutase activity increased with cumulative oxygen exposure and was statistically significantly elevated over the two other experimental groups. In contrast, animals treated with vitamin E demonstrated only small increases in lung superoxide dismutase activity in response to oxygen exposure.

Results for lung glutathione peroxidase activity are shown in Figure 4. Though results were more variable for this enzyme, statistical analysis also revealed that enzyme activity for the 100% oxygen group was significantly elevated over the other groups. Activity for the vitamin-E-treated animals exposed to oxygen was essentially the same as the room air group.

Data for lung glutathione reductase activity are depicted in Figure 5. The activity of this enzyme in the 100% oxygen group showed a tendency towards elevation over that of the other groups at 72 hr, results which suggest that the hyperoxia-induced increase in lung glutathione reductase activity was diminished with vitamin E treatment in parallel with the observations for lung superoxide dismutase and glutathione peroxidase.

Injection of the solubilizing vehicle for vitamin E was without effect on either *in vitro* lipid peroxidation or enzyme activity in animals exposed to oxygen.

Preliminary studies have been carried out on the effects of vitamin E on

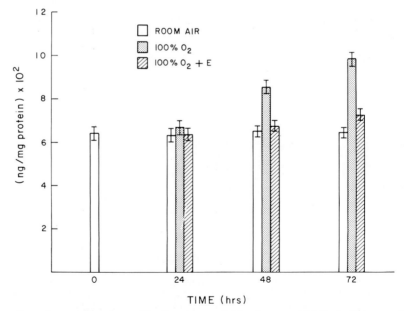

Fig. 3. Lung homogenate superoxide dismutase activities (mean ± SEM). At 72 hr, results for the 100% oxygen group were significantly elevated over the other experimental groups ($p < 0.01$).

lung histology. In animals exposed to 100% oxygen for 72 hr but not treated with vitamin E, lung light microscopic specimens showed morphologic evidence of early lung epithelial injury characterized by patchy atelectasis with adjacent zones of overexpansion of alveoli and dilation of small airways. When lungs from rabbits receiving 2 mg/100 g/day vitamin E were examined, there was not consistent evidence of protection from oxidant injury. However, lungs from animals receiving 6 mg/100 g/day vitamin E appeared to be protected. Alveoli were of uniform size, alveolar walls were delicate, and no atelectasis or alveolar overdistension was observed. Despite 72 hr of continuous exposure to 100% oxygen, specimens from animals treated with 6 mg/100 g/day vitamin E were histologically indistinguishable from room air controls.

DISCUSSION

Among mechanisms protective against oxidant injury at the cellular level, a series of pulmonary antioxidant enzymes are of central significance. This group of enzymes includes superoxide dismutase and the glutathione system. Superoxide dismutase, in effect, removes damaging superoxide anions before cell constituents are damaged. Superoxide dismutase which catalyzes the reaction $O_2^- + O_2^- + 2H^+ \rightarrow H_2O_2 + O_2$ appears to be a primary cellular defense against the superoxide radical.[12] The glutathione system through the regeneration of reduced glutathione has a reparative role and helps to maintain the cell in a

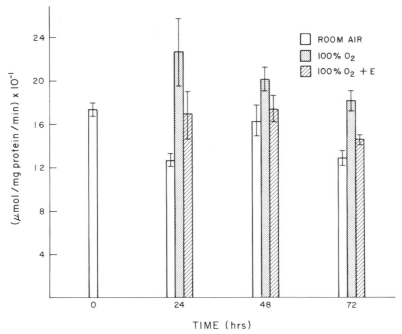

Fig. 4. Lung cytosol glutathione peroxidase activities (mean ± SEM). At 72 hr, results for the 100% oxygen group were significantly higher than the other experimental groups ($p < 0.05$).

reduced state. In the glutathione system, glutathione peroxidase inhibits lipid peroxidation by reducing peroxy fatty acids while simultaneously oxidizing glutathione. In a reaction linked to an NADPH-generating system, glutathione reductase then replenishes reduced glutathione.[16] The increase in activity of enzymes seen in response to prolonged oxygen exposure[17-19] is thought to represent an adaptive response to protect tissues from oxidant injury.

Among chemical antioxidants which may protect the lung from oxidant injury is vitamin E. Several investigators have demonstrated that vitamin E deficiency enhances the toxic effects of oxygen upon the lung,[20-22] and Taylor[23] has shown that vitamin E treatment of vitamin E deficient rats significantly decreases lung damage in animals exposed to oxidant stress. Evidence that vitamin E ameliorates bronchopulmonary dysplasia in human infants has also been reported.[5]

Though the precise mechanism by which vitamin E functions as an antioxidant has yet to be determined, speculation on its mechanism of antioxidant protection has centered on at least two areas. Lucy[24] has speculated that vitamin E may be a structural component of membranes which makes membrane polyunsaturated fatty acid more resistant to oxidant injury. Alternatively, others have provided evidence for a more direct antioxidant for vitamin E as a tissue free radical scavenger.[25]

Our findings of low serum vitamin E levels and increased erythrocyte

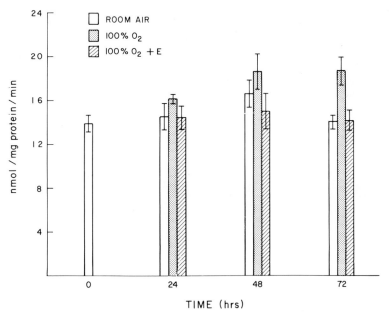

Fig. 5. Lung homogenate glutathione reductase activities (mean ± SEM). Though enzyme activity in the 100% oxygen group at 72 hr was not significantly elevated over the other groups ($p = 0.18$), results suggest that with vitamin E treatment, the hyperoxia-induced increase in lung glutathione reductase activity was diminished in parallel to the observations for superoxide dismutase and glutathione peroxidase.

sensitivity to H_2O_2 hemolysis in non-vitamin-E-treated animals suggest that newborn rabbits fed a diet high in polyunsaturated fatty acids become vitamin E deficient. When such animals are treated with vitamin E while being exposed to 100% oxygen, the lung biochemical response to hyperoxia is affected. Characteristic hyperoxia-induced increases in pulmonary antioxidant enzymes are diminished, and the susceptibility of lung tissue to *in vitro* lipid peroxidation is dramatically reduced. These findings lead us to speculate that vitamin E provides sufficient antioxidant protection to blunt the adaptive increase in antioxidant enzyme activity by decreasing the likely inductive signal, oxygen-free radicals.

While 2 mg/100 g/day vitamin E blunted the lung biochemical response to hyperoxia, we did not observe a protective effect on lung morphology at that dose. Both qualitative and quantitative morphological evidence for protection was observed at a dose of 6 mg/100 g/day. The discrepancy between the biochemical and morphological response is interesting and suggests that, although vitamin E scavenges sufficient free radicals to blunt the biochemical response to hyperoxia, structural damage continues, perhaps because of free radicals present in excess of available vitamin E. Alternatively, vitamin E may be compartmentalized within the cell so as to cause selective effects at low doses. While more work needs to be done to clarify these relationships, the work reported here provides further evidence that vitamin E is important for protection from oxidant injury.

SUMMARY

The effects of vitamin E treatment on the lung response to hyperoxic insult were studied in the newborn rabbit. In animals treated with vitamin E, lungs were more resistant to lipid peroxide formation *in vitro* and were protected from the acute epithelial injury seen in animals exposed to 100% oxygen but not treated with vitamin E. In addition, vitamin E administration diminished the hyperoxia induced increases in the pulmonary antioxidant enzymes super-oxide dismutase, glutathione peroxidase, and glutathione reductase. The findings provide evidence of antioxidant protection of lung by vitamin E and suggest that this antioxidant effect involves an inactivation of the likely stimulus for antioxidant enzyme induction, oxygen-free radicals.

REFERENCES

1. Clark, J. M., and Lambertsen, C. J., Pulmonary oxygen toxicity: a review. *Pharmacol. Rev.* **23**, 37–133 (1971).
2. Philip, A. G. S., Oxygen plus pressure plus time: the etiology of bronchopulmonary dysplasia. *Pediatrics* **55**, 44–50 (1975).
3. Edwards, D. K., Dyer, W. M., and Northway, W. H., Jr., Twelve years experience with bronchopulmonary dysplasia. *Pediatrics* **59**, 839–846 (1977).
4. Brown, E. R., Stark, A., Sosenko, I., Lawson, E. E., and Avery, M. E., Bronchopulmonary dysplasia: Possible relationship to pulmonary edema. *J. Pediatr.* **92**, 982–984 (1978).
5. Ehrenkranz, R. A., Bonta, B. W., Ablow, R. C., and Warshaw, J. B., Amelioration of

bronchopulmonary dysplasia after vitamin E administration. *N. Engl. J. Med.* **299,** 564–569 (1978).

6. Aprille, J. R., and Rulfs, J., A convenient neonatal model for developmental studies requiring artificial diets. *Biol. Neonate* **30,** 109–115 (1976).

7. Fabianek, J., DeFilippi, J., Rickards, T., and Herp, A., Micromethod for tocopherol determinations in blood serum. *Clin. Chem.* **14,** 456–462 (1968).

8. Horwitt, M. K., Harvey, C. C., Duncan, G. D., and Wilson, W. C., Effects of limited tocopherol intake in man with relationships to erythrocyte hemolysis and lipid oxidations. *Am. J. Clin. Nutr.* **4,** 408–418 (1956).

9. Taylor, S. L., Lamden, M. P., and Tappel, A. L., Sensitive fluorometric method for tissue tocopherol analysis. *Lipids* **11,** 530–538 (1976).

10. Sinnhuber, R. O., and Yu, T. C., 2-Thiobarbituric acid method for the measurement of rancidity in fishery products. *Food Technol.* **12,** 9–12 (1958).

11. Lowry, O. H., Rosebrough, N. J., Farr, A. L., and Randall, R. J.: Protein measurement with the folin phenol reagent. *J. Biol. Chem.* **193,** 265–275 (1951).

12. Misra, H. P., and Fridovich, I., The role of superoxide anion in the autoxidation of epinephrine and a simple assay for superoxide dismutase. *J. Biol. Chem.* **247,** 3170–3175 (1972).

13. Horn, H. D., Glutathione Reductase, in *Methods of Enzymatic Analysis.* H. U. Bergmeyer, Ed. Academic Press, New York, 1965, pp. 875–879.

14. Paglia, D. E., and Valentine, W. N., Studies on the quantitative and qualitative characterization of erythrocyte glutathione peroxidase. *J. Lab. Clin. Med.* **70,** 158–159 (1967).

15. Weibel, E. R., Stereological Techniques for Electron Microscopic Morphometry, in *Principles and Techniques of Electron Microscopy,* M. A. Hayat, Ed. van Nostrand-Reinhold, New York, 1973, Vol. 3, pp. 237–296.

16. Kimball, R. E., Reddy, K., Peirce, T. H., Schwartz, L. W., Mustafa, M. G., and Cross, C. E., Oxygen toxicity: Augmentation of antioxidant defense mechanisms in rat lung. *Am. J. Physiol.* **230,** 1425–1431 (1976).

17. Yam, J., Frank, L., and Roberts, R. J., Oxygen toxicity: Comparison of lung biochemical responses in neonatal and adult rats. *Pediatr. Res.* **12,** 115–119 (1978).

18. Nishiki, K., Jameson, D., Oshino, N., and Chance, B., Oxygen toxicity in the perfused rat liver and lung under hyperbaric conditions. *Biochem. J.* **160,** 343–355 (1976).

19. Crapo, J. D., and Tierney, D. F.: Superoxide dismutase and pulmonary oxygen toxicity. *Am. J. Physiol.* **226,** 1401–1407 (1974).

20. Kann, H. E., Jr., Mengel, C. E., Smith, W., and Horton, B.: Oxygen toxicity and vitamin E. *Aerospace Med.* **35,** 840–844 (1964).

21. Poland, R. L., Bollinger, R. O., Bozynski, M. E., Karna, P., and Perrin, E. V. D., Effect of vitamin E deficiency in pulmonary oxygen toxicity. *Pediatr. Res.* **11,** 577A (1977).

22. Taylor, D. W., The effects of vitamin E deficiency on oxygen toxicity in the rat. *J. Physiol.* **121,** 47p (1953).

23. Taylor, D. W., The effects of vitamin E and of methylene blue on the manifestations of oxygen poisoning on the rat. *J. Physiol.* **131,** 200–206 (1956).

24. Lucy, J. A., Functional and structural aspects of biological membranes: A suggested structural role for vitamin E in the control of membrane permeability and stability. *Ann. N.Y. Acad. Sci.* **203,** 4–11 (1972).

25. Tappel, A. L., Vitamin E as the biological lipid antioxidant. *Vitam. Horm.* **20,** 493–510 (1962).

31

Hyaline Membrane Disease Course/ Management Models

ROBERT S. GREEN, M.D., JORGE ROJAS, M.D., DANIEL P. LINDSTROM, Ph.D., SUSAN NIERMEYER, M.D., TORSTEN OLSSON, Ph.D., and ROBERT B. COTTON, M.D.

INTRODUCTION

The clinical course of hyaline membrane disease (HMD) has been classically described as one of increasing severity during the first 24–48 hr of life followed by improvement thereafter.[1] During the disease course, the pulmonary status is expressed traditionally in terms of oxygen requirement and degree of ventilatory assistance needed to maintain normal arterial blood gases. The neonatologist's skill to make appropriate changes in the inspired oxygen concentration (F_IO_2) and airway pressure results from an appreciation of this course attained from past experience. However, in practice, the experienced neonatologist is not available at the bedside 24 hr a day. It is usually the less experienced house officer, nurse clinician, or respiratory therapist who has to react to changes in the patient's clinical or blood gas status. Under these circumstances, a quantitative model projecting the expected disease course might serve as a guide by which the front line newborn intensive care unit team could anticipate F_IO_2 and ventilator adjustments.

The purpose of this report is to describe several models that may serve this application. In their construction, right-to-left intra- and extrapulmonary shunting was considered as the mechanism of hypoxemia in HMD. Two expressions of the hypoxemia were incorporated into models: (1) the alveolar-arterial oxygen tension difference ($AaDO_2$), and (2) the percent venous admix-

Department of Pediatrics, Vanderbilt University School of Medicine, Nashville, Tennessee, and the Department of Applied Medical Electronics, Chalmers University of Technology, Gothenburg, Sweden
Supported by a NHLI SCOR Grant-HL 14214

ture (VA). Since VA varies inversely over the beneficial range of mean applied proximal airway pressure (MAPAP), the arithmetic product of these two variables was used as the basis of a third model.[2-5] A fourth model was constructed from MAPAP as a single variable.

METHODS

Thirty-one premature infants with HMD who were judged appropriately managed were selected to form the model population. The diagnosis of HMD was based on previously published criteria.[6] All infants were managed with some form of distending airway pressure, either nasal CPAP or mechanical ventilation, beginning within 6 hr after birth. Indications for nasal CPAP were the presence of grunting, retracting, and an unstable chest wall along with radiographic evidence of HMD and an F_IO_2 requirement of 0.4 or greater to maintain the arterial PO_2 above 60 Torr. Mechanical ventilation using orotracheal intubation and a BABYbird respirator was begun if the arterial PCO_2 was greater than 50 Torr, if the F_IO_2 requirement on nasal CPAP exceeded 0.70, if there was apnea, or if chest wall instability and severe respiratory distress were not relieved by nasal CPAP.

Infants whose course within 72 hr following birth was complicated by pneumothorax, pulmonary air dissection, pulmonary hemorrhage, symptomatic patent ductus arteriosus, intraventricular hemorrhage, or sepsis were not included in the model population.

The HMD course models were developed for the 72-hr period beginning at birth, during which time arterial blood gases, MAPAP, and F_IO_2 were recorded. Blood gas determinations were made from blood taken from the umbilical arterial catheter. The times of blood gas measurement were determined by the house officers and were based on the clinical condition of the infant and the times of changes in F_IO_2 or ventilator settings. For the entire model population, blood gases were measured approximately every 3 hr. Blood gas determinations were performed by the hospital service laboratories. Proximal applied airway pressure was measured with a Statham P23Gb air-filled transducer connected to the proximal airway pressure monitor line extending from the endotracheal tube connection piece of the ventilator. A three-way stopcock open to all three positions was used so that pressures would appear on the manometer of the ventilator and simultaneously be transmitted to the Statham transducer. The signal from the transducer was recorded on a Hewlett-Packard 7754B polygraph system and transmitted to a PDP 11/34 laboratory minicomputer system (Digital Equipment Corp.), which was programmed to calculate inspiratory time, expiratory time, I/E ratio, peak and valley airway pressures, and integrated mean airway pressure. For patients on nasal CPAP, the respirator manometer value of the CPAP was recorded as MAPAP.

The alveolar-arterial PO_2 difference was calculated using the following equation[7] for alveolar PO_2:

$$PAO_2 = [(760 - 47)*F_IO_2] - (PaCO_2*\{F_IO_2 + [(1 - F_IO_2)/0.9]\})$$

The percent venous admixture was derived using the standard shunt equation[7]:

$$VA = 100\%(Q_s/Q_t) = 100\%(CaO_2 - Cc'O_2)/(C\bar{v}O_2 - Cc'O_2)$$

where

Q_s = shunted blood flow,
Q_t = total systemic blood flow,
CaO_2 = oxygen content of descending aortic blood,
$Cc'O_2$ = oxygen content of pulmonary capillary blood,
$C\bar{v}O_2$ = oxygen content of mixed venous blood.

In these calculations, alveolar PCO_2 is assumed equal to arterial PCO_2, the respiratory quotient is assumed to be 0.9, the hemoglobin concentration is assumed to be 15 g/dl with 80% fetal hemoglobin, the arterial-venous oxygen content difference is assumed to be 4 ml/dl, and pulmonary capillary blood oxygen tension is assumed to be in equilibrium with alveolar gas. The Severinghaus mathmetical model for oxygen-hemoglobin binding[8] was used to calculate the oxygen content of arterial blood.

All alveolar-arterial PO_2 differences and percent venous admixture calculations were performed by the computer. For each infant, the values of $AaDO_2$, VA, and MAPAP were averaged over 6-hr intervals by a time-weighted averaging program. The product of VA × MAPAP was calculated for each 6-hr interval based on the time-weighted values. For each interval, the mean and standard deviation of each of the above four functions was calculated. The computer was used to perform these calculations and store the results. The 72-hr time course of these four functions provided four course/management models of HMD.

RESULTS

The clinical characteristics of the study population are shown in Table I. Figure 1 shows the graphical representation of the model functions. The mean ± 1.28 standard deviations (SD), representing the 90th and 10th percentiles in a normally distributed population, are shown. The course/management trajectories of individual patients may then be plotted on these graphical models.

TABLE I
Study Population Characteristics

Number of patients	31
Gestational age (weeks)	31.9 ± 2.3[a]
Birth weight (g)	1702 ± 448[a]
1-min Apgar score	5.1 ± 2.6[a]
5-min Apgar score	6.8 ± 1.9[a]
Sex (male/female)	17/14
Inborn/outborn	12/19
Lived/died	31/0

[a] Mean ± standard deviation.

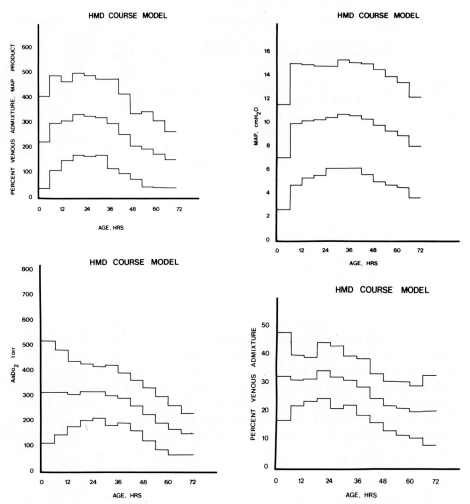

Fig. 1. Graphical representation of the four HMD course/management models. The mean ± 1.28 SD of each of the four model functions is shown for the initial 72-hr course experienced by the model population of 31 infants with HMD.

Two of these model functions, $AaDO_2$ and VA, are direct expressions of hypoxemia and reflect the disease course as influenced by management. The mean values of these functions remain relatively constant during the first 24 hr after birth and express the expected serious degree of oxygenation impairment, with VA ranging between 31% and 34% and $AaDO_2$ between 305 and 313 Torr. According to these functions, improvement is projected to begin at approximately 30 hr after birth.

The MAPAP model function reflects management as a response to the patient's course and is directly influenced by the neonatologist's perception of optimal management.

The remaining function expresses both management and course by combining MAPAP with VA as an arithmetic product. This function projects peak values between 18 and 30 hr after birth followed by improvement.

The wide range of values taken by these model functions during the initial 12 hr is attributed to the inclusion of outborn infants in the model population. Nineteen of the 31 model subjects were outborn and characteristically had markedly elevated values of VA and $AaDO_2$ at the time when management was initiated by the tertiary center team. Inborn infants, whose intrapartum and early postpartum management was more closely controlled, began with lower values of VA and $AaDO_2$ and then increased to peak values in accordance with the traditional concept of HMD course.

DISCUSSION

These course/management models are intended to serve as a reference for less experienced personnel who are beginning to participate in the management of HMD. These models allow one to place the course and management of an individual patient in the perspective of a model population. In addition, these models may be used as a quantitative basis for population comparisons and management assessment.

In the selection of model functions, an attempt was made to use variables which are routinely available in the newborn intensive care unit, or which can be derived without sophisticated instrumentation. MAPAP can be closely estimated from the manometer reading of proximal airway pressure if one knows inspiratory time and rate. A ventilator monitor (Novametrix) is now commercially available which displays an electrically integrated MAPAP. The oxygen content of blood can be derived for the estimation of VA using the Severinghaus blood gas calculator.[8] This calculation can be simplified further in those units with direct assess to computer support.

The interpretation of a single VA value is limited by the several assumptions involved in its derivation, especially the arterio-venous oxygen content difference. However, the behavior of this model function as it changes in response to MAPAP is a useful illustration of the effect of distending airway pressure on venous admixture.

There is no uniform agreement among NICUs as to what combination of F_1O_2 and MAPAP is optimal. These models can be readily constructed to fit the prevailing management practice and patient population at individual units by defining and monitoring the local model population. This approach would also enable comparative statements between units based on model parameters.

The models presented do not represent all infants with HMD. Mildly affected infants not requiring early distending airway pressure and infants with complications within the first 72 hr were excluded. Application of the models to infants with interstitial air dissection or pneumothorax and to infants who subsequently develop chronic lung disease may help identify factors aggravating these conditions. In addition, the model approach would facilitate experimental studies assessing the prevention of chronic lung disease where highly comparable study groups are essential.

By expressing ventilatory management protocols in terms of these models, management from patient to patient would become more consistent. A domain of safe or optimal model function values could be defined as a target for pressure and F_IO_2 adjustments. Similarly, combinations of model function values that are regarded as dangerous could be established to prompt front-line NICU personnel to request assistance.

In summary, four course/management models of HMD have been constructed from routinely available or readily accessible measurements of F_IO_2, airway pressure, and blood gases. These models can be adapted to the patient population and management practice of individual NICUs. Application of the models should prove useful in teaching, patient care, and clinical research.

REFERENCES

1. Stahlman, M. T., Acute Respiratory Disorders in the Newborn, in *Neonatology, Pathophysiology and Management of the Newborn*, Gordon B. Avery, Ed. Philadelphia, Lippincott, 1975.
2. Reynolds, E. O. R., Effect of alteration in mechanical ventilator settings on pulmonary gas exchange in hyaline membrane disease. *Arch. Dis. Child.* **46,** 152–159 (1971).
3. Herman, S., and Reynolds, E. O. R., Methods for improving oxygenation in infants mechanically ventilated for severe hyaline membrane diease. *Arch. Dis. Child.* **48,** 612–617 (1973).
4. Boros, S. J., Metalon, S. V., Ewald, R., Leonard, A. S., and Hunt, C. E., The effect of independent variations in inspiratory-expiratory ratio and end expiratory pressure during mechanical ventilation in hyaline membrane disease: the significance of mean airway pressure. *J. Pediatr.* **91,** 794–798 (1977).
5. Boros, S. J., Variations in inspiratory:expiratory ratio and airway pressure wave form during mechanical ventilation: the significance of mean airway pressure. *J. Pediatr.* **94,** 114–117 (1979).
6. Cotton, R. B., Stahlman, M. T., Kovar, I., and Catterton, W. Z., Medical management of small preterm infants with symptomatic patent ductus arteriosus. *J. Pediatr.* **92,** 467–473 (1978).
7. Comroe, J. H., Forston, R. E., Dubois, A. B., Briscoe, W. A., and Carlsen, E., *The Lung*, 2nd ed. Yearbook, Chicago, 1962.
8. Severinghaus, J. H., Blood gas calculator. *J. Appl. Physiol.* **21,** 1108–1116 (1966).

32

Phenobarbital and Testicular Function in Male Premature Infants

MAGUELONE G. FOREST, ANNICK LECOQ, BERNARD SALLE,* and JEAN BERTRAND

INTRODUCTION

Since the demonstration that phenobarbital (PB) decreases serum bilirubin concentrations in newborn infants,[1] this drug has been widely used in the prophylaxis of neonatal jaundice. Indeed, PB seems not only to increase the activity of several hepatic enzymes such as glycuronyl-transferase but also to activate the hepatic metabolism of unconjugated bilirubin.[2, 3] However PB is also known to have depressing effects on luteinizing hormone (LH) release and/or secretion,[4, 5] thus disrupting normal gonadal function. PB would appear rather to act at the hypothalalic level since the injection of LHRH is able to counteract the blocking effect of PB on LH.[6]

On the other hand, in full-term[7] as well as in premature[8] male infants plasma testosterone levels elevated at birth decrease rapidly in the first week of life. There is then a postnatal activation of the hypothalamo-pituitary complex responsible for a marked testicular activity as reflected by elevated plasma levels of LH[9, 10] and testosterone (T).[8, 10, 11]

The present study was undertaken with the aim to investigate whether PB treatment had a suppressive effect on the neonatal hypothalamo-pituitary-testicular axis and whether the synthesis of the specific steroid binding proteins—testosterone, estradiol-binding globulin (TeBg), and cortisol-binding globulin (CBG)—were also affected by the drug. A longitudinal study was made in 12 premature males from birth to six months of life. Plasma levels of T and cortisol as well as the binding of T and cortisol to plasma proteins were

INSERM U 34, Hôpital Debrousse, 69322 Lyon Cedex 1 and *Centre de Néonatologie, Hôpital Edouard-Herriot, 69645 Lyon Cedex 3

estimated. The results were compared to those obtained in two untreated control groups of premature and full-term male infants.

MATERIAL AND METHODS

Subjects and Protocols

Twelve premature male newborns whose mean gestational age was 35.8 ± 1.3 weeks and mean birth weight was 2200 ± 285 g were studied (group I). A first blood sample was obtained from a peripheral antecubital vein 1–21 hr after birth (mean 4–5 hr), before PB therapy. Treatment was given as a single IM injection of 10 mg/kg of PB.[12] Heparinized blood samples were then obtained, whenever possible, twice weekly, then monthly for 6 months at the occasion of health controls. A total of 68 blood samples were obtained.

Two control groups were also studied consisting of subjects who did not receive any PB therapy: Blood was obtained in the same conditions in 61 prematures (group II) and 144 full-term infants (group III) matched for age.

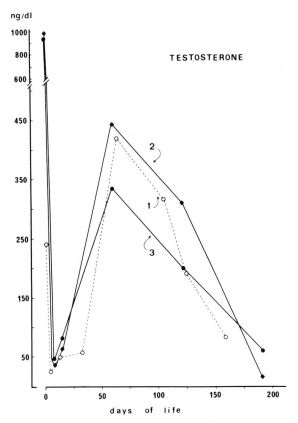

Fig. 1a. Longitudinal study of the plasma concentrations of T in 12 premature male infants given a single injection of phenobarbital on the day of birth (after the first measurement of T).

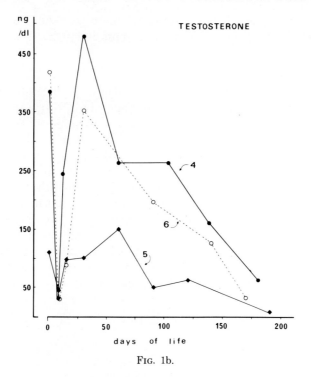

Fig. 1b.

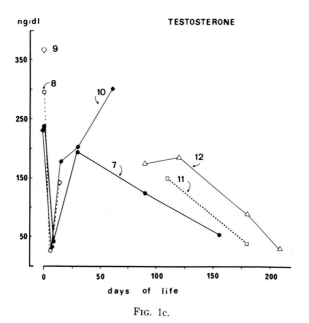

Fig. 1c.

Plasmas were immediately decanted and stored at $-20°C$ until analyzed. Informed consent was obtained from the parents and pediatricians in all cases.

Hormone Measurements

Plasma concentrations of T were determined by a specific radioimmunoassay (RIA) previously described after chromatographic purification on celite column chromatography.[13] Plasma cortisol levels were measured by RIA on unchromatographed dichloromethane extracts (Forest, unpublished). Limits of sensitivity were ≥ 1 ng/dl. Interassay coefficients of variation were 5.6% for T and 12% for cortisol. The percentages of T and cortisol bound to plasma proteins were measured by equilibrium dialysis at $37°C$ on one-fifth diluted plasma as reported earlier.[14] Their results are given without correcting for plasma dilution. However an adequate correction was used for the calculation of the unbound fractions and that of the unbound concentrations of T and cortisol.[15] All results are expressed as mean $\pm$ SD. The unpaired t test as well as analysis of variance and the mean square method were used for statistical analysis. Differences were considered significant when $p < 0.05$.

RESULTS

Plasma Concentrations of T

Longitudinal T levels observed in the premature infants treated with PB are illustrated in Figure 1. A triphasic pattern was observed as in full-term and untreated premature infants.[7-9, 11] For statistical analysis of the absolute levels reached in relation to age and/or their temporal evolution, individual values have been separated in subsequent age groups.

At birth and before PB therapy, T levels showed a wide range (100–962 ng/dl). However, mean T levels (396 ± 286) were not significantly different from those observed in 37 full-term newborns (270 ± 153 ng/dl) or in another group of 12 prematures males (232 ± 100 ng/dl). There was no correlation between T levels and either gestational age or time during the first 24 hr of life.

A rapid decrease in plasma T levels occurred during the first week of life. It

TABLE I

Evolution with Age in the Plasma Levels (ng/dl) of Testosterone in Phenobarbital-Treated (group I), Untreated Prematures (group II), and Full-Term (group III) Infants[a]

Group I				Group II				Group III			
Age (days)	n	mean ± SD	(range)	Age (days)	n	mean ± SD	(range)	Age (days)	n	mean ± SD	(range)
4–8	10	34 ± 8	(24–48)	5–8	8	37 ± 30	(5–104)	5–8	13	32 ± 14	(12–57)
11–15	8	117 ± 65	(49–247)[b]	14–17	12	214 ± 162	(25–559)	11–19	10	178 ± 23	(151–205)
29–61	12	274 ± 138	(56–478)[a]	31–58	11	167 ± 92	(68–322)[c]	31–60	31	243 ± 88	(107–461)
89–140	14	178 ± 79	(47–316)[ab]	90–130	8	299 ± 125	(214–526)[c]	90–120	22	121 ± 69	(26–245)
156–180	6	59 ± 23	(31–87)[ab]	150–180	5	120 ± 110	(48–307)[c]	150–180	14	21 ± 15	(4–53)
190–201	4	28 ± 24	(7–60)	180–210	5	128 ± 107	(48–307)[c]	180–210	17	14 ± 13	(5–49)

[a] $p < 0.05$: a = group I vs. group II; b = group I vs. group II; c = group II vs. group III.

was similar to that observed in untreated prematures as well as in full-term infants, mean (± SD) levels at 5–7 days of age being comparable in the three groups (Table I).

The postnatal activation of the hypothalamo-hypophyso-testicular axis, which manifests by the secondary rise in plasma T was also observed in PB-treated infants (Fig. 1). However, the rise was somewhat delayed as compared with the control group of full-term infants (Fig. 2): mean T levels were significantly less in PB-treated infants than in untreated full-term boys at 11–17 days of age (Table I). The apparent difference in mean T levels between groups I and II at the same age was not significant.

Peak T levels had similar values and range in the three groups, but they were observed at a older age in group II. This slight but significant delay to reach peak values in premature infants was also observed in a previous study.[11] This pattern was not found in the group of PB-treated prematures.

The decline in T levels differed significantly between control groups: T levels remained significantly higher for a long period of time up to 7 months in untreated premature as compared to full-term infants (Table I). In PB-treated infants, the temporal pattern in plasma T was intermediate to those exhibited by groups II and III, the decline being more rapid than in prematures but still slower than in full-term infants. The three groups were significantly different from each other between 89 and 180 days of age.

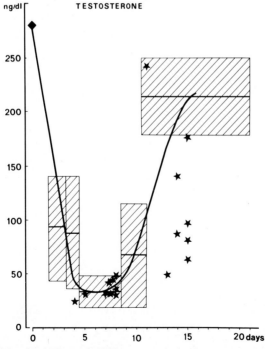

Fig. 2. Individual T levels of PB treated infants as compared to mean ± 1 S.D. levels observed in untreated full-term boys (hatched areas).

Percentage Binding of T and Plasma Concentrations of Unbound T

The longitudinal study of the percentage of T bound to plasma proteins is illustrated in Figure 3. The binding of T was very low at birth and rose progressively and significantly during the time of the study.

At birth, i.e., before treatment, the percentage binding of T in PB-treated infants (80.2 ± 6.3%) was not significantly lower than in control groups I and II (respectively, 84.7 ± 3.3 and 85.6 ± 3%).

Absolute values and temporal pattern were thereafter strikingly similar between groups II and III. In both the percentage binding of T rose very rapidly in the first week of life and then more slowly reaching by 1 month of age mean values (96.2 ± 1.4 and 96.1 ± 1.1%, respectively) which were not different of that observed later on in infancy or in a group of 47 prepubertal children (97 ± 1%). In contrast, the rise in percentage binding of T was significantly slower in PB-treated infants, reaching values of 95.2 ± 1.8%, comparable to those in the control groups only after 3 months of age.

Results of the determination of the plasma concentrations of unbound T are given in Table II. Peak values were observed at the same age as for total plasma T in the three groups. However, as a result of the significant decrease in T binding for the first 2 months of life, unbound T levels in PB-treated infants were considerably more elevated than in control groups during this period, in particular at 29–61 days of age.

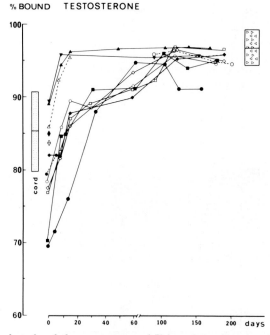

Fig. 3. Longitudinal study of the percentages of T bound to plasma proteins in PB-treated infants. Mean levels and 95% confidence limits of the values observed in the cord of full-term infants (left) and those in normal prepubertal boys (right) are given for comparison.

Plasma Concentrations of Cortisol

The results are given in Table III. Statistical analysis showed no difference in mean levels or temporal patterns among the three groups.

Percentage Binding of F and Unbound Concentrations of Cortisol

The evolution with age in the percentage of F bound to plasma proteins in PB-treated infants is illustrated in Figure 4. The percentage binding of T was low at birth and rose rapidly within a month to the values observed in older infants or prepubertal children. Statistical analysis showed no difference between PB-treated and full-term untreated infants. Both mean values and temporal patterns were strikingly similar. The same observation was made for the unbound concentrations of cortisol (not shown).

DISCUSSION

This study shows that PB treatment does not seem to affect testicular function in infancy as evidenced by comparable postnatal rise in T levels observed in treated and untreated infants. Because of ethical limitation in the volume of blood collected from these babies it has not been possible to also

TABLE II

Mean (± SD) Plasma Concentrations of Unbound Testosterone (ng/dl) in PB-Treated and Untreated Male Infants[a]

Age (days)	Group I	Group II	Group III
4–8	0.94 ± 0.50	0.72 ± 0.48	0.47 ± 0.18
11–15	2.69 ± 2.1	1.17 ± 0.6	1.11 ± 0.43
29–61	4.13 ± 2.3[ab]	1.18 ± 0.39[c]	1.43 ± 0.29
89–140	1.67 ± 0.9[b]	1.60 ± 0.42[c]	0.65 ± 0.38
156–180	0.67 ± 0.44[b]	1.15 ± 1[c]	0.18 ± 0.13
190–201	0.26 ± 0.20	0.38 ± 0.13[c]	0.07 ± 0.01

[a] Cf. Table I for definition of group, age group and number of subjects. $p < 0.05$: a = group I vs. group II, b = group I vs. group III, c = group II vs. group III.

TABLE III

Mean (± 1 SD) Plasma Concentrations of Cortisol (µg/dl) in PB-Treated and Untreated Male Infants[a]

Age (days)	Group I	Group II	Group III
First	18 ± 11.1	18.9 ± 4.3	16.7 ± 6.5
	(12)[b]	(4)	(8)
4–8	9.7 ± 5.3	6.8 ± 3.9	10.2 ± 4.5
	(10)	(7)	(13)
11–60	7.3 ± 4.5	9.3 ± 4.5	9.1 ± 5.6
	(20)	(24)	(41)
89–200	11.2 ± 5.1	10.4 ± 4.62	11.0 ± 5.7
	(23)	(15)	(19)

[a] Cf. Table I for definition of groups.
[b] Number of subjects in parentheses.

measure plasma LH. However, the elevated level of plasma T concentrations maintained for at least 3 months postnatally is indirect evidence that a significant secretion of pituitary LH did occur in the PB-treated infants. It would thus appear that PB does not block the postnatal activation of the hypothalamo-pituitary complex.

Although these results are reassuring for the future of these infants they are apparently in discordance with experimental studies showing that PB or PB derivatives block the spontaneous or provoked LH surge in rats[4, 16, 17] or hamsters.[18] These discrepancies might well be only apparent. They are probably not dose effects since the dosages of PB used in the prophylactic treatment of our infants were relatively similar to that used in the above experiments. It is also possible that the effect of PB varies among species. Indeed the blocking effect of PB on LH is not observed in monkeys.[19]

However, these experimental studies have been made in females and not in males and secondly it would appear that PB (or related compounds) rather block the positive feedback effect of sex steroids, mainly that of progesterone,[20] than have a negative feed-back effect *per se*. It is thus postulated that PB might have selective and different effects on the neuroendocrine structures involved in negative and positive feedback controls of pituitary secretions.

From our results it would appear that the temporal pattern of T levels is

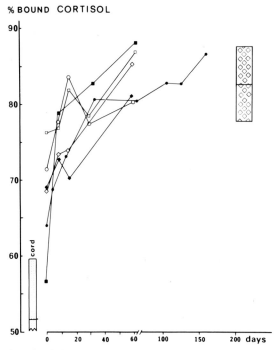

Fig. 4. Longitudinal study of the percentage of cortisol bound to plasma proteins in PB-treated infants. Mean values and 95% confidence limits in the cord of full-term infants (left) and in normal pubertal children (right) are given for comparison.

somewhat different in PB-treated and untreated premature infants. A faster decline in T levels was observed in the former group. This could be interpreted as a positive effect of PB on the maturation of the hypothalamo-pituitary axis, i.e., acquiring more rapidly a low threshold of sensitivity to the negative feedback effect of sex steroids.[21] Although significant in the present series, these differences in temporal pattern should however be interpreted with caution since other irrelevant factors might be responsible.

The third and unexpected finding was the significantly higher levels of unbound T found in PB-treated infants as compared to the two control groups. This was not due to higher total T levels but to a slower postnatal increase in the binding of T. The method used only determines the fraction of T bound to plasma proteins. T and cortisol are bound to specific proteins, respectively, TeBg and CBG, and both to albumin. The fact that the percentage of cortisol bound to plasma proteins had normal levels and a normal temporal pattern while the rise in the percentage binding of T was significantly delayed in PB-treated infants would suggest that TeBg levels but not that of CBG were affected. More specific studies are required to show direct evidence of decreased levels of TeBg as well as the specific role of PB on its hepatic synthesis.

The role of androgens in the early neonatal period is well documented in rodents. They "masculinize" for life the neural structures mediating LH release and sex behaviour in adulthood. They also irreversibly program certain liver enzymes implicated in steroid metabolism.[21, 22] The role of the postnatal surge in T levels is not yet known in the human. It is thus very uncertain to predict if the exposure to very high levels of unbound T (the biological active moiety) for several weeks in PB treated infants may have any consequence for long-term expression.

ACKNOWLEDGMENTS

This work was supported by INSERM grants (ATP 33.76.65). The authors thank Miss J. Bois for her expert secretarial help.

REFERENCES

1. Trolle, D., Decrease of total serum bilirubin concentration in newborn infants after phenobarbitone treatment. *Lancet* **II**, 705–708 (1968).
2. Catz, C., and Yaffe S. J., Pharmacological modification of bilirubin conjugation in the newborn. *Amer. J. Dis. Child.* **104**, 516–520 (1962).
3. Catz, C., and Jaffe S. J., Barbiturate enhancement of bilirubin conjugation in young and adult animals. *Pediat. Res.* **2**, 361–366 (1968).
4. Karavolas, H. J., Gupta C., and Meyer R. K., Steroid biosynthesis and metabolism during phenobarbital (PB). Block of PMS induced ovulation in immature rats. *Endocrinology* **91**, 157–167 (1972).
5. Siegel, H. I., Bast J. D., and Greenwald G. S., The effects of phenobarbital and gonadal steroids on periovulatory serum levels of luteinizing hormone and follicle-stimulating hormone in the hamster. *Endocrinology* **98**, 48–55 (1976).
6. Blake, C. A., Simulation of the proestrous luteinizing hormone (LH) surge after infusion of LH-releasing hormone in phenobarbital blocked rats. *Endocrinology* **98**, 451–460 (1976).
7. Forest, M. G., and Cathiard A. M., Pattern of plasma testosterone and Δ^4-androstenedione in

normal newborns. Evidence for testicular activity at birth. *J. Clin. Endocrinol. Metab.* **41,** 977–980 (1975).

8. Forest, M. G., Cathiard A. M., Bourgeois, J., and Genoud, J., Androgènes plasmatiques chez le nourrisson normal et prématuré. Relation avec la maturation de l'axe hypothalamo-hypophyso-gonadique. *Endocrinologie Sexuelle de la Période Périnatale*, M. G. Forest and J. Bertrand (eds.), Colloques INSERM, Paris, 1974, Vol. 32, pp. 315–336.

9. Forest, M. G., Sizonenko, P. C., Cathiard A. M., and Bertrand J., Hypophysogonadal function in human during the first year of life. I. Evidence for testicular activity in early infancy. *J. Clin. Invest.* **53,** 819–828 (1974).

10. Winter, J. S. D., Faiman, C., Hobson, W. C., Prasad A. V., and Reyes, F. I., Pituitary gonadal relations in infancy. I. Patterns of serum gonadotrophin concentrations from birth to four years of age in man and chimpanzee. *J. Clin. Endocrinol. Metab.* **40,** 545–551 (1975).

11. Forest, M. G., de Peretti, E., and Bertrand, J., Testicular and adrenal androgens and their binding to plasma proteins in the perinatal period: developmental patterns of plasma testosterone, 4-Androstenedione, dehydroepiandrosterone and its sulfate in premature and small for date infants as compared with that of full-term infants. *J. Steroid Biochem.* **12,** 25–36 (1980).

12. Salle, B., Pasquier, P., Desebre, Cl., Rouzious, J. M., and Baronty B., Phenobarbital in prophylaxis of neonatal jaundice: a control trial of two regimens. *Helvet. Pediat. Acta* **32,** 221–226 (1977).

13. Forest, M. G., Cathiard, A. M., and Bertrand, J., Total and unbound testosterone levels in newborns and normal and hypogonadal children: use of a sensitive radioimmunoassay for testosterone. *J. Clin. Endocrinol. Metab.* **36,** 1132–1142 (1973).

14. Forest, M. G., Rivarola, M. A., and Migeon, C. J., Percentage binding of testosterone, androstenedione and dehydroepiandrosterone in human plasma. *Steroids* **12,** 323–343 (1968).

15. Forest, M. G., Ances, I. G., Tapper A. J., and Migeon, C. J., Percentage binding of testosterone, androstenedione and dehydroepiandrosterone in plasma at the time of delivery. *J. Clin. Endocrinol. Metab.* **32,** 417–425 (1971).

16. Everett, J. W., and Sawyer, C. H., A 24 hour periodicity in the "LH-release apparates" of female rats, disclosed by barbiturate sedation. *Endocrinology* **47,** 198–206 (1950).

17. Kobayashi, F., Hara, K., and Miyaka, T., Facilitation by progesterone of ovulating hormone in sodium pento-barbital-blocked proestrus rat. *Endocrinol. Jpn.* **20,** 175 (1973).

18. Greenwald, G. S., Preovulatory changes in ovulating hormone in the cyclic hamster *Endocrinology* **88,** 671–677 (1971).

19. Knobil, E., On the control of gonadotropin secretion in the rhesus monkey. *Recent Progress Hormone Res.* **30,** 1–36 (1974).

20. Terasawa, E., King, M. K., Wiegand, S. J., Bridson W. E., and Gay, R. W., Barbiturate anesthesia blocks the positive feed-back effect of progesterone, but not of estrogen, on luteinizing hormone release in ovariectomized guinea pigs. *Endocrinology* **104,** 687–692 (1979).

21. Forest, M. G., de Peretti, E., and Bertrand, J., Hypothalamic-pituitary-gonadal relationships in man from birth to puberty. *Clin. Endocrinol.* **5,** 551–569 (1976).

22. de Moor, P., Verhoeven, G., and Heyns, W., Permanent effects of foetal and neonatal testosterone secretion on steroid metabolism and binding. *Differentiation* **1,** 241–253 (1973).

23. Gustafsson, J. A., Eneroth, P., Pousette, A., Skett, P., Sonnenschein, C., Stenberg A., and Attlen, A., Programming and differentiation of rat liver enzymes. *J. Steroid Biochem* **8,** 429–443 (1977).

33

Effects of Respiratory Alkalosis on Plasma Levels of Phenobarbital in the Newborn Piglet

P. MONIN,[1] P. VERT,[1] C. SANJUAN,[2] M. VIBERT,[1] and V. ROVEI[2]

The distribution of phenobarbital (PB) *in vivo* is affected by changes in blood pH.[1,2] The amplitude of these changes, because of the low pK of this drug may be of some clinical relevance[3-6] in patients treated for neurological disorders.

In the newborn baby, changes in plasma levels of PB associated with fluctuation in blood pH have been observed.[7,8] However, their effect on the course of treatment remained questionable.

Previous experimental studies[2-5] in dogs have been concerned with the effect of blood pH changes on plasma PB levels over long periods of time (30 min to 1 hr) but, little is known about this phenomenon over shorter periods. To study the magnitude of changes in plasma levels of PB related to acutes variations of pH and the rapidity of their occurrence, the following experiment on the newborn piglet was designed.

MATERIAL AND METHODS

The determination of the elimination half-life ($T_{1/2}$) of PB in the piglet was previously determined in three animals of 1, 3, and 10 days of age, following a single dose of 10 mg/kg injected intravenously. $T_{1/2}$ was, respectively, 49.1, 78.1, and 78.6 hr for these three animals, and, from these results, we have considered plasma PB levels sufficiently stable in the newborn piglet over periods of time of 4–6 hr for the effect of elimination to be ignored. Therefore,

[1] Service de Médecine Néonatale, Maternité Universitaire, 54042 Nancy, France
[2] Département de Recherche Clinique, Laboratoire LERS, Synthelabo, Paris, France

303

in the following experimental study concerned with acute changes in blood pH a single dose of PB was used.

Five newborn piglets, less than 10 days of age (Table I) were studied 20–24 hr after the administration of a single intravenous dose of PB of 10 mg/kg. The animals were anesthetized with urethane (10–15 ml/kg of a 12.5% solution injected intraperitoneally). After endotracheal intubation, the piglets were hyperventilated manually in order to keep blood pH above 7.60. Hyperventilation was continued for a period of 83 ± 23 min (range: 60–120 min) and then stopped. Venous blood samples of 0.5 ml were drawn through a polyethylene catheter, previously placed in one internal jugular vein, before hyperventilation and then every 5 or 10 min for determination of pH, PCO_2, and PB plasma levels. Blood sampling was continued until pH returned to normal. Blood pH and PCO_2 were measured on an ABL_2 radiometer blood gas analyzer; PB levels were determined by high performance liquid chromatography (HPLC) with a sensitivity of 1 μg/ml.

RESULTS

In all cases except one, the pH increased sharply within a few minutes of the beginning of hyperventilation (Fig. 1). During the alkalosis there were only small variations in pH. After stopping hyperventilation there was always a period of mixed metabolic and respiratory acidosis probably related to ventilatory depression and to a partial (or complete) occlusion of the endotracheal tube by secretions. Removal of the tube always led to a prompt recovery with normalization of pH and PCO_2. In case 1, hyperventilation never induced significant alkalosis (Table I). Instead, after stopping ventilation the animal developed a metabolic acidosis which persisted, after removal of the tube until death. In case 3, during the alkalotic period, a generalized seizure was accompanied by a transient drop in pH from 7.6 to 7.35 (Fig. 2).

The rise in blood pH related to hyperventilation was always associated with a significant elevation of plasma level of PB (Fig. 1), which remained high until hyperventilation was stopped. When pH fell, plasma PB levels fell correspondingly; acidotic pH was associated with PB levels below control values. When

TABLE I

Influence of Respiratory Alkalosis on the Plasma Level of Phenobarbital in the Newborn Piglet

No.	Weight (g)	Postnatal Age (days)	Hyperventilation (min)	pH	Phenobarbital μg/ml, %
P_1	1300	5	75	—	—
P_2	1700	6	60	7.65	2.4, 25.5
P_3	1600	7	120	7.62	1.72, 23
P_4	1750	8	70	7.66	1.23, 20
P_5	2900	9	90	7.77	2.7, 36
n = 5	1850 ± 612	7 ± 1.5	83 ± 23	—	2.01 ± 0.66

pH eventually returned to normal, plasma PB levels also returned to the control levels.

These parallel variations are very constant and for each individual, plasma PB levels are directly related to pH and inversely related to pCO_2 (Fig. 3). When the changes in PB concentrations (expressed as percentage of previous values, Δ PB%) between the different phases of the experiment (control period, respiratory alkalosis, mixed acidosis, recovery) are compared with the corresponding changes in hydrogen ion concentration (ΔH + nmol/liter), there is a

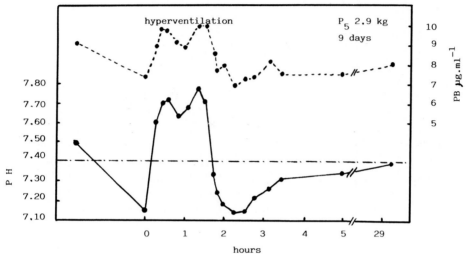

Fig. 1. Changes in blood pH and plasma level of phenobarbital (mg/ml) during hyperventilation and thereafter in piglet no. 5.

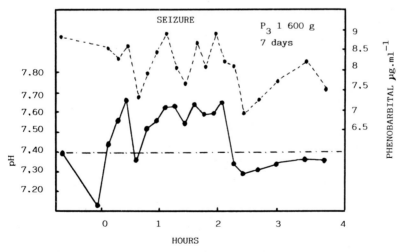

Fig. 2. Plasma level of phenobarbital and pH changes in piglet no. 3. There is a parallel and sharp drop of PB level occurring with a seizure (arrow).

significant inverse correlation ($r = -0.89$, $p < 0.01$, Fig. 4). It is interesting to note that changes in plasma PB happened very quickly within a few minutes of the change in pH. This is particularly well shown first when hyperventilation is discontinued, following which samples were drawn every 5 min (Fig. 5) and secondly after the generalized seizure in piglet no. 3, where, with a drop of pH from 7.66 to 7.35, PB levels decreased from 8.61 to 7.25 mg/ml (-16%).

The variations of pH in this study were induced initially by hyperventilation.

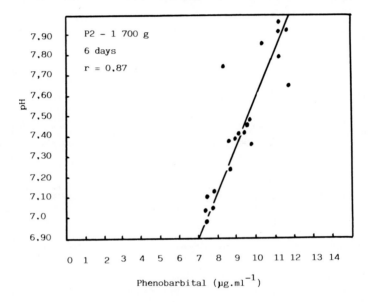

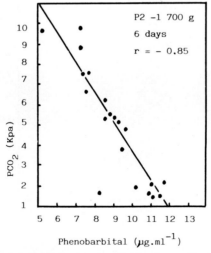

Fig. 3. For each individual, phenobarbital levels are directly related to blood pH ($r = 0.87$) and inversely related to PCO_2 ($r = -0.85$).

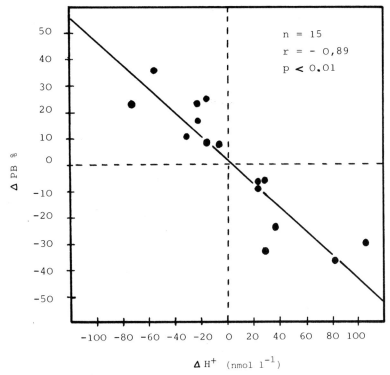

Fig. 4. Changes in PB plasma levels (Δ PB%) related to hydrogen ion concentration (nmol/liter) between the different periods of the procedure: control, alkalotic, mixed acidosis, and recovery.

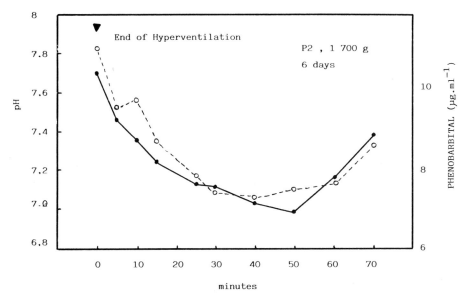

Fig. 5. When hyperventilation is discontinued, the changes in phenobarbital plasma levels occur concomitantly with the reduction of blood pH.

Consequently, PCO_2 was decreased sharply and regularly until a steady state was obtained. However, the changes in pH were not always constantly related to the fall in PCO_2. Analysis of the values of pH and PCO_2 point by point, for any rise in pH until the plateau was reached following the beginning of hyperventilation, shows that for similar pH changes, the drop in PCO_2 varied widely. This may be related to changes in other parameters such as PaO_2. These differences in PCO_2 drops influenced the magnitude of the changes in plasma PB levels. As shown in Figure 6 for similar (small) pH variations the rise in PB is inversely related to corresponding changes in PCO_2. On the other hand, changes in PB levels remained rather small for large pH variations when PCO_2 was greatly decreased.

DISCUSSION

Several studies have been published in the past about PB distribution *in*

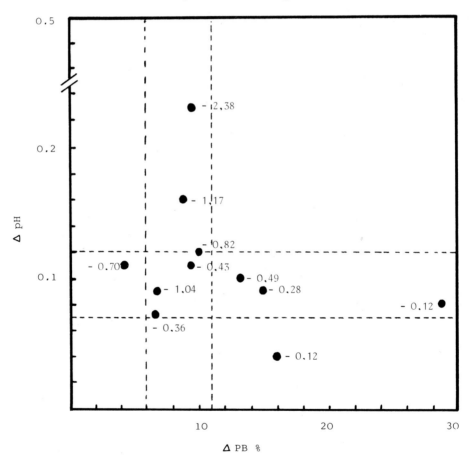

Fig. 6. Influence of changes in PCO_2 (Kpa) on the effect of the variations of blood pH on plasma levels of phenobarbital: for similar pH changes (i.e., 0.1) changes in PB (Δ PB%) are inversely related to the magnitude of PCO_2 drop (numbers represent the drop of PCO_2 in Kpa).

vivo.[2, 5] These studies were, however, specifically concerned with changes in drug distribution over relatively long periods of time, and little is known about the acute effect of short-term biological changes. PB dissociation is affected by variations in blood *p*H *in vivo*, and this gives rise to changes in distribution between intra- and extracellular compartments. Changes in PB plasma levels

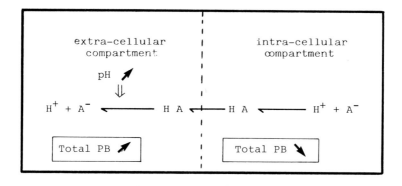

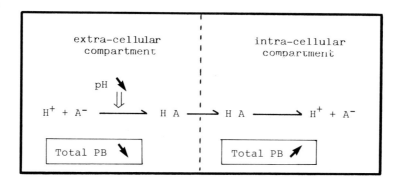

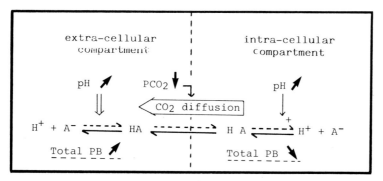

Fig. 7. Effects of changes in intra- and extracellular *p*H on the distribution of phenobarbital (for explanation, see the text).

are related to the difference between the pH inside and outside the cell.[3] Undissociated PB in extracellular fluid decreases as pH rises, and there is a diffusion of undissociated PB from within the cells until a new equilibrium is reached. Dissociated PB does not diffuse freely. As a result, any rise in extracellular pH is accompanied by an elevation of total drug concentration in the extracellular compartment (Fig. 7). This effect has been utilized for the treatment of PB poisoning by forced alkaline diuresis.[6] Urinary excretion was not measured in our study, but return of PB levels to initial values shows that this short-term alkalosis did not induce significant PB excretion.

The comparison of pH and PB according to the corresponding drop in PCO_2 (ΔPCO_2) shows the effect of PCO_2 on the magnitude of PB changes. Any drop in PCO_2 in the extracellular compartment will induce a diffusion of CO_2 from inside to outside the cell. This diffusion will increase intra cellular pH and induce dissociation of PB. As shown in Figure 6, this effect limits the rise in plasma PB concentration during respiratory alkalosis.[3]

From these data it is obvious that even with short-term pH changes, the corresponding variations in PCO_2 influence the plasma PB level; but we can assume that this "protective effect" of PCO_2 on the magnitude of PB changes during respiratory alkalosis is enhanced with slower acid-base status fluctuations than in the present study.

The different ΔPCO_2 seen in this study, despite the hyperventilation, could be explained by some degree of metabolic acidosis occurring during the procedure. The vasoactive effect of CO_2 is responsible for vasoconstriction during hypocapnia; this could have produced, during the alkalotic period, some degree of tissue ischemia with lactacidemia.

This acute release of PB which occurs during short-term alkalosis is the result of drug exchange between the different tissue compartments, but the part due to brain release can be assessed as tissue concentration measurements in such acute circumstances would necessarily be required. However, such changes in PB plasma levels can be considered as a possible explanation for some therapeutic failures and difficulties in achieving a stable therapeutic level.

The occurrence of a seizure in case 3 shows clearly how any acute alkalosis or increase in blood pH (rapid correction of acidosis, start of assisted ventilation) may facilitate new seizures in a patient already treated and with PB plasma levels previously considered as therapeutic. On the other hand, acute acidosis such as may occur during apnea may facilitate central depression by promoting diffusion of undissociated PB into the cells.

CONCLUSION

PB plasma levels are significantly affected *in vivo* by acute changes in blood pH in newborn piglets, and this experimental model seems appropriate for studying similar phenomena which occur clinically. The observed data may have clinical relevance in view of the very frequent instability of acid-base status in the neonatal period in babies treated for respiratory distress and/or neurological injury.[7]

Plasma levels do not reflect accurately drug distribution and need to be interpreted together with the blood pH at sampling.

Further studies are required to appreciate the changes in brain concentration.

REFERENCES

1. Butler, T. C., Mahaffee, C., and Waddell, W. J., Phenobarbital: studies of elimination, accumulation, tolerance and dosages schedules. *J. Pharmacol. Exp. Ther.* **3,** 425–435 (1954).
2. Waddell, W. J., and Butler, T. C., The distribution and excretion of phenobarbital. *J. Clin. Invest.* **36,** 1217–1226 (1957).
3. Butler, T. C., Some Quantitative Aspects of the Pharmacology of Phenobarbital, in *Antiepileptic Drugs: Quantitative Analysis and Interpretation.* Pippenger, C. F., Penry, J. K., and Kutt, H., Eds. Raven Press, New York, 1978, pp. 261–271.
4. Mollaret, P., Monsallier, J. F., Pocidalo, J. J., and Rapin, M., Etudes sur l'intoxication barbiturique aigue. I. Les effets des variations de l'équilibre acido-basique sur la répartition du phénobarbital dans l'arganisme du chien néphectomisé. *Rev. Fr. Etudes Clin. Biol.* **4,** 575–581 (1959).
5. Jalling, B., Plasma and cerebro-spinal fluid concentrations of phenobarbital in infants given singles doses. *Dev. Med. Child. Neurol.* **16,** 781–793 (1974).
6. Lous, P., Barbituric acid concentration in serum from patients with severe acute poisoning. *Acta Pharmacol. Toxical. (Kbh.)* **10,** 261–280 (1954).
7. Monin, P., Vert, P., André, M., and Vibert, M., Acid base status and blood gases during seizures in neonates with birth asphyxia. *Pediatr. Res.* **13,** 527 (1979).
8. Vert, P., Monin, P., Vibert, M., Morselli, P. L., and André, M., Acid-Base Changes and Monitoring of Plasma Levels of Phenobarbital and Clonazepam in the Newborn Treated for Postasphyxic Seizures, in *Intensive Care of the Newborn III*, Stern, L., Ed., Masson, New York, 1980.

34

Blood Gases, Acid-Base Changes, and Monitoring of Plasma Levels of Phenobarbital and Clonazepam in the Newborn Treated for Postasphyxic Seizures

P. VERT,[1] P. MONIN,[1] P. L. MORSELLI,[2] M. VIBERT,[1] and M. ANDRE[1]

The concept of brain damage secondary to neonatal seizures is well established, but generally severity of convulsions and sequelae is supposed to be related to the same common cause. There is now experimental evidence showing that convulsions themselves have a deleterious effect on brain development, regardless of their cause. These data published by Westerlain[10] led us to examine some of the biochemical changes occurring during convulsions, particularly those of blood gas levels, and acid-base balance. Since pH variations are known to influence the distribution and the excretion of drugs, plasma levels of phenobarbital and clonazepam were monitored in the same patients.

SUBJECTS AND METHODS

Thirty term newborns, 16 boys and 14 girls, presenting with seizures were studied (Table I). All had a history of acute fetal distress after a normal pregnancy. The mean gestational age $\pm$ SD was 39.8 $\pm$ 1.3 weeks and the infants birth weights were appropriate for the term: 3,106 $\pm$ 425 g. The mean Apgar scores were 4.2 $\pm$ 3.3 at 1 min and 6.0 $\pm$ 3.0 at 5 min. At the time of the

[1] Service de Médecine Néonatale, Maternité Universitaire, 54042 Nancy, France
[2] Département de Recherche Clinique, LERS, Synthelabo Paris, France

313

study 19 infants were breathing spontaneously and 11 needed intermittent positive pressure ventilation (IPPV).

The infants entered the study after a first tonic and/or clonic convulsion and were studied during at least one further episode. At the same time EEG recordings were done routinely and confirmed patterns of paroxysmal activity. Capillary blood samples for pH, PCO_2 (ABL2 Radiometer) and drug levels were taken by heel prick before therapy, every 6 hr and during convulsive episodes. Transcutaneous PO_2 recordings were made in nine infants (54 episodes) using a Huch electrode.[3] Heart rate and respiratory mouvements were monitored (Hewlett-Packard Respirograph), and for infants receiving IPPV the ventilator settings were regularly adjusted according to the results of blood gases and pH assessments.

The therapeutic protocol for convulsions was to give first phenobarbital at a loading dose of 10 mg/kg and a daily maintenance dose of 5 mg/kg. In cases where convulsive episodes persisted 6 hr after the first dose of phenobarbital, clonazepam was prescribed at a loading dose of 0.1 mg/kg and daily maintenance dose of 0.2 mg/kg.

Plasma levels of phenobarbital and clonazepam were measured by high performance liquid chromatography[8] with a limit of confidence of 6 and 10%, respectively.

RESULTS

Transcutaneous PO_2

During 14 tonic-clonic seizures observed in four infants $tc PO_2$ fell from a mean initial value $\pm$ 1 SD of 83 $\pm$ 13 mmHg to a mean of 42 $\pm$ 15 mmHg (p

TABLE I

Postasphyxic Convulsions: N 30, F 14, M 16

	Mean $\pm$ SD
GA	39.8 $\pm$ 1.3
BW	3106 $\pm$ 425 g
Apgar	
1 min	4.2 $\pm$ 3.3
5 min	6.0 $\pm$ 3.0
Age 1st convulsion	36.5 $\pm$ 49.3 H

Spontaneous breathing (19)—IPPV (11).

TABLE II

Changes during Convulsions

	Tonic-Clonic (14 Episodes)	Clonic (40 Episodes)
Initial $tc PO_2$ (mmHg $\pm$ SD)	83.2 $\pm$ 13.4	81.4 $\pm$ 21.5
Change $tc PO_2$	−41.5 $\pm$ 18.4	+5.15 $\pm$ 5.8
p	<0.05	NS

< 0.05). In contrast, during 40 clonic episodes there was no significant change in $tcPO_2$ (Table II). The impedance pneumogram showed apnea during tonic-clonic episodes with a mean duration of 78 ± 47 sec. No apnea was observed during clonic episodes. On the contrary the respiratory rate was increased during all but one clonic episode (39/40). Figure 1 shows a scheme of the course of the hypoxic phase showing a mean recovery time of 227 ± 101 sec, significantly longer that the mean time of fall (108 ± 60 sec) ($p < 0.05$).

pH and PCO$_2$

Blood pH was measured during 74 distinct episodes of convulsions, 36 in infants breathing spontaneously (BS) and 38 in infants on IPPV (Fig. 2). In both groups there is a significant number of episodes where the infants were in an alkalotic state with pH over 7.40: 16 out of 36 for those breathing spontaneously and 26 out of 38 for infants on IPPV. There are only six episodes with a blood pH below 7.30; in two of them there was clinical and radiological evidence of meconium aspiration (pH 7.21 and 7.02). PCO_2 measurements were made simultaneously with blood pH during convulsions (Fig. 2). Hypocapnia below 35 mmHg was present in 38 cases (13 BS and 25 IPPV). Hypercapnia over 40 mmHg was observed in 18 episodes, 10 SB and 8 IPPV. These results confirm that respiratory alkalosis is common during neonatal seizures.

In some cases in whom routine pH and PCO_2 measurements had been made in the 6 hr preceding a convulsion, the effect of convulsions on pH and PCO_2 could be more precisely appreciated.

In 12 convulsive episodes in infants breathing spontaneously there were no

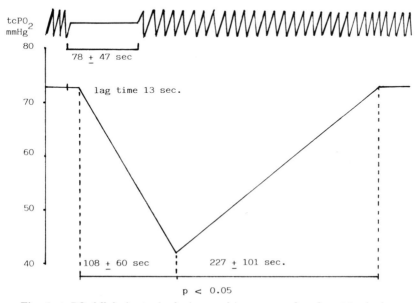

Fig. 1. $tcPO_2$ fall during tonic-clonic convulsions mean values from 14 episodes.

significant pH changes in four, a decrease in two, and an increase in six (Fig. 3). PCO_2 measured at the same time in 11 cases, had decreased in eight. Since it was observed in babies breathing spontaneously, this unexpected trend towards respiratory alkalosis during convulsions is of particular importance in explaining the alkalotic pH found in 42 episodes of seizures. During 10 episodes of convulsions in infants on IPPV, blood pH increased in four, decreased in four, and was unchanged in two, while pH was increased in seven, decreased in two, and unchanged in one. Blood pH and PCO_2 changes in these artificially ventilated infants are more scattered than for infants BS, as would be expected from complex regulatory changes both in the patient and in the ventilator resulting in a disorganized pattern.

The relationship between the number of convulsive episodes and blood pH was considered. Maximum pH changes $\pm$ SD (ΔpH) were 0.14 ± 0.9 in infants presenting with one or two convulsive episodes and 0.25 ± 0.8 in those having more than two convulsions ($p < 0.05$). Comparing these two groups of infants for phenobarbital plasma levels there was no significant difference (Table III). Furthermore, alkalosis was significantly linked with the risk of recurrence of

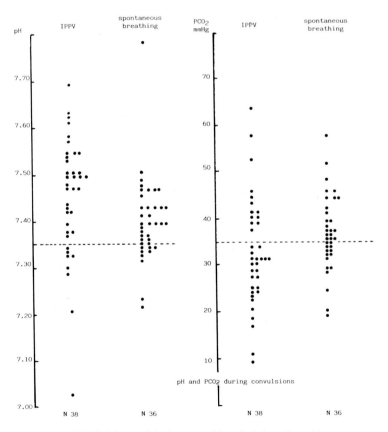

Fig. 2. Blood pH and PCO_2 observed during convulsions in infants breathing spontaneously and in infants artificially ventilated (IPPV).

convulsions (Table IV). In blood samples taken 6 hr after the first convulsion six infants who did not have a second episode had a mean $pH \pm SD$ of 7.36 ± 0.04 whereas 15 infants who experienced a recurrence had a mean pH of 7.45 ± 0.07 ($p < 0.05$). Again there was no significant difference in plasma phenobarbital levels in the two groups of infants.

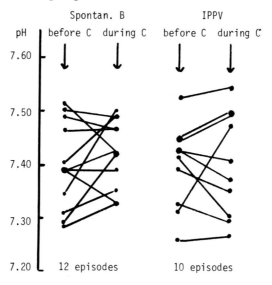

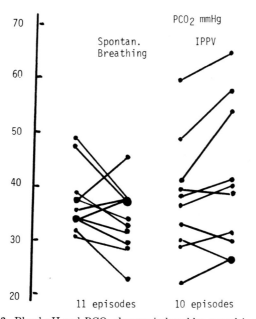

Fig. 3. Blood pH and PCO_2 changes induced by convulsions.

Plasma Levels of Phenobarbital and Clonazepam

In 18 cases plasma levels of phenobarbital could be assessed before and during convulsive episodes (Table V). Significant changes of more than 5% of the initial levels were found in 12 cases with a mean increase of 28.6% in four cases and a mean decrease of 25.4% in eight cases.

Plasma phenobarbital level changes (ΔPB) could be correlated to pH changes (ΔH$^+$) in 12 cases (Fig. 4). Phenobarbital levels increased with pH, or, in other words, there was an inverse correlation between the concentration of H$^+$ and the concentration of phenobarbital ($r = -0.84$). In the same way Figure 5 shows an inverse relationship between changes in PCO$_2$ (ΔPCO$_2$), and ΔPB observed in 18 cases ($r = -0.60$).

Plasma levels of clonazepam were measured before and during convulsions in 11 episodes (Table VI). There was a significant change of more than 5% of the initial level in 10 cases; a mean increase of 68.5% was observed in six cases and a mean decrease of 15.7% in four cases. But there was no detectable relationship between clonazepam level changes and pH or PCO$_2$ variations during convulsions.

TABLE III

Maximum pH Variations and Recurrence of Convulsions

Convulsions	Plasma Phenobarbital (μg/ml) (mean ± SD)	pH (mean ± SD)
1 or 2 episodes	14.7 ± 2.6	0.14 ± 0.9
>2 episodes	18.0 ± 5.5	0.25 ± 0.8
p	NS	<0.05

TABLE IV

Alkalosis and Recurrence of Convulsions. Blood Samples 6 Hrs after 1st Convulsion

Evolution of Convulsions	Plasma Phenobarbital (μg/ml ± SD)	pH (±SD)
No recurrence N 6	11.7 ± 5.0	7.36 ± 0.04
Recurrence N 15	12.1 ± 5.8	7.45 ± 0.07
p	NS	<0.05

TABLE V

Changes (%) of Plasma Phenobarbital during Convulsions: N 18

	N	Mean	Range
Increase ≥ 5%	4	+28.6	+6.5-+92
Decrease ≥ 5%	8	-25.4	-7.4--50
Not significant	6	-1.0	+1.2--2

COMMENTS

When this study was designed, the expected blood gas and pH changes were hypoxemia, hypercapnia, and acidosis as shown by Meldrum in monkeys.[4, 5] tcPO_2 recordings showed the expected hypoxemia in cases of tonic-clonic convulsions which included an apneic phase. Clonic seizures did not induce any significant change in tcPO_2, since they were not accompanied by apnea. The duration of apnea and the long time for recovery even after the restarting of respiration prolonged the hypoxemic episode, to a mean time of 335 sec (108 + 227) (Fig. 1). These apneic attacks might be severe enough to explain any resultant brain damage.

The frequent observation of a respiratory alkalosis both during convulsions and during the interictal period is unexpected and raises questions about its causes or mechanism and its consequences. The design of the study does not permit us to know whether alkalosis precedes or follows the first episode of

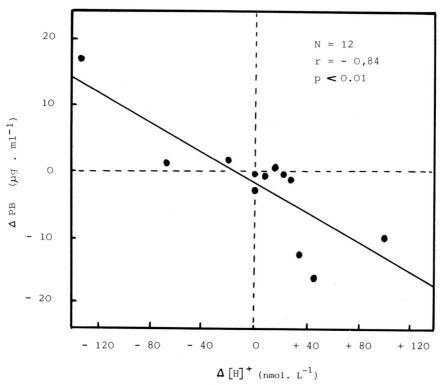

Δ Phenobarbital / $\Delta[\text{H}]^+$

During convulsions

Fig. 4. Plasma phenobarbital changes inversely correlated to H$^+$ concentration changes in the blood during 12 convulsive episodes.

convulsions. For infants breathing spontaneously two main causes could be suggested: (a) A delay in the normalization of CSF pH following a metabolic acidosis as described, for example, in the recovery phase of diabetic acidosis.[11] All the infants are assumed to have passed through a metabolic acidosis during their acute intrapartum asphyxia. (b) Another mechanism involved is the observed increase in respiratory rate during the clonic phase of convulsions. Since the respiratory recording was an impedance pneumogram, we have no

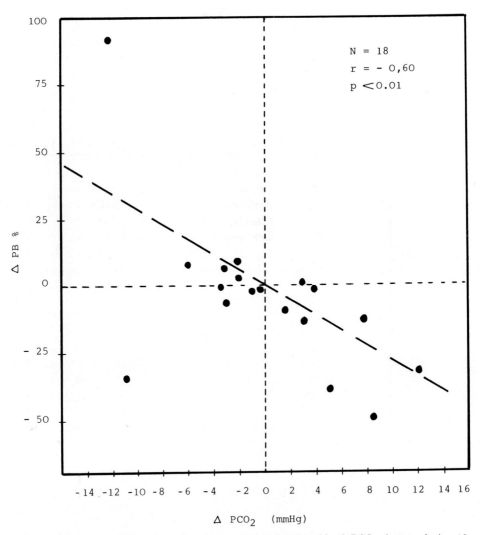

Fig. 5. Plasma phenobarbital changes inversely correlated to blood PCO_2 changes during 18 convulsive episodes.

further evidence supporting true hyperventilation. Infants who were treated by IPPV could have been overventilated and put into respiratory alkalosis because of increased thoracic compliance induced by muscular hypotonia.

The consequences of alkalosis in the newborn are not well documented. Experimentally a respiratory alkalosis reduces cerebral blood flow.[2] The shift to the left of the oxyhemoglobin dissociation curve by alkalosis (Bohr effect) can also impair oxygen transport to the tissues.

The most striking consequence of respiratory alkalosis is the observation of an increased risk for recurrence of convulsions. This fact is consistently related to the well-known effect of alkalosis in lowering the threshold of neuromuscular excitability.

We have as yet no data concerning preventive or therapeutic measures against postasphyxic respiratory alkalosis.

The relationship between blood pH and plasma phenobarbital levels was documented long ago in connection with the treatment of barbiturate intoxication by alkalinization. In nephrectomised dogs induced ventilatory alkalosis produces a rise and acidosis a fall in plasma phenobarbital levels.[6] The pKa of phenobarbital, at 7.4, is close to the range of pH changes observed in human blood, and, consequently, these induce major variations in the ionization of the drug. The same effect of pH variations on plasma phenobarbital levels has been observed in dogs[6] and in newborn piglets.[7]

Figure 6 shows one example of plasma phenobarbital level fluctuations in relation to pH changes during recurrent convulsions. Such fluctuations over short periods of time cannot be related to significant changes in the elimination of the drug since the elimination half-life for phenobarbital is around 100 hr.[1,9] The variations observed in plasma levels suggest that pH changes alter the distribution of the drug between intra- and extracellular spaces.

When evaluating the significance of a given phenobarbital level during convulsions or status epilepticus, it would be inaccurate and misleading to draw any definite conclusions. The erroneous interpretation of a given level of phenobarbital results from the paradoxical situation of an increased plasma level masking a decreased tissue level. Solely because of a pH change, plasma phenobarbital may rise from a therapeutic to a toxic level or from an ineffective level to one usually accepted as effective. These variations could also be a cause of ineffectiveness of the treatment and one of the causes of the recurrence of convulsions. Although not related to pH changes, the fluctuations of plasma clonazepam levels during convulsions lead to similar doubts about the usefulness of this measurement in an unstable biological situation.

We conclude that the tendency to ventilatory alkalosis during postasphyxic

TABLE VI

Changes (%) of Plasma Clonazepam during Convulsions: N 11

	N	Mean	Range
Increase ⩾ 5%	6	+68.5	+5–+120
Decrease ⩾ 5%	4	−15.7	−10–−28
Not significant	1	—	+3.5

seizures suggests at least two possible mechanisms for the recurrence of convulsions: (a) lowering of the threshold of neuromuscular excitability; (b) the displacement of phenobarbital from its intracellular site of action.

SUMMARY

Blood gases and pH changes occurring during convulsions were studied in 30 term newborns presenting with postasphyxic seizures. Hypoxemia measured by tcPO_2, monitoring was observed only during tonic-clonic episodes(ΔtcPO_2, 41.5 ± 18.4 mmHg) and not during clonic seizures. pH and PCO_2 measurements during convulsions showed that respiratory alkalosis is a common finding, both in infants breathing spontaneously and in those treated by IPPV. There was a close relationship between blood alkalosis and the recurrence of convulsions. Plasma phenobarbital levels monitored in 18 cases during convulsions showed

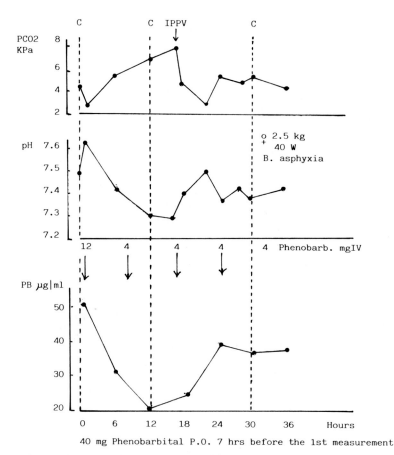

Fig. 6. Plasma phenobarbital changes observed in a newborn in relation to pH and PCO_2 changes. During the first 12 hr of observation plasma levels of phenobarbital were decreasing in spite of two additional doses of the drug. C = convulsions. Because of alkalosis the initial level of phenobarbital was in the toxic range.

variations correlated to pH changes. Phenobarbital levels increased with alkalosis ($r = -0.84$). In the same way in 12 cases there was an inverse relationship between changes in PCO_2 and in phenobarbital levels ($r = -0.60$). During convulsions significant changes in plasma clonazepam levels were observed in 10 episodes out of 11, but did not correlate with pH changes. These data suggest two possible mechanisms involved in the recurrence of convulsions: (a) lowering of the threshold of neuromuscular excitability by alkalosis; (b) displacement of phenobarbital from its intracellular site of action.

ACKNOWLEDGMENT

We are grateful to Doctor Simon Tuck for his collaboration.

REFERENCES

1. Boreus, L. O., Jalling, B., and Kallberg, N., Phenobarbital metabolism in adults and in newborn infants. *Acta Paediatr. Scand.* **67,** 193–200 (1978).
2. Gotoh, F., Meyer, J. S., and Takagi, Y., Cerebral effects of hyperventilation in man. *Arch. Neurol.* **12,** 410–424 (1964).
3. Huch, R., Lubbers, D. W., and Huch, A., Reliability of transcutaneous monitoring of arterial PO_2 in newborn infants. *Arch. Dis. Child.* **49,** 213–218 (1974).
4. Meldrum, B. S., and Horton, R. W., Physiology of status epilepticus in primates. *Arch. Neurol.* **28,** 1–9 (1973).
5. Meldrum, B., Physiological changes during prolonged seizures and epileptic brain damage. *Neuropädiatrie* **9,** 203–212 (1978).
6. Mollaret, P., Monsallier, J. F., Pocidalo, J. J., and Rapin, M., Etudes sur l'intoxication barbiturique aiguë. I Les effets des variations de l'équilibre acido-basique sur la répartition du phënobarbital dans l'organisme du chien néphrectomisé. *Rev. Fr. Etude Clin. Biol.* **4,** 575–581 (1959).
7. Monin, P., Vert, P., Sanjuan, C., Vibert, M., and Rovei, V., Effects of Respiratory Alkalosis on Plasma Levels of Phenobarbital in the Newborn Piglet, in *Intensive Care in the Newborn* III, Stern, L., Salle, B., and Friis-Hansen, B., Eds. Masson, New York, 1981.
8. Rovei, V., Sanjuan, C., and Morselli, P. L., Comparison between HPLC and GLC-ND: Analytical Methods for the Determination of AED in Plasma and Blood of Patients, in *Antiepileptic Therapy: Advances in Drug Monitoring*, Sohannessen, S. I., Morselli, P. L., Pippenger, C. E., Richens, A., Schmidt, D., and Meinardi, H., Eds. Raven Press, New York, 1980, pp. 349–356.
9. Royer, R. J., Vert, P., Mur, J. M., Pladys, J. C., Humbert, F., and Royer-Morrot, M. J., Données pharmacocinétiques sur le phénobarbital. Etude de l'influence de l'âge gestationnel et de la dysmaturité. *Arch. Fr. Pediatr.* **33,** 905–913 (1976).
10. Westerlain, C. G., Neonatal seizures and brain growth. *Neuropädiatrie* **9,** 213–228 (1978).
11. Winters, R. W., Lowder, J. A., and Ordway, N. K., Observations on the plasma carbon dioxide tension during recovery from metabolic acidosis. *J. Clin. Invest.* **37,** 640–645 (1958).

35

The Glucocorticoids in Normal, Premature, and Small for Dates Newborn Infants throughout the Neonatal Period

WŁADYSŁAW ROKICKI and JEAN BERTRAND

In many handbooks of pediatrics one can find the opinion that the great frequency of hypoglycemic states in premature newborns, still greater in the infants suffering from intrauterine growth retardation, is the result of deteriorated adrenal activity.[21] On the other hand, investigators who have studied glucocorticoid levels in cord blood or in peripheral blood of premature infants have more often found it increased[4, 13, 15, 25] than decreased.[18, 37] It is also difficult to explain why a tendency toward hypoglycemic states appears only at a certain period of neonatal age.

The previous suggestions of adrenal cortex insufficiency in small for dates (SFD) infants, based on the determinations of plasma electrolytes, glucose metabolism, and acidophilic leucocytes[30] or on the assay of cortisol production rate and excretion of 17-hydroxycorticoids[12] have not been supported by more recent studies.[15, 37]

The differential adrenal cortex activity in premature or in SFD infants as compared with full-term subjects could be suspected on the basis of morphological findings (different histological picture of adrenal glands in prematures,[33] greater reduction of adrenals than of the other organs in newborns with intrauterine growth retardation[21]).

Unité de Recherches Endocriniennes et Metaboliques chez l'Enfant, U-34 Lyon, France, and Clinic of Pathology Pregnancy, Institute of Obstetrics and Gynecology, Silesian Academy of Medicine, Bytom, Poland

In fact, our knowledge about newborn adrenal function is still very poor, particularly in neonatal pathological states.

No data are available concerning the changes of adrenal function in the neonatal period of premature or SFD infant. There are only a few such studies in full-term neonates. During those studies the plasma content of cortisol, sometimes of cortisone, and very rarely of corticosterone was determined from birth throughout the first several days of life.[1, 10, 32, 40] We do not know of any data concerning the plasma content changes in the neonatal period either of the oxidized derivative of corticosterone—11-dehydrocorticosterone or of the immediate precursor of cortisol—11-deoxycortisol.

THE AIM OF THE WORK

In order to be able to undertake the studies of glucocorticoid hormones in hypoglycemic states of newborns, we were obliged to first determine the norms of the studied hormones not only just after delivery but also during the entire neonatal period. The norms have been prepared separately for full-term, premature, and intra-uterine growth retarded newborn infants.

MATERIAL AND METHODS

Plasma content of cortisol (F), cortisone (E), corticosterone (B), 11-dehydrocorticosterone (A), and 11-deoxycortisol (S) was determined in 77 full-term, 93 premature, and 49 SFD newborns from birth up to the third month of life. Infants severely distressed were excluded from our material. All the studied infants were born vaginally and were considered to be in satisfactory clinical condition, at least in relation to their body weight. None of the mothers was treated with glucocorticoids.

The mean body birth weight of the studied infants was: for the full-term 2520–4300 g, averaging 3219 ± 423 g; for the prematurely born 780–2500 g, averaging 1820 g ± 468 g (fetal age of 27–36 weeks); and of SFD newborns 1350–2480 g, averaging 2096 ± 313 g. All the infants with intrauterine growth retardation were born as a result of pregnancies lasting 38–41 weeks and their birth weight was always below two standard deviations for gestation and the newborn's sex. The studied infants were born in the Clinic of Pathological Pregnancy, Institute of Obstetrics and Gynecology, Silesian Medical Academy, Poland, in some others hospitals of Upper Silesia, Poland, as well as in Clinique St. Charles, Hospital of the University of Montpellier, France. The Polish children were compared with the norms established by Brzozowska[3] and the French ones with the norms published by Sempé and Masse.[28] The newborns were divided into the following age groups: 0–6 hr after birth, 7–12 hr, 13–24 hr, 2nd day of life, 3rd–5th day, 6th–12th day, 13th–30th day, and 2nd–3rd month.

The glucocorticoid plasma contents have been determined using a modified radioimmunological method separately described by the authors.[27]

During routine blood collection (in order to study bilirubin level, electrolytes contents, etc.) 0.5–1 ml of the newborn's blood was additionally taken into dry heparin and immediately centrifuged. After addition of 1000–2000 cpm of the labeled hormones (in order to calculate the recoveries) the studied hormones were extracted from 0.1–0.25 ml of plasma diluted with 1 ml of distilled water. The extraction was performed by vigorous manual shaking with methylene chloride. After centrifugation the aqueous phase as well as the protein precipitate were carefully discarded. The methylene chloride phase was blown to dryness, and the residue was redissolved in a small volume of 2% methanol in methylene chloride (which was always used as a solvent) and subjected to column chromatography. Sephadex LH-20 columns (48 × 1 cm) were used. All the separations were performed at a temperature 26 ± 1°C with a solvent passage speed of about 25 ml/hr. The following fractions of the column eluates were used to determine the Kendall's A, B, S, E, and F compound contents: 20–22 ml, 26–31 ml, 33–38 ml, 41–53 ml, and 58–83 ml, respectively. These fractions were blown to dryness and immediately assayed or stored (−30°C) for further study as an alcohol solution. All the hormone assays were performed three times utilizing phosphate buffer to the same volume one-, two-, and threefold quantities of the material studied. As a final result the mean value of those three determinations have been calculated. The nonspecific antibodies used in this work were raised in the rabbit against cortisone-21-BSA and kindly donated to us by Dr. Bidlingmayer (Children's Hospital, München). They gave cross reactions with cortisol as following: F—100%, E—59.3%, B—14.4%, S—45%, A—34%.

RESULTS AND DISCUSSION

The obtained results ± one standard deviation are presented in Figures 1–8 and Tables I–VIII.

In the full-term newborns the high plasma levels at the beginning of extrauterine life of the biologically most important glucocorticoid in a human being—cortisol—declined abruptly within the first 12 hr after birth and remained low up to the 3rd–5th day. Afterwards the mean cortisol level started to rise (from the 6th–12th day) and in the 2nd–3rd month reached the value corresponding with that observed at a more advanced age.[13]

In contrast, the plasma levels of cortisol in premature infants during first 5 days of life were significantly higher than in full-term neonates (except in the age group of 0–6 hr, in which the difference was not yet significant). During the next few days in preterm infants a decrease in cortisol was observed but at a more advanced age than in the control group (full-term newborns). Thus the diminution of cortisol plasma content started from the age group of 6th–12th day, and the lowest levels of this hormone were found in preterm newborns at the second month of life. In the third month an increase of plasma cortisol content in premature infants was demonstrated.

In the studied newborns with intrauterine growth retardation the mean cortisol plasma level was lower during the first 6 hours of life than in full-term infants. However, this result should be interpreted very carefully because the difference was not statistically significant. Later on in SFD newborns an increase of plasma cortisol level was observed (significantly exceeding the value found in full-term infant). Beginning from the age group 6th–12th day the mean cortisol content in SFD infants declined and was not statistically different from that observed in full-term newborns.

The mean plasma content of cortisone (oxidated, biologically inactive derivative of cortisol) in full-term infants was highest in the first 6 hr after birth. Its continuous subsequent decrease was observed during the studied period. However the mean value of this hormone in the 2nd–3rd month of life in full-term infants was still higher than that known from the literature,[13] cortisone level in the adult (which is about 2 µg/dl of plasma).

The mean cortisone plasma contents in all the groups but one (3rd–5th day) of premature newborns were not significantly different from those observed in the full-term infants. Thus, the gradual decrease of cortisone level in preterm newborns was also demonstrated (with the exception of its peak in 3rd–5th day).

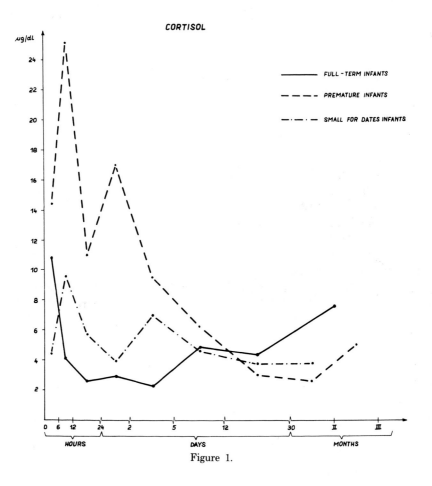

Figure 1.

The mean cortisone plasma level in SFD newborns was significantly lower as compared with full-term infants in the first 6 hr of life. Afterwards its values were not significantly different from those observed in full-term subjects with the exception of the age group 3rd–5th day in which the plasma content of the studied hormone was higher than in the full-term infants.

The neonatal pattern of the second biologically active studied hormone—corticosterone—was similar to the one of cortisol. Thus, one can observe in full-term infants the abrupt decline of corticosterone after birth followed by its low plasma concentrations up to the 3rd–5th day, and its subsequent increase.

In the preterm newborns the average corticosterone plasma levels starting after birth from nonsignificantly higher values than in full-term subjects declined during the first month of life. However, their values too on the second day as in the 3rd–5th day group significantly exceeded the plasma concentrations of this hormone observed in the full-term infants at corresponding ages. The lowest level of hormone was found in prematures in the second month of life. In the third month its plasma content rose, which closely corresponds with the observation concerning cortisol in these children.

In the SFD newborns the mean corticosterone plasma level during the first 6 hr of life was not significantly lower as compared with full-term infants and significantly lower as compared with the preterm subjects. Afterwards its averages were not statistically different from those observed in full-term newborns, with the exception of the 3rd–5th day, in which group the plasma level of corticosterone was significantly higher in SFD infants. Significantly

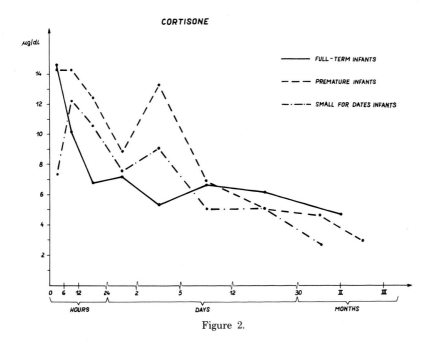

Figure 2.

lower corticosterone level in SFD newborns as compared with preterm subjects were observed on the second day of life.

The neonatal pattern of the inactive derivative of corticosterone, 11-dehydrocorticosterone, was not very different from the one of cortisone in full-term as well as in preterm infants, indicating a diminution of this hormone's plasma content during newborn development.

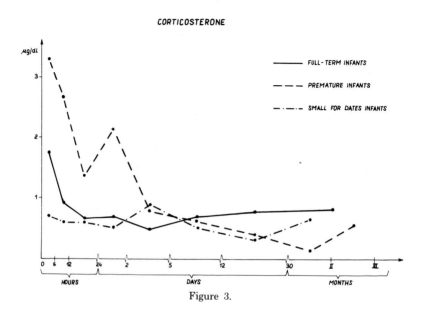

Figure 3.

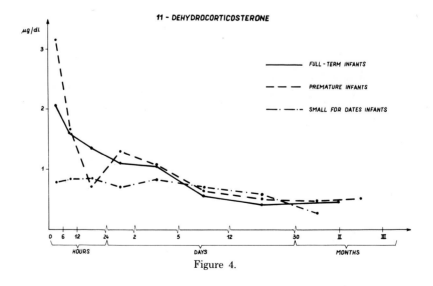

Figure 4.

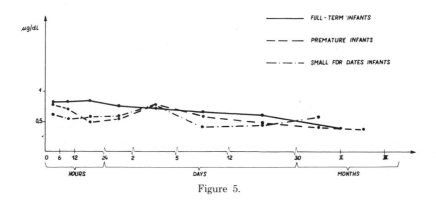

Figure 5.

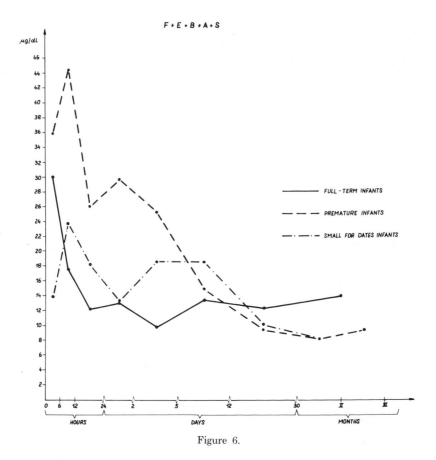

Figure 6.

On the other hand in the SFD newborns the plasma level of 11-dehydrocorticosterone was significantly lower in the first 6 hr of life than in full-term or preterm subjects.

The neonatal pattern of the fifth hormone studied, 11-deoxycortisol, was quite different from the patterns of the glucocorticoids already discussed both in the full-term as well as in premature and SFD infants. The mean plasma value of this hormone in full-term newborns decreased during the period studied very slowly but continuously. Its average in the 2nd–3rd month of life exceeded the norm in adults (0.1–0.2 μg/dl).[5, 14]

The 11-deoxycortisol patterns in premature and SFD infants were not very different from the ones in full-term newborns, with the exception of the 13–24-hr and 2nd day of life groups of prematures, in which the observed values were slightly but significantly lower than in the control subjects.

Up to the present time one can find in the literature results concerning so-called "total corticoids" determinations.[25] These results should be more similar to the total of the hormones assayed in this work than to the cortisol level. On the other hand the total of the studied hormones perhaps represents good adrenal cortex activity.

Studying the neonatal pattern of presented total levels one can redetermine the rapid and statistically significant diminution of adrenal cortex activity after birth in the full-term infants with its lowest value in the 3rd–5th day group and its increase afterwards.

In the premature newborns during the first 5 days of life the total of assayed hormones was significantly higher than in full-term infants, with the exception of the first 6 hr after birth. Afterwards its decrease reaching the minimum in the second month was observed.

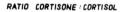

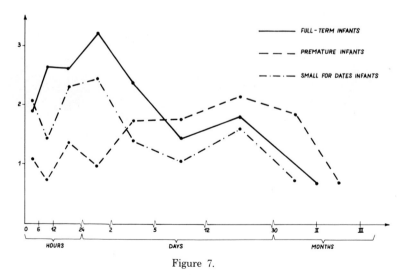

Figure 7.

In the SFD infants the mean value of the studied glucocorticoid total was significantly lower during the first 6 hr after birth compared with full-term as well as with premature subjects. Afterwards the hormonal total in the SFD newborns was not very different from the one in the full-term infants with exception of the 3rd–5th day in which group its value was significantly higher.

The ratios of inactive to active forms of the studied hormones have been also calculated. The E/F ratio in the adult is about 0.2.[13] In placenta and in fetal tissues, except the lung,[6, 34] the large amounts of cortisol coming from the mother are about 80% oxidized to cortisone,[19] which is considered to be the mechanism protecting the fetal pituitary-adrenal axis. This rapid conversion, probably extrahepatic,[24] has also been demonstrated in our material in the newborn. Thus, in our full-term infants the mean values of E/F and A/B during the first 5 days of life were between 2 and 3, except in the first 6 hours after birth when they were slightly below 2. In the groups of full-term infants at more advanced ages than the 3rd–5th day of life the studied ratios decreased. In the second month both ratios were already below 1 and in the third month a still stronger advantage of the active forms was found.

In the prematurely born infants the both studied ratios were significantly lower in the first 5 days of life than in the full-term subjects. Afterwards their mean values rose in the prematures reaching the maximum much later than in the control groups: (E/F on 13th–30th day and A/B in the second month of life). In the third month the averages of both ratios were below 1.

In the SFD newborns the E/F and A/B neonatal patterns were not very different from those in full-term infants. However, in the age group 3rd–5th

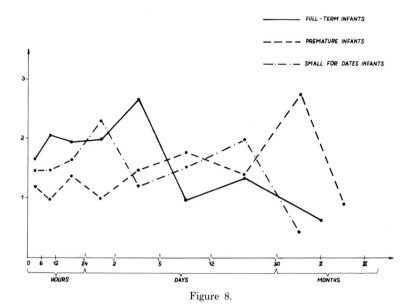

Figure 8.

day the conversion of active hormones to their oxidized derivatives was significantly less as compared with full-term subjects.

In the full-term, premature, and SFD infants there was a highly significant positive correlation ($P < 0.001$) between cortisol and corticosterone as well as between cortisone and 11-dehydrocorticosterone content. The E/F and A/B ratios were also positively correlated.

The results presented above, excluding those concerning 11-dehydrocorticosterone and 11-deoxycortisol level changes not previously studied during neonatal development even in full-term subjects, are in good agreement with the results obtained in human-beings as well as in animals, with respect to the rapid plasma fall in biologically active glucocorticoids immediately after birth and their subsequent increase.[1, 10, 13, 17, 35, 36, 40] In this same time period a continuous deterioration of plasma cortisone content was observed.[10, 32]

The view that in normal circumstances in the perinatal period it is not ACTH or not only ACTH that controls adrenal cortex activity can be supported by present results, e.g., rapid reduction of plasma levels of the determined glucocorticoids after birth in full-term infants in spite of known high plasma contents of ACTH in this period.[11, 41]

Bertrand, *et al.* observed that newborn infants responded normally to ACTH but that this response was reduced in the first 24–36 hr of life.[2]

TABLE I

Mean Values of Cortisol (F) in the Plasma (μg/dl $\pm$ 1 SD)
(Number in Brackets = Number of Observations)

Age	(Hr)			(Days)				(Months)	
	0–6	7–12	13–24	2nd	3rd–5th	6th–12th	13th–30th	2nd	3rd
Full-term newborns	(6) 10.83 ±6.97	(8) 4.05 ±0.98	(6) 2.58 ±0.84	(16) 2.93 ±1.92	(19) 2.29 ±0.83	(10) 4.87 ±1.92	(6) 4.38 ±2.47	(6) 7.59 ±3.23	
	⟵⟶ $P < 0.01$	⟵⟶ $P < 0.02$		⟵ $P < 0.001$ ⟶					
Premature newborns	(7) 14.43 ±3.16	(3) 25.09[c] ±18.6	(5) 10.99[b] ±7.15	(7) 16.88[d] ±11.55	(16) 9.47[d] ±6.95	(23) 6.21 ±4.68	(21) 3.07 ±2.65	(8) 2.65 ±1.07	(3) 5.05 ±5
	$P < 0.001$ ↕			$P < 0.01$ ↕		⟵ $P < 0.01$ ⟶			
Small for dates newborns	(4) 4.48 ±1.99	(3) 9.56[c] ±3.83	(4) 5.71[a] ±2.89	(9) 3.92 ±1.98	(7) 7.0[d] ±2.98	(6) 4.67 ±2.09	(13) 3.8 ±2.7	(1) 3.84	
	⟵⟶ $P < 0.05$			⟵⟶ $P < 0.05$					

Statistical significance as compared with full-term newborns at corresponding age:
[a] $P < 0.05$.
[b] $P < 0.02$.
[c] $P < 0.01$.
[d] $P < 0.001$.

TABLE II

Mean Values of Cortisone (E) in the Plasma (μg/dl $\pm$ 1 SD)
(Number in Brackets = Number of Observations)

Age	(Hr)			(Days)				(Months)	
	0–6	7–12	13–24	2nd	3rd–5th	6th–12th	13th–30th	2nd	3rd
Full-term newborns	(6) 14.57 ±3.48	(8) 10.14 ±3.81	(6) 6.79 ±2.83	(16) 7.2 ±3.29	(19) 5.35 ±2.8	(10) 6.65 ±3.0	(6) 6.18 ±1.81	(6) 4.7 ±1.83	
	←——→ $P < 0.05$								
Premature newborns	(7) 14.3 ±8.02	(3) 14.27 ±2.37	(5) 12.43 ±6.35	(7) 8.82 ±3.38	(16) 13.23[b] ±9.69	(23) 6.83 ±3.14	(21) 5.08 ±3.74	(8) 4.63 ±3.27	(3) 2.98 ±2.25
				←——————→ $P < 0.01$					
Small for dates newborns	(4) 7.32[a] ±5.47	(3) 12.21 ±2.33	(4) 10.54 ±5.03	(9) 7.54 ±2.94	(7) 9.05[b] ±3.23	(8) 5.07 ±2.19	(13) 5.12 ±3.67	(1) 2.86	

Statistical significance as compared with full-term newborns at corresponding age:
[a] $P < 0.05$.
[b] $P < 0.01$.

TABLE III

Mean Values of Corticosterone (B) in the Plasma (μg/dl $\pm$ 1 SD)
(Number in Brackets = Number of Observations)

Age	(Hr)			(Days)				(Months)	
	0–6	7–12	13–24	2nd	3rd–5th	6th–12th	13th–30th	2nd	3rd
Full-term newborns	(6) 1.75 ±1.14	(8) 0.94 ±0.29	(6) 0.67 ±0.18	(16) 0.71 ±0.45	(19) 0.5 ±0.25	(10) 0.7 ±0.54	(6) 0.79 ±1.09	(6) 0.84 ±0.43	
	←——————→ $P < 0.05$								
Premature newborns	(7) 3.3 ±1.53	(3) 2.68 ±2.62	(5) 1.37 ±1.69	(7) 2.14[b] ±1.85	(16) 0.79[a] ±0.54	(23) 0.66 ±0.6	(21) 0.41 ±0.21	(8) 0.15[c] ±0.07	(3) 0.57 ±0.41
	$P < 0.02$			$P < 0.05$ ←——→ $P < 0.02$			←——→ $P < 0.01$	←——→ $P < 0.02$	
Small for dates newborns	(4) 0.71 ±0.6	(3) 0.62 ±0.36	(4) 0.61 ±0.38	(9) 0.53 ±0.46	(7) 0.9[a] ±0.73	(8) 0.53 ±0.54	(12) 0.33 ±0.24	(1) 0.66	
				←——————→ $P < 0.05$					

Statistical significance as compared with full-term newborns at corresponding age:
[a] $P < 0.05$.
[b] $P < 0.01$.
[c] $P < 0.001$.

In our studies in the premature newborns the high glucocorticoid levels were demonstrated in the first 5 days of life. It could be suggested on this basis that the adrenal cortex of preterm neonates is able to react with increased hormone production to the stress of the premature's extrauterine life. The high levels of cortisol in preterm newborns have already been reported.[4, 13, 15] Burton, *et al.* studied cord blood cortisol and cortisone levels and found higher concentrations of both assayed hormones in prematures as compared with full-term infants.[4] The good response of the adrenal cortex of prematurely born neonates to the stress of exchange transfusion was reported by Milner, *et al.*[16] Klein, *et*

TABLE IV

Mean Values of 11-Dehydrocorticosterone (A) in the Plasma (μg/dl $\pm$ 1 SD)
(Number in Brackets = Number of Observations)

Age	(Hr)			(Days)				(Months)	
	0–6	7–12	13–24	2nd	3rd–5th	6th–12th	13th–30th	2nd	3rd
Full-term newborns	(6) 2.07 ±0.88	(8) 1.61 ±1.6	(6) 1.36 ±0.81	(16) 1.11 ±0.59	(19) 1.06 ±0.48	(10) 0.57 ±0.49	(6) 0.43 ±0.22	(6) 0.48 ±0.17	
Premature newborns	(7) 3.16 ±0.98	(3) 1.67 ±0.53	(5) 0.72 ±0.33	(7) 1.3 ±1.16	(16) 1.08 ±1.1	(23) 0.65 ±0.38	(21) 0.51 ±0.3	(8) 0.49 ±0.37	(3) 0.52 ±0.43
	$P < 0.05$ $\rightarrow$	$\leftarrow$ $P < 0.02$ $\rightarrow$			$\leftarrow$	$P < 0.05$	$\rightarrow$		
	$P < 0.01$				$\leftarrow$	$P < 0.05$	$\rightarrow$		
Small for dates newborns	(4) 0.79[a] ±0.43	(3) 0.83 ±0.37	(4) 0.85 ±0.25	(9) 0.72 ±0.32	(7) 0.83 ±0.34	(8) 0.71 ±0.52	(13) 0.57 ±0.35	(1) 0.29	

[a] Statistical significance as compared with full-term newborns at corresponding age: $P < 0.05$.

TABLE V

Mean Values of 11-Deoxycortisol (S) in the Plasma (μg/dl $\pm$ 1 SD)
(Number in Brackets = Number of Observations)

Age	(Hr)			(Days)				(Months)	
	0–6	7–12	13–24	2nd	3rd–5th	6th–12th	13th–30th	2nd	3rd
Full-term newborns	(6) 0.82 ±0.22	(8) 0.83 ±0.23	(6) 0.85 ±0.24	(15) 0.76 ±0.21	(19) 0.73 ±0.38	(10) 0.66 ±0.22	(6) 0.61 ±0.22	(6) 0.39 ±0.19	
Premature newborns	(7) 0.79 ±0.27	(3) 0.72 ±0.23	(5) 0.5[a] ±0.22	(7) 0.55[a] ±0.1	(16) 0.76 ±0.62	(23) 0.58 ±0.28	(21) 0.49 ±0.19	(8) 0.41 ±0.15	(3) 0.38 ±0.11
Small for dates newborns	(4) 0.62 ±0.49	(3) 0.55 ±0.12	(4) 0.58 ±0.15	(9) 0.58 ±0.24	(7) 0.78 ±0.42	(8) 0.42[a] ±0.19	(13) 0.46 ±0.25	(1) 0.58	

[a] Statistical significance as compared with full-term newborns at corresponding age: $P < 0.05$.

al.[13] studied cortisol, cortisone, and corticosterone contents in cord and peripheral blood in the case of preterm births and found increased adrenal function in premature suffering from the respiratory distress syndrome. In the premature infants reported by Klein, *et al.* low cortisone/cortisol ratios were found,[13] which corresponds very closely with our results. Reynolds demonstrated higher levels of cortisol and so-called total corticoids in preterm newborns suffering from the respiratory distress syndrome who survived as compared with those who died.[25] Malan, *et al.*[15] found higher cortisol levels in cord blood plasma in infected preterm neonates than in noninfected subjects. Nwosu, *et al.* reported higher cortisol concentrations in amniotic fluid in preterm births as compared with full-term or post-term ones.[22]

Our results seem to be in good agreement with all of these findings.

On the other hand Gutai, *et al.* considered that low birth weight alone did not appear to affect cortisol concentration in newborn infant plasma.[8] Murphy[18] and Sybulski[37] found low cortisol levels in cord plasma in the cases of prematures suffering from respiratory distress syndrome. Similarly Taeusch, *et al.* reported in the rabbit an absent or very weak response of premature adrenals to adrenocorticotrophin.[38]

Our results concerning the second 11-β-dehydrogenase—dependent hormonal system, corticosterone: 11-dehydrocorticosterone can be compared with only a few papers. Klein, *et al.* in the work already cited[13] reported in the peripheral blood of premature newborns corticosterone concentration values

TABLE VI

Mean Values of the Totals of the Studied Hormones (F + E + B + A + S) in the Plasma (μg/dl ± 1 SD)

(Number in Brackets = Number of Observations)

Age	(Hr)			(Days)				(Months)	
	0–6	7–12	13–24	2nd	3rd–5th	6th–12th	13th–30th	2nd	3rd
Full-term newborns	(6) 30.05 ±10.04	(8) 17.57 ±4.36	(6) 12.17 ±3.95	(15) 13.05 ±4.29	(19) 9.91 ±3.73	(10) 13.45 ±4.02	(6) 12.39 ±3.34	(6) 13.97 ±4.31	
	←$P < 0.01$→	←$P < 0.05$→		←$P < 0.05$→	←$P < 0.05$→				
Premature newborns	(7) 35.98 ±7.7	(3) 44.42^c ±23.87	(5) 26.01^a ±13.29	(7) 29.69^d ±16.03	(16) 25.34^d ±16.56	(23) 14.92 ±7.47	(21) 9.57 ±5.3	(8) 8.32 ±3.94	(3) 9.5 ±8.61
	↕ $P < 0.001$			↕ $P < 0.02$					
Small for dates newborns	(4) 13.92^b ±5.34	(3) 23.78 ±4.12	(4) 18.28 ±7.36	(9) 13.29 ±4.48	(7) 18.56^d ±6.02	(8) 18.62 ±14.85	(12) 10.14 ±6.7	(1) 8.23	

Statistical significance as compared with full-term newborns at the same age:

[a] $P < 0.05$.
[b] $P < 0.02$.
[c] $P < 0.01$.
[d] $P < 0.001$.

slightly lower than ours (1.1–1.2 µg/dl in infants aged 1–32 hr). It is known that cortisol and corticosterone are secreted in parallel.[20] On the other hand, it is also known that corticosterone as well as its metabolites are secreted in important quantities in the neonatal period.[9, 29, 31] According to Savage, et al.[29] the excretion of 17-hydroxycorticosteroids and the α-ketolic metabolites of cortisol gradually rises with age and correlates with body weight. On the other hand the α-ketolic metabolites of corticosterone are relatively high in infancy, but after the age of 4 years their excretion also correlates with the infant's body weight. The ratio of α-ketolic metabolites of cortisol to the α-ketolic metabolites of corticosterone is approximately 5:1 in the first 2 years of life, but thereafter is 15:1, reflecting the higher excretion of corticosterone in infancy.[29]

In the literature we have found only one paper concerning 11-dehydrocorticosterone content in the blood plasma.[31] In this paper Schweitzer, et al. demonstrated the presence of 11-dehydrocorticosterone in the maternal circulation as well as in cord plasma, but in the latter in considerably higher concentration. As reported by Schweitzer, cord blood plasma 11-dehydrocorticosterone content in seven cases of full-term pregnancies averaging 1.3 µg/dl seems to be in close relation with our results concerning peripheral newborn plasma in the first 6 hr after birth which equals 2.07 µg/dl. Demonstrated in our work is the gradual decrease of 11-dehydrocorticosterone during the infant's development also in agreement with Schweitzer's observations.

In our material of premature infants the decrease of glucocorticoid hormones,

TABLE VII

Mean Values ± 1 SD of Cortisone/Cortisol Ratio
(Number in Brackets = Number of Observations)

Age	(Hr)			(Days)				(Months)	
	0–6	7–12	13–24	2nd	3rd–5th	6th–12th	13th–30th	2nd	3rd
Full-term newborns	(6) 1.88 ±1.17	(8) 2.63 ±1.12	(6) 2.62 ±0.68	(16) 3.2 ±1.85	(19) 2.35 ±1.03	(10) 1.45 ±0.61	(6) 1.8 ±0.92	(6) 0.69 ±0.33	
Premature newborns	(7) 1.08 ±0.77	(3) 0.73[a] ±0.32	(5) 1.36[b] ±0.59	(7) 0.97[c] ±0.9	(16) 1.73 ±0.85	(23) 1.76 ±1.52	(21) 2.15 ±1.76	(8) 1.85 ±1.37	(3) 0.77 ±0.2
Small for dates newborns	(4) 2.06 ±2.23	(3) 1.43 ±0.58	(4) 2.3 ±1.29	(9) 2.43 ±1.48	(7) 1.4[a] ±0.37	(8) 1.05 ±0.6	(13) 1.6 ±0.8	(1) 0.74	

$P < 0.05$ (between Premature 2nd day and 3rd–5th days)

$P < 0.05$ (Small for dates, 2nd day to 6th–12th days)

Statistical significance as compared with full-term newborns at corresponding age:
[a] $P < 0.05$.
[b] $P < 0.02$.
[c] $P < 0.01$.

particularly of their active forms, after the first 5 days of life could be understood as a result of improved clinical conditions; a newborn is already better adapted to extrauterine life. However, it is surprising that the lowest plasma values of these hormones (F, B) were observed in second month followed by their increase in the third month. Thus, it could be considered that in spite of higher plasma concentrations of the studied hormones during the first 5 days of premature life their neonatal pattern is in its general outline not very different from the one observed in full-term newborns, but is "displaced" in time. A similar phenomenon was reported by Forest, et al.[7] who have studied the changes of testosterone levels in premature and full-term neonates.

It is also surprisingly demonstrated in our material of premature newborns less conversion of the active hormones (F, B) to their inactive forms (E, A) during the first 5 days of life. Until now no attention was paid to this phenomenon, though it is perceptible in the work of Klein, et al.[13]

It is known that many enzymatic systems are not yet matured in preterm infants. If this would involve 17-hydroxysteroid 11-β-dehydrogenase, the diminished conversion of studied active hormones to their derivatives could be understood. On the other hand, this observation may be considered as an additional factor which facilitates the adaptation of premature infant to extrauterine life. In consequence of lower oxidation of active hormones to their inactive derivatives the tissue concentration of cortisol and corticosterone rises, and the beneficial influence of active glucocorticoids on tissue (primarily lung) maturation is assured.

It is difficult to discuss the 11-deoxycortisol neonatal pattern, which is different from every other one studied in this work. It should be noticed, however, that Cawson, et al. studying 11-deoxycortisol content in cord plasma in relation to onset of labour did find its value relatively constant, with the exception of elective cesarian section, whereas the value of concomitantly

TABLE VIII

Mean Values ± 1 SD of 11-Dehydrocorticosterone/Corticosterone Ratio
(Number in Brackets = Number of Observations)

Age	(Hr)			(Days)				(Months)	
	0–6	7–12	13–24	2nd	3rd–5th	6th–12th	13th–30th	2nd	3rd
Full-term	(6)	(8)	(6)	(16)	(19)	(10)	(6)	(6)	
newborns	1.65	2.05	1.94	1.98	2.65	0.97	1.33	0.63	
	±1.11	±2.37	±0.96	±1.09	±1.73	±0.5	±1.18	±0.18	
Premature	(7)	(3)	(5)	(7)	(16)	(23)	(21)	(8)	(3)
newborns	1.18	0.98	1.37	1.0	1.46[a]	1.76	1.4	2.74	0.9
	±0.68	±0.61	±1.46	±0.9	±1.2	±1.92	±0.81	±1.88	±0.26
Small for	(4)	(3)	(4)	(9)	(7)	(8)	(12)	(1)	
dates	1.46	1.46	1.63	2.29	1.2[a]	1.52	1.98	0.44	
newborns	±1.05	±0.76	±0.57	±2.28	±0.59	±1.32	±1.58		

[a] Statistical significance as compared with full-term newborns at corresponding age: $P < 0.05$.

assayed cortisol changed considerably.[5] Ducharme, et al.[6] came to the conclusion that metabolism of 11-deoxycortisol was effected exclusively by adrenal tissue preparations. At the same time conversion of cortisol to cortisone was effected by all the tissues, except perhaps the lung.[6] As well, Oddie, et al.,[23] as did Kolanowski,[14] reported increase of cortisol, corticosterone and 11-deoxycortisol plasma levels in adults after adrenocorticotrophin administration. It should be noted, however, that in the work of Kolanowski the urinary cortisol excretion for 24 hr increased about 40 times after ACTH injection and the simultaneously determined 11-deoxycortisol, only six times. Thomas, et al.[39] in the lamb studied the cortisol/11-deoxycortisol ratio in the fetus as well as in the newborn and found the significant changes of its value that indicates the changes of 11-β-hydroxylase activity in the perinatal period. It was also suggested that metabolic clearance of deoxycortisol is different than that of cortisol.[14]

It is not easy to discuss our data concerning glucocorticoid hormones in infants suffering from intrauterine growth retardation. In the literature we have found only two references concerning cortisol levels in cord plasma in the cases of small for dates newborns.[15, 37] In both these papers the authors reported higher cortisol levels than in controls. It should be noted, however, that the infants were prematurely born neonates with a body weight below the 10th percentile. Thus, these results can hardly be compared with ours concerning peripheral blood hormones levels of full-term newborns with body weight always below the 5th percentile. Reynolds, et al.[26] demonstrated that the urinary excretion of 16-α-hydroxyepiandrosterone was significantly reduced in infants with intrauterine growth retardation, while the excretion of THE and 6-β-OH-F was normal.

Our results concerning SFD infants who showed slightly reduced adrenal activity at the beginning of extrauterine life (0–6 hr after birth) followed by a proper or even increased adrenal function in the further neonatal period are in good agreement with those of Forest, et al. (personal communication), who demonstrated that the neonatal pattern of sexual hormones in SFD infants was "in between" those of full-term and premature newborns.

ACKNOWLEDGMENTS

The kindness of Doctor Bonnet of Clinique St. Charles in Montpellier (France), who has provided us with blood plasma samples is very much appreciated. The authors are also very thankful to Dr. Bidlingmayer from Childrens Hospital in München for the antibodies utilised in this work.

REFERENCES

1. Anders, T., Sachar, E., Kream, J., Roffwarg, H., and Hellman, L., Behavioral state and plasma cortisol response in the human newborn. *Pediatrics* **46**(4), 532 (1970).
2. Bertrand, J., Loras, B., Gilly, R., and Cautenet, B., Contribution à l'etude de la sècretion et du metabolism du cortisol chez le nouveau-né et le nourisson de moins de 3 mois. *Pathol. Biol.* **11,** 997 (1963).

3. Brzozowska, I., Kształtowanie się wielkości parametrow rozwoju fizycznego noworodków w Polsce. *Probl. Med. Wieku Rozwoj.* **3**, 83 (1973).

4. Burton, A., McClellan, D., Drummond, M., Mah, T., Thomson, M., Wong, W., and Turnell, R., Corticosteroids in premature cord blood determined fluorometrically by enzymatic reduction of cortisone. *J. Clin. Endocrinol. Metab.* **39**(5), 950 (1974).

5. Cawson, M., Anderson, A., Turnbull, A., and Lampe, L., Cortisol, cortisone and 11-deoxycortisol levels in human umbilical and maternal plasma in relation to the onset of labour. *J. Obstet. Gynecol. Br. Commw.* **81**(10), 737 (1974).

6. Ducharme, J., Limal, J., Antic, B., and Sandor, T. C_{21} steroid metabolism and conjugation in the human premature neonate. *Acta Endocrinol.* **72**, 63 (1973).

7. Forest, M., de Peretti, E., and Bertrand, J., Testosterone and adrenal androgens and their binding to plasma proteins in the perinatal period: developmental patterns of plasma testosterone, 4-ene-androstendione, dehydroepiandrosterone and its sulfate in premature and small for date infants as compared with that of full-term infants. *J. Steroid Biochem.* **12**, 25 (1980).

8. Gutai, J., George, R., Koeff, S., and Bacon, G., Adrenal response to physical stress and the effect of adrenocorticotrophic hormone in newborn infants. *J. Pediatr.* **81**(4), 719 (1972).

9. Hall, C., Branchaud, C., Klein, G., Loras, B., Rothman, S., Stern, L., and Giroud, C., Secretion rate and metabolism of the sulfates of cortisol and corticosterone in newborn infants. *J. Clin. Endocrinol. Metab.* **33**(1), 98 (1971).

10. Hillman, D., and Giroud, C., Plasma cortisone and cortisol levels at birth and during the neonatal period. *J. Clin. Endocrinol. Metab.* **25**, 243 (1965).

11. Kauppila, A., Simila, S., Ylikorkala, O., Koivisto, M., Makela, P., and Haapalakti, J., ACTH levels in maternal, fetal and neonatal plasma after short-term prenatal dexamethazone therapy. *Br. J. Obstet. Gynaecol.* **84**(2), 124 (1976).

12. Kenny, F., and Preeyasombat, C., Cortisol production rate. VI. Hypoglycemia in the neonatal and postneonatal period, and its association with dwarfism. *J. Pediatr.* **70**, 65 (1967).

13. Klein, G., Baden, M., and Giroud, C., Quantitative measurement and significance of five plasma corticosteroids during the perinatal period. *J. Clin. Endocrinol. Metab.* **36**(5), 944 (1973).

14. Kolanowski, J., Simultaneous determination of cortisol, deoxycortisol and corticosterone in plasma and urine by competitive protein binding assay. Response of normal subjects to ACTH and Metopyrone. *J. Steroid Biochem.* **5**(1), 55 (1974).

15. Malan, A., Roos, P., Woods, D., Heese, V., and Millar, R., Cord cortisol levels in relation to amniotic fluid infection and hyaline membrane disease. Materials from Intensive Care of the Newborn Meeting, 26–30 August 1979, Saint-Julien en Beaujolais, France, p. 34.

16. Milner, R., Goode, M., Cser, A., and Ratcliffe, J., Glucocorticoid and corticotrophin response in the newborn child undergoing exchange transfusion. *J. Endocrinol.* **67**(2), 30P (1975).

17. Morikawa, Y., and Hashimoto, Y., Rise of plasma corticosterone concentrations in rats immediately before and after birth and in fetal rats after the ligation of maternal uterine blood vessels or of the umbilical cord. *Endocrinology* **100**(5), 1443 (1977).

18. Murphy, B., Evidence of cortisol deficiency at birth in infants with respiratory distress syndrome. *J. Clin. Endocrinol. Metab.* **38**(1), 158 (1974).

19. Murphy, B., Cortisol economy in the human fetus and neonate. Materials from the symposium: The Endocrine Function of the Human Adrenal Cortex, Florence, 4–7 October 1977, p. 22.

20. Nabors, C., West, C., Mahajan, D., and Tyler, F.: Radioimmunoassay of human plasma corticosterone: method, measurement of episodic secretion and adrenal suppression and stimulation. *Steroids* **23**(3), 363 (1974).

21. Nelson, W., Vaughan, V., and McKay, R., Eds. *Textbook of Pediatrics.* Saunders Co., Philadelphia-London-Toronto, 1969, p. 367.

22. Nwosu, U., Bolognese, R., Wallach, E., and Bongiovanni, A. Amniotic fluid cortisol concentrations in normal labor, premature labor, and postmature pregnancy. *Obstet. Gynecol.* **49**(6), 715 (1977).

23. Oddie, C., Coghlan, J., and Scoggins, B.: Plasma deoxycorticosterone levels in man with

simultaneous measurement of aldosterone, corticosterone, cortisol and 11-deoxycortisol. *J. Clin. Endocrinol. Metab.* **34**(6), 1039 (1972).

24. Pepe, G., and Townsley, J.: Catabolic regulation of blood cortisol in premature and term baboon neonates. *J. Steroid Biochem.* **8**, 187 (1977).

25. Reynolds, J., Serum total corticoid and cortisol levels in premature infants with respiratory distress syndrome. *Pediatrics* **51**(5), 884 (1973).

26. Reynolds, J., Turnipseed, M., and Mirkin, B., Adrenal cortical function in abnormal newborn infants. *J. Steroid Biochem.* **6**(5), 669 (1975).

27. Rokicki, W., Loras, B., and Bertrand, J.: The simple radioimmunoassay method of simultaneous determination of cortisol (F), cortisone (E), corticosterone (B), 11-dehydrocorticosterone (A) and 11-deoxycortisol (S) in the small aliquots of plasma using a single set of reagents. In preparation.

28. Sempé, M., and Masse, N., La croissance normale. Méthodes de mesure et resultats. XXe Congrès de Pédiatres de Langue Française, Nancy, 1965.

29. Savage, D., Forsyth, C., McCafferty, E., and Cameron, J.: The excretion of individual adrenocortical steroids during normal childhood and adolescence. *Acta Endocrinol.* **79**(3), 551 (1975).

30. Schwarz-Tiene, E., La funzionalita cortico-surrenale negli stati distrofici del lattante. *Ann. Ital. Pediatr.* **3**(5), 409 (1950).

31. Schweitzer, M., Branchaud, C., and Giroud, C.: Maternal and umbilical cord plasma concentrations of steroids of the pregn-4-ene C-21-yl sulfate series at term. *Steroids* **14**(5), 519 (1969).

32. Sippel, W., Becker, H., Versmold, H., Bidlingmaier, F., and Knorr, D., Longitudinal studies of plasma aldosterone, corticosterone, deoxycorticosterone, progesterone, 17-hydroxyprogesterone, cortisol and cortisone determined simultaneously in mother and child at birth and during the early neonatal period. I. Spontaneous delivery. *J. Clin. Endocrinol. Metab.* **46**(6), 971 (1978).

33. Skałba, H. Zmiany histofizjopatologiczne w nadnerczach płodów i noworodków w związku ze śmiertelnością okołoporodową. *Ginekol. Pol.* **29**(3), 325 (1958).

34. Smith, B., Tanswell, A., Worthington, D., and Piercy, W. Local control of glucocorticoid levels by individual tissues in the fetus: Commonality among foregut derivatives. Materials from: Intensive Care of the Newborn Meeting, 26–30 August 1979, Saint-Julien en Beaujolais, France, p. 58.

35. Stahl, F., Hubl, W., Schnorr, D., and Dörner, G., Evoluation of a competitive binding assay for cortisol using horse transcortin. *Endokrinologie* **72**(2), 214 (1978).

36. Stevens, J., Plasma cortisol levels in the neonatal period. *Arch. Dis. Child.* **45**(242), 592 (1970).

37. Sybulski, S., Umbilical cord plasma cortisol levels in association with pregnancy complications. *Obstet. Gynecol.* **50**(3), 308 (1977).

38. Taeusch, H., Patterson, A., Williams, L., and Colle, E., Plasma glucocorticoid concentrations after injections of heroin, corticotrophin, saline and cortisol in fetal and neonatal rabbits. *Biol. Neonat.* **30**(1–4), 131 (1976).

39. Thomas, S., Wilson, D., Pierrepoint, C., Cameron, E., and Griffiths, K., Measurement of cortisol, cortisone, 11-deoxycortisol and corticosterone in foetal sheep plasma during the perinatal period. *J. Endocrinol.,* **68**(2), 181 (1976).

40. Ulstrom, R., Colle, E., Reynolds, J., and Burley, J., Adrenocortical steroid metabolism in newborn infants. IV. Plasma concentrations of cortisol in the early neonatal period. *J. Clin. Endocrinol. Metab.* **21**, 414 (1961).

41. Winters, A., Oliver, C., Colston, C., MacDonald, P., and Porter, J., Plasma ACTH levels in the human fetus and neonate as related to age and parturition. *J. Clin. Endocrinol. Metab.* **39**(2), 269 (1974).

36

Cord Cortisol Levels in Relation to Amniotic Fluid Infection and Hyaline Membrane Disease

ATTIES F. MALAN, M.D., M.MED.(PAED.), DIP. MID.C.O.G.(S.A.), PETER J. ROOS, M.B. Ch.B., M.R.C.O.G., DAVID L. WOODS, M.B. Ch.B., M.R.C.P., D.C.H., ROBERT P. MILLAR, Ph.D., and H. DE V. HEESE, M.D., B.Sc., F.R.C.P., D.C.H.

INTRODUCTION

Although very little data are available on the incidence of hyaline membrane disease (HMD) in the Third World, it is the general experience that HMD is seen less frequently than in developed countries. Autopsy studies certainly show a lower incidence of HMD associated with poorer fetal growth, and in less affluent population groups.[1, 2] In Cape Town the incidence of HMD was 4.4% in the poorer communities,[3] much lower than the 14% reported in a review of the literature.[4] It is thought that chronic fetal deprivation may act as a stress factor leading to earlier lung maturation.

Several studies have shown that amniotic fluid infection (AFI), conventionally diagnosed histologically as placental inflammation, is high in the local indigent population.[5, 6] This may be due to lack of hygiene, but analyses have shown that the antibacterial properties of amniotic fluid (AF) are less than optimal.[7] Only 9% of samples were bacteriocidal at 6 hr. The antibacterial property of AF has been ascribed to a specific polypeptide linked to zinc.[8] The latter appeared to be deficient in the mothers studied by Woods, et al.[7]

It was postulated that AFI could be another factor responsible for enhanced lung maturation, and this was therefore investigated.

Departments of Paediatrics and Child Health, Obstetrics and Gynaecology, and Chemical Pathology, University of Cape Town, Observatory 7925, Republic of South Africa

343

PHYSIOLOGICAL CONSIDERATIONS

In the scheme of events leading to the onset of labour,[3] fetal cortisol plays an important role. It is responsible for influencing the placenta with reversal of the progesterone dominance. At the same time it acts on receptor sites in the fetal lung stimulating surfactant production and/or release. Naeye, et al.[9] have shown that infection before birth results in enlarged adrenal glands and increased fetal cortisol levels might be expected.

The placental membranes are a rich source of prostaglandins and these could be released due to the effect of bacteria in the AF. A possible pathway would be activation of the complement system with C3a in turn stimulating prostaglandin release. Both prostaglandins and cortisol will initiate labour.

In this study, cord plasma cortisol levels were correlated to bacteriological evidence of intrauterine colonization and to events around delivery.

PATIENTS AND METHODS

Infants born before the 37th week of gestation were the subjects of the study. They were delivered in the hospitals of the Peninsula Maternity and Neonatal Services, and were predominantly of the Cape coloured population group.

All infants were seen by the same investigator (P.J.R.) within a half hour of birth, when the following specimens were obtained for bacteriological culture as described by Roos, et al.[6]:

(i) Placental blood: This specimen was taken from the vessels on the fetal surface of the placenta, as described by Wolf and Olinsky,[10] and placed in thioglycolate diphasic blood culture medium (Castenada) and Stuart's medium for later culture on mycoplasma media.

(ii) Placental tissue: Using sterile surgical gloves and a mask, the operator stripped the amnion off the fetal aspect of the placenta. Once this was done, clean gloves were used, and a surgically sterile blade excised a portion of placenta ($2 \times 1 \times \frac{1}{2}$ cm) uncontaminated by the maternal genital tract. This was then placed in cooked meat broth.

(iii) Gastric aspirate: This was taken by means of a sterile feeding tube, and put into Stuart's transport medium.

(iv) External ear swab: The external auditory meatus was swabbed, using a conventional cotton swab, which was placed in Stuart's transport medium.

All specimens were sent directly to the bacteriological laboratories, or incubated overnight at 37°C. Routine aerobic and anaerobic culture methods were used in all cases. The placental blood was also cultured for mycoplasma.

Cord blood was taken at delivery, centrifuged, and the plasma stored at −20°C until radioimmunoassay for plasma cortisol.[11] The various obstetric events were ascertained and recorded. Where possible, placentae, membranes, and cords were examined histologically for inflammation. All infants were scored for their gestational age and their weight compared with the weight for gestation standards of Lubchenco, et al.[12] The presence or absence of HMD was determined using standard criteria. Student's t and Wilcoxon's Rand Sum tests were used in the analyses.

RESULTS

Of 56 infants with complete bacteriological collections, 40 (72%) showed positive cultures from at least one of the previously mentioned sites. Table I shows the organisms cultured and the sites from which they were obtained.

Placental tissue gave the highest positive return on cultures, i.e., 65%. Of these, one-quarter were anaerobes, confined to placental tissue and blood. In general, there was good correlation between the placental tissue and the other sites, especially placental blood. In contrast, the predominant culture in the gastric aspirate was E. coli.

There was histological evidence of infection in 53% of cases. Extraplacental membranitis was the commonest finding and was virtually confined to those cases in which positive cultures were obtained.

Plasma from four infants was not included in the cortisol analyses because of congenital infections in two (herpes and syphilis, respectively), abruptio placentae in one, and a lost specimen in the fourth. Eight mothers had received dexamethasone, and data from their infants were considered separately (Table II).

Where antenatal dexamethasone (12 mg/day for two doses) had been given to the mother, the cortisol levels were significantly depressed. It should be pointed out that in only two of these infants were the cultures positive. One of these was the only vaginal delivery in this group, the others all delivering via elective caesarian section prior to the onset of spontaneous labour. Dexameth-

TABLE I

Details of Number and Sites of Organisms Isolated

	Placental Blood	Placental Tissue	Gastric Aspirate	Ear Swab
Acinotobacter	—	—	—	1
Bacteroides	5	6	—	—
Bacillus sp	1	1	3	1
Diphtheroids	3	6	1	—
E. coli	2	4	8	3
Haemophilus	2	—	—	—
Klebsiella	1	1	—	1
Mycoplasma	2	—	—	—
Proteus sp	1	—	—	—
Peptostreptococcus	1	3	—	—
Staphylococcus:				
aureus	2	3	1	1
epidermidis	4	6	5	3
Streptococcus:				
alpha haemolytic	—	1	2	1
beta haemolytic Gp. A	—	2	1	1
beta haemolytic Gp. B	1	1	1	1
nonhaemolytic (anhaemolytic)	—	3	1	—

asone levels were not determined in maternal or cord blood. Table III gives the main finding of the study. The remaining 44 infants were all delivered vaginally after spontaneous onset of preterm labour. Those with positive bacterial cultures had significantly raised plasma cortisol levels (519 ± 158 nm/ liter), as compared to infants with negative cultures (325 ± 134 nm/liter). There was no difference in gestational age or sex distribution between the two groups. Only two infants developed HMD, and both were negative for bacterial growth with low levels of cord cortisol (231 and 238 nm/liter).

Table IV shows the relation between prolonged rupture of membranes (arbitrarily defined as 18 hr or longer) and cortisol levels. There is no significant association. A correlation coefficient between the duration of membrane rupture and cortisol levels was not significant ($r = -0.06$). There was similarly no correlation between the duration of labour and cortisol levels ($r = -0.15$).

A surprising finding was that the cortisol levels did not correlate with the placental histological results (Table V). Infants with fetal growth retardation had significantly raised cord cortisol levels when compared to those between the 10th and 90th percentile on a weight basis (Table VI). The mean cortisol value of the growth retarded infants was the highest recorded. Seven of these nine infants, however, also had positive bacteriology.

DISCUSSION

The bacteriological findings are discussed more fully elsewhere,[6] but the incidence of positive cultures were considerably higher than recorded studies.[10, 13] Although overt clinical infection was rare, it does point to an infected environment and diminished ability to cope with bacteria ascending through the cervix and membranes.

The type II pneumocytes in the lung have receptor sites for cortisol,[14] and the latter rises as pregnancy advances.[15] This, together with the finding of advanced pulmonary maturity after corticosteroid therapy,[16] suggests that cortisol plays an important role in pulmonary surfactant production and

TABLE II

Cord Cortisol Levels (Mean ± SD) in Relation to Dexamethasone Therapy

	Number	Cortisol (nm/liter)	Gestation (weeks)
Treated	8	197 ± 76[a]	34.2 ± 1.5
Untreated	44	489 ± 203[a]	34.2 ± 2.4

[a] $p < 0.001$.

TABLE III

Cord Cortisol Level (Mean ± SD) in Relation to Bacteriological Cultures

	Number	Cortisol (nm/liter)	Gestation (weeks)
Positive	33	519 ± 158[a]	34.1 ± 2.4
Negative	11	325 ± 134[a]	34.2 ± 2.5

[a] $p < 0.001$.

protection against HMD. Infants who develop HMD have low cord cortisol levels at birth,[17, 18] while fetal "stress" results in increased adrenal response.[9, 19]

The present study clearly showed that, in the presence of intrauterine bacteria, cord cortisol levels were significantly raised. This has not previously been recorded, but is not unexpected in view of the autopsy findings of Naeye, *et al.*[9] Of great interest is the fact that the cortisol levels did not correlate with either duration of membrane rupture or labour, throwing new light on the controversy regarding the association of prolonged membrane rupture with respiratory distress syndrome.[20, 21] Obviously, the presence or absence of intra-uterine bacterial colonization is the key factor.

An infected environment, or amniotic fluid infection syndrome as this is also called, is very common in the infants studied, confirming previous findings. It is possible that amniotic infection *preceded* labour and membrane rupture. In this event it would in part explain the high rate of preterm delivery, with a lower incidence of HMD in our community.[3]

The depressant effect of exogenous steroids on cord cortisol levels[22] was confirmed in this study. Only one mother was in labour, however,[18] and there was a low rate of bacterial growth in this group. Although cord cortisol levels correlated with bacterial isolations, we are at a loss to explain why the placental histology did not correlate with the cortisol levels. Histological changes were only seen in two-thirds of infants with bacterial isolation. Perhaps bacterial culture is a more sensitive index of amniotic fluid infection, and bacterial invasion precedes placental inflammatory changes. Sybulski[23] has previously recorded increased levels of cord cortisol in fetal growth retardation. It is generally accepted that growth retarded infants are not candidates for HMD.

TABLE IV

Cord Cortisol Levels (Mean ± SD) in Relation to Time of Membrane Rupture

	Number	Cortisol (nm/liter)	Gestation (weeks)
<18 hr	34	477 ± 164	34.5 ± 2.5
≥18 hr	10	464 ± 204	33.2 ± 2.4

TABLE V

Cord Cortisol Levels (Mean ± SD) in Relation to Placental Histology

	Number	Cortisol (nm/liter)	Gestation (weeks)
Positive	18	465 ± 173	34.1 ± 2.1
Negative	14	490 ± 181	34.4 ± 3.1

TABLE VI

Cord Cortisol Levels (Mean ± SD) in Relation to Fetal Growth

	Number	Cortisol (nm/liter)	Gestation (weeks)
<10th percentile	9	555 ± 207[a]	34.4 ± 3.0
10th–90th percentile	35	449 ± 159[a]	34.0 ± 2.3

[a] $p < 0.05$.

SUMMARY

Amniotic fluid infection, defined as positive bacterial cultures in this study, was very prevalent in hospital patients and was associated with preterm labour. We think it is a cause of labour explaining, in part, the high incidence of preterm labour in less advantaged communities.

Cord plasma cortisol was elevated in infants with positive cultures, supporting the concept that intrauterine bacterial colonization protects against HMD by stimulating fetal cortisol production. Cortisol levels were not related to duration of membrane rupture or labour.

REFERENCES

1. Naeye, R. L., Freeman, R. K., and Blanc, W. A., Nutrition, sex and fetal lung maturation. *Pediatr. Res.* **8,** 200 (1974).
2. Farrell, P. M., and Wood, R. E., Epidemiology of hyaline membrane disease in the United States: Analysis of national mortality statistics. *Pediatrics* **58,** 167 (1976).
3. Malan, A. F., Antenatal factors in relation to hyaline membrane disease. *Paediatrician* **5,** 292 (1976).
4. Farrell, P. M., and Avery, M. E., Hyaline membrane disease. *Am. Rev. Respir. Dis.* **111,** 657 (1975).
5. Higgs, S. C., Malan, A. F., and Heese, H. de V., The perinatal infective environment of infants of very low birth weight. *S. Afr. Med. J.* **51,** 574 (1977).
6. Roos, P. J., Malan, A. F., Woods, D. L., Botha, P., Hyland, J., and Heese, H. de V., The bacteriological environment of preterm infants. *S. Afr. Med. J.* (accepted for publication).
7. Woods, D. L., Malan, A. F., Gunston, K. D., Steyn, D. L., Meyer, J., and Dempster, W. S., Antibacterial activity of amniotic fluid. *S. Afr. Med. J.* **55,** 1059 (1979).
8. Schlievert, P., Johnson, W., and Galask, R. P., Bacterial growth inhibition by amniotic fluid. VI Evidence for a zinc-peptide antibacterial system. *Am. J. Obstet. Gynecol.* **125,** 906 (1976).
9. Naeye, R. L., Harcke, H. T., and Blanc, W. A., Adrenal gland structure and the development of hyaline membrane disease. *Pediatrics* **47,** 650 (1971).
10. Wolf, R. L., and Olinsky, A., Prolonged rupture of membranes and neonatal infection. *S. Afr. Med. J.* **50,** 574 (1976).
11. Carr, P. J., Millar, R. P., and Crowley, H., A simple radioimmunoassay for plasma cortisol: comparison with the fluorimetric method of determination. *Ann. Clin. Biochem.* **14,** 207 (1977).
12. Lubchenco, L. O., Hansman, C., and Boyd, E. Intra-uterine growth in length and head circumference as estimated from live births at gestational ages from 26 to 42 weeks. *Pediatrics* **37,** 403 (1966).
13. Maudsley, R. F., Brix, G. A., Hinton, N. A., *et al.*, Placental infection and inflammation: Prospective bacteriological and histological study. *Am. J. Obstet. Gynecol.* **95,** 648 (1966).
14. Ballard, P. A., and Ballard, R. A., Cytoplasmic receptor for glucosteroids in lung of the human fetus and neonate. *J. Clin. Invest.* **53,** 477 (1974).
15. Murphy, B. E. P., Patrick, J. Denton, R. L., *et al.*, Cortisol in amniotic fluid in human gestation. *J. Clin. Endocrinol. Metab.* **40,** 164 (1975).
16. Liggins, G. C., Prenatal glucocorticoid treatment: Prevention of Respiratory Distress Syndrome, in *Report of the 70th Ross Conference on Pediatric Research*, Stern, L., Ed.
17. Murphy, B. E. P., Cortisol and cortisone levels in the cord blood at delivery of infants with and without the respiratory distress syndrome. *Am. J. Obstet. Gynecol.* **119,** 1112 (1974).
18. Sybulski, S., and Maughan, G. B., Relationship between cortisol levels in umbilical cord plasma and development of the respiratory distress syndrome in premature newborn infants. *Am. J. Obstet. Gynecol.* **125,** 239 (1976).
19. Gould, B., and Gluck, L., The relationship between accelerated pulmonary and neurological maturity in certain clinically stressed pregnancies. *Am. J. Obstet. Gynecol.* **127,** 181 (1977).

20. Bauer, C. R., Stern, L., and Colle, E., Prolonged rupture of membranes associated with a decreased incidence of respiratory distress syndrome. *Pediatrics* **53,** 7 (1974).

21. Jones, M. D., Burd, L. I., Bowes, W. A., *et al.*, Failure of association of premature rupture of membranes with respiratory distress syndrome. *N. Engl. J. Med.* **292,** 1253 (1975).

22. Ballard, P. A., Granberg, P., and Ballard, R. A., Glucocorticoid levels in maternal and cord serum after prenatal betamethasone therapy to prevent respiratory distress syndrome. *J. Clin. Invest.* **56,** 1548 (1974).

23. Sybulski, S., Umbilical cord plasma cortisol levels in association with pregnancy complications. *Obstet. Gynecol.* **50,** 308 (1977).

37

Pharmacokinetics of Indomethacin in Premature Infants with Symptomatic Patent Ductus Arteriosus

ROBERT B. COTTON, M.D., DOCIA HICKEY, M.D., and
ALAN R. BRASH, Ph.D.

Indomethacin, an inhibitor of prostaglandin synthesis, has been used since 1976 to constrict the ductus of premature infants with symptomatic patent ductus arteriosus (PDA).[1,2] The use of this drug has proceeded with only limited documentation of its pharmacokinetic behavior in the early neonatal period of premature infants. Other than preliminary reports[3-6] indicating that the drug's half-life in these infants is considerably longer than in adults, little information is available on which to base a dosage schedule which achieves the desired pharmacologic effect without an unnecessary and potentially dangerous accumulation of the drug.

In order to characterize further the pharmacokinetic behavior of indomethacin, serial plasma levels were measured following the intravenous administration of 0.2 mg/kg of the drug* to 11 preterm infants with symptomatic PDA. One infant received two doses of indomethacin at 3 and 9 days after birth. The remaining 10 infants received only a single dose.

As a prerequisite for study, informed consent was obtained from the patients' parents. In addition, each patient had documentation of a platelet count >100,000 mm³ and a serum creatinine level ≤1.5 mg/dl immediately prior to study entry.

* Kindly supplied by Morton Rosenberg, M.D., of Merck, Sharp & Dohme

Departments of Pediatrics and Clinical Pharmacology, Vanderbilt University School of Medicine, Nashville, Tennessee

Supported by a NHLI SCOR Grant HL 14214

The diagnosis of symptomatic PDA was based on previously described criteria[7] and was substantiated by echo[8] and impedance cardiography.[9] The gestational age of these patients ranged from 28 to 32 weeks, with birth weights of 1100–1620 g. Seven of the 11 infants had hyaline membrane disease as an initial cause of respiratory distress. Nine infants were requiring mechanical ventilation via an endotracheal tube at the time of indomethacin administration. The postnatal age of indomethacin administration ranged between 2 and 14 days.

After receiving indomethacin, 10 of the 11 patients had clinical evidence of major ductus constriction, demonstrated by a marked diminution in murmur intensity and precordial activity and a striking improvement in peripheral perfusion. Diminished left-to-right shunting in these infants was also documented by echo and impedance cardiography. The ductus of one of the 10 responders subsequently reopened sufficiently to require a second dose of indomethacin 6 days later. Following the second dose, ductus constriction was sustained, and mechanical ventilation was discontinued successfully.

The patient whose ductus had little or no response to indomethacin was a 1.2-kg, 29-week gestational age infant without HMD who had a massive intraventricular hemorrhage 3 days after birth followed by the onset of symptomatic PDA. Following a course of conventional anticongestive measures, indomethacin was given to this patient 8 days after birth.

As a group, urine output fell during the 24-h period following indomethacin to 66% of the previous 24-hr volume. Four patients, including the nonresponder, had little or no decrease in urine output following indomethacin. Serum creatinine levels did not change significantly.

Blood samples anticoagulated with solid EDTA were taken for plasma indomethacin analysis at 10 min, 40 min, 2 hr, 6 hr, 12 hr, 24 hr, and daily through the fifth day after the drug was given. A preindomethacin sample was taken as a blank. Plasma indomethacin concentration was measured using combined gas chromatography-mass spectometry. The plasma half-life ($T_{1/2}$), clearance (C), and volume of distribution (V_d) were derived using the beta phase of the biexponential disappearance curve.

The pharmacokinetic behavior of indomethacin during the 11 studies of the 10 responders is summarized in Table I. The results obtained from the nonresponder are tabulated separately for comparison. Examples of individual clearance curves are shown in Figure 1.

The half-life of indomethacin was more prolonged when administered at an early postnatal age. When indomethacin was given before 7 days after birth, $T_{1/2}$ exceeded 35 hr in five of six studies. When the drug was given between 7 and 14 days after birth, $T_{1/2}$ was less than 35 hr in five of six studies. No correlation was observed between $T_{1/2}$ and sex, birth weight, gestational age, postconceptual age, serum creatinine level, baseline urine output, or magnitude of decrease in urine output.

The $T_{1/2}$ observed in the responders was considerably longer than the previously reported[3-6] values of 11–24 hr, which were obtained from studies made beyond the first week after birth. Half of our studies were carried out within the first postnatal week, when $T_{1/2}$ values as long as 86 hr were observed. It is likely that the more rapid elimination of the drug during the second week is due to improving renal and hepatic function during that period.

The patient who had no demonstrable ductus constriction following indomethacin at 8 days also eliminated the drug more rapidly than the responders, and consequently had considerably lower plasma levels, especially at 12 hr and

TABLE I

Indomethacin Pharmacokinetics

	Responders (11 studies)		Nonresponder (1 study)
	Mean	Range	
$T_{1/2}$ (hr)	43.0	20.8–86.0	12.3
V_d (ml/kg)	322	252–373	430
C (ml/kg/hr)	6.1	2.4–10.3	24.3
6-hr level (ng/ml)	625	520–780	465
24-hr level (ng/ml)	471	316–635	150

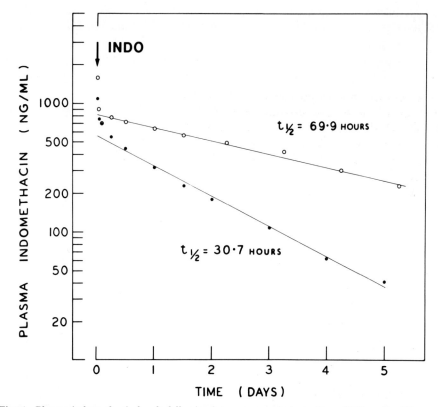

Fig. 1. Plasma indomethacin levels following intravenous adminstration of 0.2 mg/kg. The open circles are levels from a 1.2-kg, 29-week gestational age infant who received indomethacin 3 days after birth. $T_{1/2}$ was 69.9 hr in this patient. The closed circles are levels from a 1.0-kg, 28-week gestational age infant with a $T_{1/2}$ of 30.7 hr following administration of the drug 13 days after birth.

beyond. In a previous study,[10] no difference was found between plasma levels of responders and nonresponders when measured up to 2½ hr after receiving the drug orally or rectally. Based on their findings, it appears that the duration of plasma level above a critical level may be more important then early peak concentrations in determining whether the desired clinical response will be achieved.

Even though an exceptionally rapid clearance of indomethacin possibly accounted for the drug's failure in one patient, the remaining patients exhibited prolonged clearance, especially when the drug was administered during the first postnatal week. These results indicate that repeated doses during that period may lead to a dangerous accumulation of the drug in many of these infants who are critically ill and who are highly vulnerable to the toxic effects of the drug such as platelet dysfunction, renal failure, and altered organ blood flow.

ACKNOWLEDGMENTS

The authors are grateful for the support, encouragement, and scientific guidance generously provided by Dr. Mildred T. Stahlman and Dr. John Oates in the design and execution of this study.

REFERENCES

1. Friedman, W. F., Hirschklau, M. J., Printz, M. P., Pitlick, P. T., and Kirkpatrick, S. E., Pharmacologic closure of patent ductus arteriosus in the premature infant. *N. Engl. J. Med.* **295,** 526–529 (1976).

2. Heymann, M. A., Rudolph, A. M., and Silverman, N. H., Closure of the ductus arteriosus in premature infants by inhibition of prostaglandin synthesis. *N. Engl. J. Med.* **295,** 530–533 (1976).

3. Friedman, Z., Whitman, V., Maisels, M. J., Berman, W., Marks, K. H., and Vesell, E. S., Indomethacin disposition and indomethacin-induced platelet dysfunction in premature infants. *J. Clin. Pharmacol.* **18,** 272–279 (1978).

4. Bhat, R., Vidyasagar, D., Vadapalli, M., Whalley, C., Fisher, E., Hastreiter, A., and Evans, M., Disposition of indomethacin in preterm infants. *J. Pediatr.* **95,** 313–316 (1979).

5. Bhat, R., Evans, M., Vidyasagar, D., Ramirez, J., Fisher, E., and Hastreiter, A., Pharmacokinetics of IV versus oral indomethacin in preterm infants. *Pediatr. Res.* **13,** 367 (1979).

6. Thalji, A., Yeh, T. F., Raval, D., and Pildes, R. S., Pharmacokinetics of intravenous indomethacin in premature infants. *Pediatr. Res.* **13,** 374 (1979).

7. Cotton, R. B., Stahlman, M. T., Kovar, I., and Catterton, W. Z., Medical management of small preterm infants with symptomatic patent ductus arteriosus. *J. Pediatr.* **92,** 467–473 (1978).

8. Baylen, B. G., Meyer, R. A., Kaplan, S., Ringerburg, W. E., and Korfhagen, J., The critically ill infant with patent ductus arteriosus and pulmonary disease—an echo cardiographic assessment. *J. Pediatr.* **86,** 423–432 (1975).

9. Cotton, R. B., Lindstrom, D. P., Olsson, T., Riha, M., Graham, T. P., Selstam, U., and Catterton, W. Z., Impedance cardiographic assessment of symptomatic patent ductus arteriosus. *J. Pediatr.* **96,** 711–715 (1980).

10. Alpert, B. S., Lewins, M. J., Rowland, D. W., Grant, M. J. A., Olley, P. M., Soldin, S. J., Swyer, P. R., Coceani, F., and Rowe, R. D., Plasma indomethacin levels in preterm newborn infants with symptomatic patent ductus arteriosus—clinical and echo cardiographic assessments of response. *J. Pediatr.* **95,** 578–582 (1979).

38

Perinatal Net Base Metabolism and Skeletal Growth

POUL KILDEBERG

At birth the human term infant contains about 850 mmol of "base," largely confined to the developing skeleton. Postnatally, the infant continues to accumulate "base" while on a milk diet with a low pH and a positive concentration of titratable acid, relative to normal extracellular fluid. In order to approach the process in quantitative terms, some definitions are needed.

DEFINITIONS

The Brønsted-Lowry definitions of *an* acid and *a* base are qualitative definitions, analogous to those of "aldehydes," "ketones," "alkohols," etc. Clearly, a corresponding definition of *an amount of acid (base)* is a prerequisite to quantitative descriptions of acid-base metabolism in system physiologic terms such as rates of gain and loss, balance, flux, distribution, concentration, control, and regulation. An amount of acid is best defined on the basis of the *extent*, ξ_{H^+}, of partial acid-base reactions, $HB^n \rightleftharpoons B^{n-1} + H^+$, i.e., as an amount of hydrogen ion donated. ξ_{H^+} depends on the amounts of substance of molecular acids, bases, and ampholytes present, on the number of acid (HB^n) and base (B^{n-1}) groups per molecule and their individual apparent strength constants, pK_{acA},[6] as well as on ionic strength, temperature, and the actual pH. We shall define an amount of acid as the *sum of changes in extent* of partial acid-base reactions between the actual system (S) and a reference system (S_{ref}) in which the amounts of substance of its components exist at reference values of pH (7.40), temperature (37°C), and ionic strength (0.170 mol/kg). This concept of "an amount of acid" may be given explicit formulations in terms of amounts of hydrogen ion *accepted by* the buffer systems of the actual system (Brønsted-Lowry terminology) or, alternatively, in terms of amounts of hydrogen ion

Odense University, Pediatric Dept. H, DK-5230 Odense M, Denmark

donated to these buffer systems by stoichiometric contents of nonionic acids and bases ("anion-cation terminology"), cf. Refs. 2, 4, and 5. The latter alternative has the advantage of permitting the identification of amounts of acid contributed by physiologically specific *kinds of* Brønsted acids and bases on the basis of stoichiometric sources of origin. For example, x mmol of Cl^- (in the reference state) indicates the presence of x mmol of hydrogen ion donated by x mmol of HCl; y mmol of Na^+ indicates the consumption of y mmol of H^+ by (dissolution of) y mmol of NaOH; and z mmol of oxidized phosphorus indicates the presence of $1.8 \cdot z$ mmol of H^+ donated by z mmol of H_3PO_4, at reference values of pH, temperature, and ionic strength. In general terms,

amount of (titratable) acid $= n$TA(S)

$$= \sum_i z_i \cdot n\mathrm{An}_i^{z^-}(S_{ref}) - \sum_j z_j \cdot n\mathrm{Cat}_j^{z^+}(S_{ref}), \quad (1)$$

where z are charge numbers and An and Cat are anionic and cationic constituents (groups) of the reference system representing preformed components of the *actual* (untitrated) system, i.e., components of the imaginary titrant are excluded.

To the organism, hydrogen ions are all alike. Therefore, differences in physiological behavior between particular hydrogen ions must be determined by the behavior of the anions by which they are accompanied or the cations for which they are exchanged. An amount of hydrogen ion associated (in the reference state) with *nonbicarbonate, nonmetabolizable anion* or exchanged for *nonmetabolizable cation* is called an amount of *net acid, nNA(S)*. For an amount of *net base, nNB(S)*, we get from Eq. (1),

$$n\mathrm{NB}(S) = -n\mathrm{NA}(S) = \sum_k z_k \cdot n\mathrm{Cat}_{nm}^{z^+}(S_{ref}) - \sum_p z_p \cdot n\mathrm{An}_{nm}^{z^-}(S_{ref}), \quad (2)$$

where subscripts "nm" refer to nonbicarbonate, nonmetabolizable species. For biological fluids, Eq. (2) reduces to

$$n\mathrm{NB}(S) = n\mathrm{NA}^+(S) + n\mathrm{K}^+(S) + 2n\mathrm{Ca}^{++}(S)$$

$$+ 2n\mathrm{Mg}^{++}(S) - n\mathrm{Cl}^-(S) - 2n\mathrm{SO}_4^{--}(S) - 1.8n\mathrm{tP}(S), \quad (3)$$

where "tP" is "total phosphorus," i.e., contributions by metabolic end products other than sulfuric acid are quantitatively unimportant.[2, 4, 5, 7]

PERINATAL NET BASE METABOLISM

Net base is largely of exogenous (dietary) origin, dynamically stored in the skeleton, and circulated at an extracellular concentration subject to *specific* renal control.[2] During growth from fetal life to adulthood, more than 30,000 mmol of NB accumulate in the human organism, about 97% of which are deposited in the skeleton—as hydroxyapatite, carbonate, and amorphous phosphate. For every mmol of hydroxyapatite deposited,

$$10Ca^{++} + 4.8HPO_4^{--} + 1.2H_2PO_4^- + 2OH^- - 7.2H^+ \rightleftharpoons$$

$$(Ca_3(PO_4)_2)_3 \cdot Ca(OH)_2, \quad (4)$$

$7.2 + 2 = 9.2$ mmol of NB are extracted from the extracellular fluid to be continuously replaced by processes of placental transfer or gastrointestinal absorption, respectively. Under normal circumstances, renal contributions to the *balance* of NB are negligible. Postnatally, excess renal NB generation (= excess renal NA *ex*cretion) replaces gastrointestinal NB absorption only when the latter process is blocked by $CaCl_2$ loading, NH_4Cl loading, food restriction, parenteral nutrition, etc.[7, 9, 10]

Applying Eq. (3) to the available data on human fetal mineral composition (whole carcass analyses) gives the rough values for fetal NB illustrated in Figure 1. It is seen that the amount of fetal NB rises exponentially from 0 to about 500 mmol at 230 days. At term, the fetus contains about 850 mmol of NB at an overall concentration of 245 mmol/kg body mass. Applying, tentatively, an "average" fetal growth curve, further preliminary information may be derived. During the first 240 days of gestation, the estimated rate of NB retention rises exponentially to about 20 mmol/day, this increase being accounted for not only by increasing fetal size but also by a rise in the rate of retention per kg body mass. The resulting change in body composition is illustrated by an exponential rise in estimated fetal NB concentration from 36 to about 240 mmol/kg—and in the concentration of NB in "new tissue" (from 45 to 310 mmol/kg). Such changes may be due to changing skeletal composition, increasing relative skeletal mass, or both.

The breast-fed human infant ingests NB at a rate of about 0.75 mmol/100 kJ, or 3.75 mmol/kg/day, of which 30–40% is absorbed. The *balance* of NB of the breast-fed term infant is about 1.0–1.3 mmol/kg/day. Concentrations of NB in cow's milk (approx. 60 mmol/liter) are about three times higher than those of mature human milk; and NB balances of infants fed cow's milk formulae are generally elevated. It appears that "appropriate daily allowances" of acid and base for the human infant need to be established. In weanling rats loaded with sodium bicarbonate, the balance of NB rose markedly; and during a subsequent 8-day recovery period the excess NB retained was *not* excreted.[8]

As already implied, milk is a rich source of *nonmetabolizable base*. The low *p*H and positive titratable acidity of milk is explained by the presence of metabolizable organic acids, such as citric acid, which are not relevant to the conception of skeletal base stores and renal acid-base control.

A 4-kg breast-fed infant may absorb NB at a rate of about 6 mmol/day. If *parenteral alimentation* is substituted for oral feedings, and if the infusate supplies NA at a rate of 4 mmol/day, the acid load will be $6 + 4 = 10$ mmol/

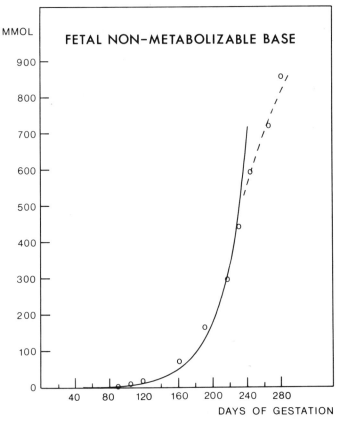

Fig. 1. Fetal nonmetabolizable base. Solid curve: exponential regression line fitted by the method of least squares (0–240 days). Stippled curve: fitted by hand.

day. In this situation, only the renal response will limit retardation of body growth—which in turn will lead to increased rates of endogenous NA production and further charges on the kidney. Concentrations of NA in solutions containing nonmetabolizable D-amino acids are difficult to calculate [Eq. (2), cf. Ref. 2], and only L-amino acids should be used. The available evidence suggests that infusates should provide *net base* at a rate of 1.5–2.0 mmol/kg/day. It is seen from Eq. (3) that if rates of infusion of Na^+, K^+, Ca^{++}, Mg^{++}, and phosphorus are 2.5, 2.5, 0.9, 0.2, and 1.25 mmol/kg/day, respectively, a rate of NB infusion of 1.75 mmol/kg/day will be achieved if Cl^- is administered at a rate of 3.2 mmol/kg/day.

REFERENCES

1. Engel, K., and Kildeberg, P., Physiological viewpoints on clinical acid-base diagnostics. *Scand. J. Clin. Lab. Invest.* **37**(*Suppl. 146*), 21–26, 1977.
2. Kildeberg, P., Quantitative acid-base physiology. System physiology and pathophysiology of renal, gastrointestinal, and skeletal acid-base metabolism. Submitted for publication.
3. Kildeberg, P., and Engel, K., A Physiological Approach to Acid-Base Diagnostics, in *Blood*

pH, Gases, and Electrolytes, National Bureau of Standards Special Publication 450, Durst R. A. Ed. U.S. Dept. of Commerce, Washington, D.C., 1977, pp. 133–141.

4. Kildeberg, P., and Engel, K., On the Concepts of Amount of Acid, Kind of Acid, and Balance of Acid, in *Blood pH and Gases*, Maas, A. H. J., Ed. University Press, Utrecht, 1979, pp. 19–23.

5. Kildeberg, P., and Winters, R. W., Balance of Net Acid: Concept, Measurement, and Applications, *Advances in Pediatrics*, 25, Barness, L. A., Ed. Yearbook Med. Publ., Chicago, 1978, pp. 349–381.

6. Siggaard-Andersen, O., *The Acid-Base Status of the Blood*, 4th rev. ed. Munksgaard, Copenhagen, 1974.

7. Wamberg, S., Kildeberg, P., and Engel, K., Balance of net base in the rat. II. Reference values in relation to growth rate. *Biol. Neonat.* **28,** 171–190 (1976).

8. Wamberg, S., Hansen, A. C., Engel, K., and Kildeberg, P., Balance of net base in the rat. III. Effects of oral sodium bicarbonate and sodium citrate loading. *Biol. Neonat.* **34,** 24–31 (1978).

9. Wamberg, S., Hansen, A. C., Engel, K., and Kildeberg, P., Balance of net base in the rat. IV. Effects of oral calcium and phosphate loading. *Biol. Neonat.* **34,** 121–128 (1978).

10. Wamberg, S., Engel, K., and Kildeberg, P.: Balance of net base in the rat. V. Effects of oral ammonium chloride loading. *Biol. Neonat.* **36,** 99–108 (1979).

39

Serum Ferritin in Preterm Infants

H.DE V. HEESE,[1] M.D., B.SC., F.R.C.P., D.C.H., S. SMITH,[2] M.B., Ch.B.,
F.C.P.(S.A.), S. WATERMEYER,[3] R.N., W. S. DEMPSTER,[4]
F.I.M.L.S.(U.K.), J. MEYER,[5] REGISTERED MEDICAL TECHNOLOGIST,
and G. J. KNIGHT,[6] F.I.S.

Iron deficiency with consequent iron deficiency anaemia is common during infancy. The foetus gains most of its iron during the last 3 months of intra-uterine life. Preterm infants are born with a lack of reserve iron and are therefore particularly at risk of developing iron deficiency after about 2 months when iron stores have been depleted.

Iron is stored as ferritin and haemosiderin. The latter is in the bone marrow and can be stained with Prussian blue. Ferritin is measurable in small amounts of serum and is a good indicator of body iron status.[9, 10, 15] An abnormally low concentration correlates with a lack of marrow iron, but bone marrow aspiration is not practicable or diagnostically helpful in the newborn.

In adults and 6–12-month-old infants, ferritin levels of 13–20 μg/liter[23] and 8–15 μg/liter,[8] respectively, indicate significant depletion of iron stores. Values

[1] Professor and Head of the Department of Paediatrics and Child Health, University of Cape Town; Chief Paediatrician, Groote Schuur Hospital Group, Red Cross War Memorial Children's Hospital, Somerset Hospital and the Princess Alice Orthopaedic Hospital, Cape Town, Republic of South Africa

[2] Research Fellow, Department of Paediatrics and Child Health, University of Cape Town, Cape Town, Republic of South Africa

[3] Research Assistant, Department of Paediatrics and Child Health, University of Cape Town, Cape Town, Republic of South Africa

[4] Chief Technologist, Institute of Child Health Laboratories, Red Cross War Memorial Children's Hospital, Rondebosch, Cape Town, Republic of South Africa

[5] Technologist, Institute of Child Health Laboratories, Red Cross War Memorial Children's Hospital, Rondebosch, Cape Town, Republic of South Africa

[6] Head, Department of Computer Services, Red Cross War Memorial Children's Hospital, Rondebosch, Cape Town, Republic of South Africa

below 12 μg/liter in adults[10] and 8 μg/liter in infants are associated with changes in red blood cell indices and indicate iron deficiency.

The values for depletion and deficiency in infants under the age of 6 months are dependent on age.[8]

A study was designed to measure serum ferritin in mother/preterm infant pairs at birth, 1 week, and 8 weeks of life and to compare the values obtained with corresponding levels at birth and 8 weeks in mother/full-term infant pairs previously studied. In some of the preterm infants serum ferritin was also studied during the first week of life at 2 hr, 24 hr, 48 hr, 72 hr, and 96 hr. These measurements were made in an attempt to define the time after birth when the highest mean ferritin value is reached.

MATERIAL AND METHODS

Subjects

Fifty-six mother and preterm infant pairs were studied.

Mothers. For entry into the study the mother had to be healthy with an apparent normal pregnancy and a haemoglobin level of more than 10 g/dl at her last antenatal clinic attendance before the onset of labour. A history of multiple pregnancy, antepartum haemorrhage, blood transfusion, or prolonged rupture of membranes were important reasons for exclusion. All mothers attended the antenatal clinic regularly from before the 20th week of pregnancy, and all received regular oral ferrous sulphate tablets. The majority of mothers belonged to social classes 4 and 5.

Preterm Infants. Infants of 30–35.9 weeks gestation and birth weights of 950–2800 g, born to mothers satisfying the foregoing criteria, were admitted to the study. The following exclusions were made as far as the infant was concerned: a history of asphyxia neonatorum at birth, respiratory distress, central nervous system disease, failure to thrive, exchange or blood transfusion, evidence that more than routine nursery care was required, and congenital infections manifested by a serum IgM of more than 30 μg/liter. All infants were scored according to the Dubowitz system[5] and were classified on the charts of Battaglia and Lubchenco[1] as well as on one constructed for infants of lower socioeconomic group Cape Town mothers.[27]

Infants were fed on a modified (humanized) milk while in the hospital nursery and thereafter on a partially modified milk fortified with either 12.7 mg or 6 mg iron per liter respectively with added vitamins. The modified milk contained 12.6 IU of vitamin E whereas the partially modified milk was not supplemented with this vitamin. The period in the nursery varied but a thriving infant was usually discharged when his weight reached 2250–2500 g. No additional iron or vitamins were given during the study period.

Serum ferritin values were measured in samples of maternal venous and cord blood at parturition and venous samples from the infant at 1 and 8 weeks after birth.

During the first week of life 50 of the preterm infants were divided into five groups of 10 infants. Serum ferritin values for each group were measured at one of the following time intervals: at 2 hr, 24 hr, 48 hr, 72 hr, and 96 hr after birth. In each infant three values were therefore available in the first week, i.e., cord blood, one of the above-mentioned time intervals, and at 1 week of age.

Full-Term Mother/Infant Pairs. Serum ferritin in 137 mother/full-term infant pairs were studied. The mother/infant pairs were selected on strict criteria to represent "normal" mothers and "normal" infants. Mothers belonged to the same social classes as the preterm mothers. The results of this study will be reported on in a separate publication.[8]

Serum Ferritin Estimation. Serum ferritin was measured by immunoradiometric assay using a modification of the method of Miles, *et al.*, with reagents prepared by the method of Addison, *et al.*[4] Informed consent was obtained from mothers, and the study was approved by the Ethical Review Committee of the Faculty of Medicine of the University of Cape Town.

RESULTS

The distribution of serum ferritin was positively skewed in all groups. All results are expressed using geometric and not arithmetic means. Correlations were calculated after logarithmic transformation of the original units. Results are graphically depicted on a logarithmic scale in Figures 1 and 2.

Mothers

Mothers of preterm infants differed significantly in parity and weight, but not in age, height, or serum ferritin from mothers with full-term infants (Table I). The mean serum ferritin level of the mothers with preterm infants was 58 μg/liter ranging from 7 to 477 μg/liter.

The mean for mothers of preterm infants and the mean for mothers of fullterm infants are shown in Table I and Figure 1. In Figure 2 the distribution of serum ferritin is shown plotted against ranges determined for Cape Town mothers at term reflecting very low, low, marginal, and acceptable levels (Table II).[8] These levels were derived from centile charts for normal mother/infant pairs followed during infancy. Forty-eight (85.7%), two (3.6%), and six (10.7%) mothers had acceptable, marginal, and low ferritin values.

Preterm Infants

In general, appropriate for gestational age preterm infants of lower socioeconomic group mothers in Cape Town are lighter, shorter, and smaller in head circumference than North American infants of similar gestational age. When weight is plotted against centiles constructed for gestational age of lower socioeconomic group Cape Town infants, the weights of all the preterm infants fall within the 10th and 90th centiles. The average values for gestational age at birth and weight, length, and skull circumference of the 56 preterm infants differed significantly from the 137 full-term infants (Table III) at birth and 8 weeks.

The mean serum ferritin in cord and venous blood at 1 week and 8 weeks of age are shown in Figure 1. Mean ferritin values in preterm infants in cord blood at 1 and 8 weeks were 170 µg/liter (range 5–1120 µg/liter), 282 µg/liter (range 42–933 µg/liter), and 151 µg/liter (range 40–891 µg/liter), respectively. For full-term infants the ferritin values in cord blood and 8 weeks were 258 µg/liter (range 50–1366 µg/liter) and 386 µg/liter (range 61–1285 µg/liter). The mean serum ferritin levels of the preterm infants were significantly lower both in cord blood ($p < 0.005$) and venous blood at 8 weeks ($p < 0.001$) from those of full-term infants (Table IV). As for the mothers in Figure 2 the distribution of serum ferritin values of the preterm infants in cord blood and in venous blood at 1 week and 8 weeks of age are plotted against ranges determined for full-term infants in Cape Town reflecting very low, low, marginal, and acceptable levels[8] (Table III). Thirty-seven and 34 infants at birth and 8 weeks had acceptable ferritin values. Seven infants (12.5%) had low and a further 12 (21.4%) marginal cord serum ferritin values. At the age of 8 weeks 15 (26.8%) infants had low and a further seven (12.5%) had marginal values.

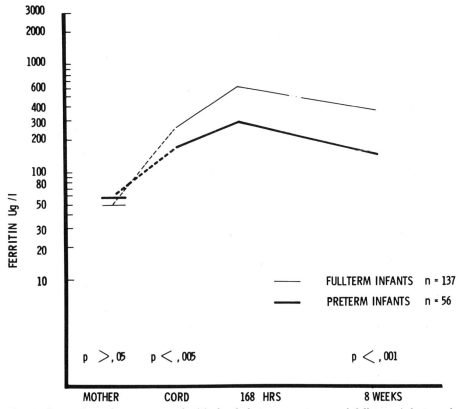

Fig. 1. Comparison of mean serum ferritin levels between preterm and full-term infants and those of their mothers.

In a series of multiple regression analyses in which the log of the preterm infant's ferritin was the dependent variable, no evidence could be demonstrated that the infant's ferritin is conditioned by the mother's ferritin level, the gestational age (range 30–35 weeks), or the birth weight of the infant, nor by any combination of these variables. In full-term infants there is also no

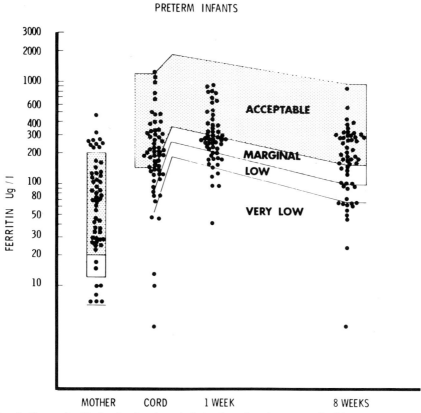

Fig. 2. Serum ferritin levels of preterm infants plotted against serum ferritin ranges determined for full-term infants.

TABLE I

Mothers of Preterm and Full-Term Infants

		Age (years)	Parity No.	Weight (kg)	Height (cm)	Ferritin (μg/liter)
Mothers of Preterm infants	Mean	23.7	1.3	54.6	155.8	58
	SD	5.83	1.3	7.32	6.21	log 0.51
	Range	16–44	1–5	43–77	144–170	7–477
Mothers of full-term infants	Mean	23.4	2.4	60.5	156.5	49
	SD	6.93	2.6	9.27	6.89	log 0.50
	Range	14–40	1–9	41–94	131–171	2–255
p		>0.05	<0.005	<0.001	>0.05	>0.05

correlation between cord and maternal serum ferritin level or the infant's birth weight.

The mean ferritin levels measured in cord blood and in venous blood at 2, 24, 48, 72, 96, 168 hr and 8 weeks are given in Table V and Figure 3. One of the 10 infants measured at 48 hr had a very low ferritin value of 13 µg/liter. This value has been omitted in the construction of the graph where the mean value of 288 µg/liter for the remaining nine infants is plotted. This value is 69.4% above the cord level. The maximum level is reached at 72 hr. The changes expressed as a percentage increase over the cord blood value are given in Table V. The level increases rapidly within the first 2 hr after birth, and at 24 and 72 hr levels are 40.6% and 108.2% above the cord blood value. At 8 weeks it is 11.2% below the latter value. The percentage increase over the cord blood value at 24 hr and 8 weeks for full-term infants are 149.2% and 49.6%, respectively.

DISCUSSION

If one believes a state of preclinical iron deficiency, i.e., depleted iron stores but no anaemia and iron deficiency anaemia, to be harmful, then the administration of iron is indicated. Animal studies indicate that iron deficiency anaemia early in postnatal development results in biochemical abnormalities of some organs, e.g., the brain, which persist long after the anaemia has been corrected.[3] But the role of iron excess or deficiency in infection continues to be a matter of debate.[18] Until such time as there is clarity on this issue, it may be inadvisable to administer iron too early, and when given this should be in

TABLE II

Serum Ferritin Ranges; Mother at Parturition and Infants during the First Year of Life

	Mother	Infant									
		Birth	Weeks					Months			
Ferritin	Parturition	Cord	4	6	8	12	18	6	9	12
Very low	≤6	≤50	≤149	≤113	≤63	≤20	≤9	≤4	≤4	≤4
Low	7–12	51–85	150–215	114–167	64–98	21–36	10–16	5–7	5–7	5–7
Marginal	13–20	86–144	216–315	168–249	99–155	37–64	17–31	8–15	8–15	8–15
Acceptable	≥21	≥145	≥316	≥250	≥156	≥65	≥32	≥16	≥16	≥16

TABLE III

Comparison of Gestational Age and Weight, Length, and Skull Circumference of Preterm and Full-Term Infants at Birth and 8 Weeks

		Birth				8 Weeks		
	No.	GA (weeks)	W (g)	L (cm)	SC (cm)	W (g)	L (cm)	SC (cm)
PT	56	34.3	1988	43.0	30.4	3477	49.3	36.2
FT	137	39.8	3037	48.7	33.8	4457	55.2	37.9
p	<0.001	<0.001	<0.001	<0.001	<0.001	<0.001	<0.001	<0.001

optimal amounts only. This is especially the case in preterm infants with their known susceptibility to infection. What constitutes optimal iron supplementation and its appropriate time and route of administration in preterm infants of mothers belonging to lower socioeconomic groups in developing countries also remains speculative. Compliance with recommended feeding practices and iron supplementation is often uncertain. In developed countries studies indicate that low birth weight infants who receive no supplemental iron may develop iron deficiency by 3 months of age.[14] Recommended iron supplementation of 2 mg/kg/day[2] from 2 weeks of age prevents the development of iron deficiency.[14]

Uncomplicated iron deficiency anaemia can be diagnosed by examination of the blood film and from red blood cell indices measured by automated equipment. Clinical anaemia, however, only becomes apparent after a significant fall in serum iron, rise in serum total iron-binding capacity and fall in transferrin saturation. A rise in free erythrocyte protoporphyrin levels takes place when the iron supply is inadequate to meet the demands of erythropoiesis.

At birth, and during the first months of life, especially in those babies born prematurely, normal values for many of the foregoing parameters are not clearly defined. Moreover, tests are expensive, require sophisticated laboratory equipment and expertise, and it is necessary to restrict the volume of blood taken for laboratory investigations in infants of low birth weight.

TABLE IV

Serum Ferritin in Preterm and Full-Term Infants at Birth and 8 Weeks

	Preterm	Full Term	
Cord blood			
n	56	136	
Mean	170	258	
SD	log 0.440	log 0.376	$p < 0.005$
Range	5–1120	50–1366	
8 weeks			
n	56	91	
Mean	151	386	
SD	log 0.370	log 0.283	$p < 0.001$
Range	40–891	61–1285	

TABLE V

Serum Ferritin (μg/liter)—Mothers and Preterm Infants

	Mother	Cord	Hr					Weeks	
			2	24	48	72	96	1	8
n	56	56	10	10	10	10	10	53	56
Av	58	170	223	239	211	354	290	282	151
Range	7–477	5–1120	72–577	64–868	13–976	272–557	173–888	42–930	4–897
% increase or decrease over cord value			+31.2	+40.6	+24.1	+108.2	+70.6	+65.9	−11.2

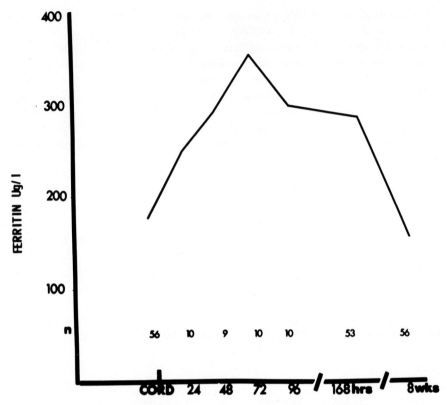

Fig. 3. Mean serum ferritin levels of preterm infants measured at different ages.

The small quantity of ferritin normally present in the serum probably comes from the breakdown of cells in iron containing tissues. Under most circumstances the concentration of serum ferritin indicates the amount of body storage iron; i.e., it will be increased if there is too much iron and lowered if there is too little iron in the tissues. Low values have been recorded only in iron deficiency.[9] It may be increased in acute and chronic liver disease,[19] occasionally in infections and in some malignant diseases.[25] It is also increased in conditions associated with an increased red blood cell turnover.[13]

In the present study special care was taken to exclude mothers and infants with any condition known to be associated with raised ferritin levels.

The mean serum ferritin of the mothers with preterm infants did not differ significantly from those whose infants were born at fullterm. These levels for pregnant mothers at term are greater than those reported in many series.[20, 24, 12, 11] Segall, *et al.* from Cape Town advanced possible reasons for these differences.[22] The levels, however, are in agreement with others determined at term in mothers who received iron supplementation from early pregnancy.[6] Six mothers (10.7%) had unacceptably low ferritin levels, and two mothers (3.69%) had levels indicative of possible iron depletion. These mothers had adequate haemoglobin levels. In iron deficiency, however, there is depletion of iron stores before there is a fall in serum iron levels, and this in turn occurs before there is a drop in haemoglobin.

Seven (12.5%) preterm infants had unacceptably low and a further 12 (21.4%) probably unacceptably low cord serum ferritin values. Isoimmunization, foetal to maternal haemorrhage, or chronic congenital infections were largely excluded as being possible causes to explain the low iron stores. These infants show evidence of a relative iron deficiency at birth, a concept advanced by Neale and Hawksley in 1933.[17] A study by Gottuso, et al.[7] in preterm infants showed that some presented with raised free erythrocyte protoporphyrin levels at birth, possibly indicating a state of relative iron deficiency. The ferritin levels of the mothers of the seven infants with unacceptably low ferritin values were all well within the normal range. This would suggest that the normal transference of iron from the mother to the foetus must have been impaired.

At the age of 8 weeks 15 (26.8%) infants had unacceptably low and a further seven (12.5%) had probably unacceptably low values for age. These infants in most instances had had low cord serum ferritin levels at 8 weeks. In general the serum ferritin level of a preterm infant during the first 8 weeks tended to follow a pattern; i.e., the infant starting with a low level remained low and vice versa. The mean serum ferritin at 8 weeks (151 µg/liter) was 11.2% lower than the level in cord blood (170 µg/liter), but the difference is not significantly different ($p > 0.05$). This mean level falls within the marginal range for age (Table III).

It would therefore appear that the iron in the milk feeds (6 or 12.7 mg/liter) either had no apparent effect on iron stores or was insufficient in a significant number of the preterm infants to satisfy the demands for iron with the infants' rapid increase in weight and expansion in blood volume. According to recommended standards for preterm infants[2] the intake of iron from the partially modified milk was probably too low. It is not possible to comment on the effects of the vitamin E content of the milks and its interaction which can result in haemolytic anaemia.[26, 16]

The mean ferritin of 170 µg/liter and 151 µg/liter of preterm infants in cord blood and venous blood at 8 weeks, respectively, differed significantly from the mean of 258 µg/liter in cord blood ($p < 0.005$) and 386 µg/liter in venous blood at 8 weeks ($p < 0.001$) in full-term infants. The mean gestational age of the preterm infants was 34.3 weeks (range 30–35.9 weeks). At 8 weeks in the preterm infants, i.e., at a mean corresponding term age of approximately 42 weeks, the mean ferritin of 151 µg/liter falls still far short of the mean cord ferritin of 258 µg/liter in the full-term infants. It is also of interest to note that the mean cord serum value of preterm infants is less than three times the maternal value; in full-term infants the corresponding value is more than five times. The preterm infant is therefore at a considerable disadvantage as far as his iron stores are concerned at a time when, after the period of reduced erythropoietic activity after birth, this activity recommences.

There is no correlation ($p > 0.05$) between the maternal serum and preterm infants' cord ferritin level at parturition or at 8 weeks, a state similar to that in full-term infants.[22] This lack of relationship was also evident in the mothers with unacceptably low serum ferritin levels; cord and ferritin levels in five of the six infants were all within acceptable ranges. The one infant with an unacceptably low level in the cord blood had a serum ferritin of only 4 μg/liter at 8 weeks.

These findings accord well with knowledge about iron stores in the preterm and full-term infant. Accumulation of iron in the foetus is independent of the mother's iron status; placental uptake of iron is independent of the foetus. The foetus gains most of his iron during the last 3 months of intrauterine life.

If the foetus gains most of its iron during the last 3 months of intrauterine life and if serum ferritin reflects iron stores, a progressive rise in serum ferritin with increase in gestational age could perhaps have been expected. Such a correlation could not be demonstrated but may well be evident in a study of a larger number of preterm infants of different gestational ages.

The part of the study designed to define the time after birth when the highest mean ferritin value is reached (Table II, Figure 3) indicated that this level is reached at 72 hr. The mean level of 354 μg/liter at this time in the preterm infants was 108.2% above the mean cord level of 170 μg/liter for the group.

Thirty of the 50 infants required phototherapy for raised bilirubin levels: in six of them this was still necessary at 96 hr. The number of infants studied at the different time intervals was small, and it was therefore not possible to analyse results in a meaningful manner. It would be difficult on ethical grounds to justify the taking of venous or capillary samples at 24-hr intervals in apparently normal preterm infants during the first week of life.

In these studies no attempt was made to define the usefulness of serum ferritin as the sole criterion of iron deficiency in the individual preterm infant. Its measurement in this respect has been suggested as being limited; on the other hand, its value in the assessment of iron nutrition in infant groups and in the differential diagnosis of severe anaemia has been confirmed.[21]

SUMMARY

Serum ferritin measurements were carried out in 56 mother/preterm infant pairs at parturition, during the first week and at 8 weeks of life. Changes recorded parallel known changes in iron metabolism during the last trimester of pregnancy and early infancy.

The findings suggest that, in spite of apparent adequate antenatal care, some of the mothers were still iron deficient or depleted at the time of parturition. Some of the preterm infants were also judged to be iron deficient or depleted at birth. At 8 weeks 27% and 12%, respectively, had ferritin levels indicative of deficiency or depletion of iron stores.

It is concluded that it is necessary to commence with the supplementation of medicinal iron in addition to that in commercial milk not later than the age of 8 weeks in preterm infants born in Cape Town to lower socioeconomic group mothers.

ACKNOWLEDGMENTS

We wish to thank the Medical Superintendent of Groote Schuur Hospital for permission to publish, staff members of the Department of Obstetrics and Gynaecology and nursing staff for their kind cooperation, the South African Medical Research Council for financial assistance, and Dr. R. McDonald and Mrs. L. G. Makepeace for help with the preparation of the manuscript.

REFERENCES

1. Battaglia, F. C. and Lubchenco, L. O., A practical classification of newborn infants by weight and gestational age. *J. Pediatr.* **71,** 159 (1967).
2. Committee on Nutrition, Iron supplementation for infants. *Pediatrics* **58,** 765 (1976).
3. Dallman, P. R., *et al.,* Brain iron: Persistent deficiency following short term iron deprivation in the young rat. *Br. J. Haematol.* **31,** 209 (1975).
4. Dempster, W. S., Steyn, D. L., Knight, G. J., and Heese, H. de V., Immunoradiometric assay of serum ferritin as a practical method for evaluating iron stores in infants and children. *Med. Lab. Sci.* **34,** 337 (1977).
5. Dubowitz, L., Dubowitz, V., and Goldberg, C., Clinical assessment of gestational age in the newborn. *J. Pediatr.* **77,** 1 (1970).
6. Fenton, V., Cavill, I., and Fisher, J., Iron stores in pregnancy. *Br. J. Haematol.* **37,** 145 (1977).
7. Gotusso, M. A., Oski, B. F., and Oski, F. A., Free erythrocyte porphyrins in cord blood. *J. Pediatr.* **92,** 810 (1978).
8. Heese, H. de V., Dewar, R., Segall, M. L., Dempster, W. S., and Knight, G. J., Serum ferritin in normal mothers and their full-term infants at birth and during infancy. Unpublished data.
9. Jacobs, A., Miller, F., Worwood, M., Beamish, M. R., and Wardrop, C. A., Ferritin in the serum of normal subjects and patients with iron deficiency and iron overload. *Br. Med. J.* **4,** 206 (1972).
10. Jacobs, A., and Worwood, M., Ferritin in serum. Clinical and biochemical implications. *N. Engl. J. Med.* **292,** 951 (1975).
11. Jenkins, D. T., Wishart, M. M., and Schenberg, C., Serum ferritin in pregnancy. *Aust. N. Z. J. Obstet. Gynaecol.* **18,** 223 (1978).
12. Kelly, A. M., Macdonald, D. J., and McNay, M. B., Ferritin as an assessment of iron stores in normal pregnancy. *Br. J. Obstet. Gynaecol.* **84,** 434 (1977).
13. Lipschitz, D. A., Cook, J. D., and Finch, C. A., A clinical evaluation of serum ferritin as an index of iron stores. *N. Engl. J. Med.* **290,** 1213 (1974).
14. Lundström, U., and Siimes, M. A., At what age does iron supplementation become necessary in low-birth-weight infants? *J. Pediatr.* **91,** 878 (1977).
15. Mazza, J., Barr, R. M., McDonald, J. W. D., and Valberg, L. S., Usefulness of the serum ferritin concentration in the detection of iron deficiency in a general hospital. *Can. Med. Assoc. J.* **119,** 884 (1978).
16. Melhorn, D. K., and Gross, S., Vitamin E dependent anaemia in the premature infant. 1. Effects of large doses of medicinal iron. *J. Pediatr.* **79,** 569 (1971).
17. Neale, A. V., and Hawksley, J. C., Studies in the anaemias of childhood. Part VI—Nutritional anaemia in mother and child. *Arch. Dis. Child.* **8,** 227 (1933).
18. Pearson, H. A., and Robinson, J. E. The Role of Iron in Host Resistance, in *Advances in Pediatrics,* Barnes, L. A., Ed. Year Book Medical Publishers, Chicago, 1976, Vol. 23, pp. 1–27.
19. Prieto, J., Barry, M., and Sherlock, S. Serum ferritin in patients with iron overload and with acute and chronic liver diseases. *Gastroenterology* **68,** 525 (1975).
20. Rios, E., Lipschitz, D. A., Cook, J. D., and Smith, N. J., Relationship of maternal and infant iron stores as assessed by determination of plasma ferritin. *Pediatrics* **55,** 694 (1975).
21. Saarinen, U. M., and Siimes, M. A., Serum ferritin in assessment of iron nutrition in healthy infants. *Acta Paediatr. Scand.* **67,** 745 (1978).

22. Segall, M. L., Heese, H. de V., Dempster, W. S., Knight, G. J., and Malan, A. F., Serum Ferritin: An Evaluation of Maternal and Infant Iron Stores, in *Intensive Care in the Newborn, II.* Stern, L., Oh, W., and Friis-Hansen, B., Eds., Masson, New York, 1978, pp. 159–170.

23. Sheehan, R. G., Newton, M. J., and Frankel, E. P., Evaluation of a packaged kit assay of serum ferritin and application to clinical diagnosis of selected anaemias. *Am. J. Clin. Pathol.* **70,** 79 (1978).

24. Valberg, L., Sorbie, J., Ludwig, J., and Pelletier, O., Serum ferritin and the iron status of Canadians. *Can. Med. Assoc. J.* **114,** 417 (1976).

25. Wands, J., Rowe, J., Mezey, S., Waterbury, L., Wright, J., Halliday, W., Isselbacher, K., and Powell, L., Normal serum ferritin concentrations in precirrhotic hemochromatosis. *N. Engl. J. Med.* **294,** 302 (1976).

26. Williams, M. L., Shott, R. J., O'Neal, P. L., and Oski, F. A., Role of dietary iron and fat on vitamin E deficiency anaemia of infancy. *N. Engl. J. Med.* **292,** 887 (1975).

27. Woods, D. L., unpublished data.

40

Computer-Assisted Monitoring of Sick Newborn Infants

A. VEILLEUX, G. PUTET, and B. SALLE

INTRODUCTION

The care of sick newborns requires multiple and increasingly complex monitoring systems. Most of these systems give instantaneous data for each physiological parameter of the monitored infant. Evaluation of data tendencies during a period of time still requires handwritten reports on an hourly basis. Therefore the application of computer technology to data handling and display is inherently appealing.[1, 6]

We have developed a computer-assisted monitoring system which is capable of recording and storing the principal physiological parameters automatically and which gives a simple and complete display of these data as either trend curves or tabulations.

We report here our experience with this system which has been working in our Unit for 12 months.

METHODOLOGY

1. Computer Based System

The system is described in Figure 1: data from each monitored bed are automatically acquired through an ASCII-coded serial interface and brought to the 28 K words memory of the processor (LSI-11 based). These data can be displayed on two bedside video screens—video display (VD) I and II. Each screen has a different purpose: VD I is a general ward status summary; VD II is fitted with a simplified interactive keyboard which allows dialogues with the

Neonatal Department, Hôpital Edouard Herriot, 69374 Lyon Cédex 2, France

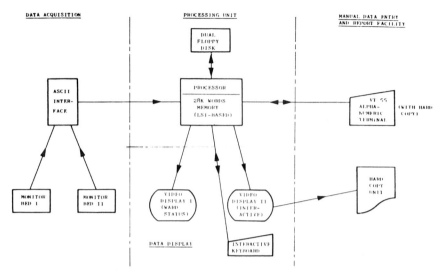

Fig. 1. Computer based system for neonatal intensive care unit; diagram (see text).

computer. A hard copy unit is connected to it. An alphanumeric terminal (VT 55 cathode-ray terminal with hard copy) is located in the Neonatal Unit and allows (1) the manual entry of clinical or biological data (blood gases) of each monitored infant and (2) communication with different programs stored in the computer's floppy diskette mass storage device such as R-L shunt using Gersony's method,[4] alveo-capillary gradient calculations, gestational age estimation, etc.

2. Data Handling

Initiation of work with a patient is done by pressing keys of the VD II keyboard, selecting the bed number, entering the infant's hospital identification number, and entering a command to begin monitoring. More clinical data about this patient can be entered through the VT 55 terminal.

Most of the parameters are automatically recorded from the classical bedside monitoring system* of each bed: EKG, respiratory rate, two temperature channels (cutaneous and core temperatures) and their gradient, FiO_2, blood pressures (systolic, diastolic, and mean) and ventilation pressures (peak, PEEP, and mean airways pressure or MAP). Each bedside monitoring system has its own visual and audio alarm devices. Pressure monitors have both a screen and a chart paper recorder system which can give continuous pressure curves visualisation.

Drugs given (up to eight for each bed) are manually entered into the computer by pressing a key on the VD II keyboard.

Blood gases (PO_2, pH, PCO_2, bicarbonate) are entered manually on the VT 55 terminal along with ventilation data (peak, PEEP, frequency, inspiratory-

---

Mennen-Greatbach

expiratory ratio, FiO₂), so that various curves of these data can be displayed by this terminal as required for comparison purposes.

All data are deposited in the floppy diskette mass storage of the computer and remembered for 72 hr. The hard copy system permits the generation of a permanent record of parts or all of these recorded data.

3. Data Display

All automatically and manually recorded parameters and entered drugs can be visualised at the bedside. VD I (Fig. 1) displays them continuously as instantaneous numerical values for all monitored infants and gives an "instant" evaluation of the infant's status (a visual alarm system is built in for each parameter). On the VD II, data can be examined in depth for any one infant, selected in a single stroke at the interactive keyboard. In the upper part of the VD II screen (Fig. 2), numerical values of the monitored parameters are displayed. In the lower part, trend curves of one or two parameters are shown; the choice of parameters as well as the period of time to be visualised (time axis adjustable from 1 to 24 hr) and of the day (backup to 3 days) is simple through the VD II keyboard. Hard copy of the displayed data is always available.

All data, automatically or manually entered on both keyboards, can be visualised on the VT 55 screen either as tabulation or as trend curves. Blood

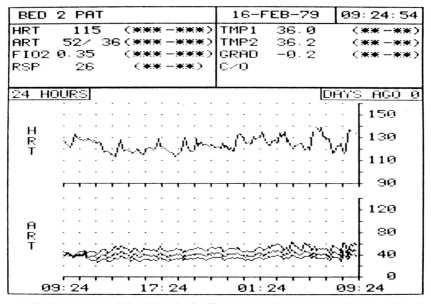

Fig. 2. Hard-copy print of the video display II screen; on the upper part is given the patient identification, date, time, and instantaneous data of monitored parameters. The lower part shows 24-hr trend curves of heart rate (beats/min) and arterial pressure (mmHg) for the previous 24 hr (an improved program gives a smaller blood pressure scale); systolic, diastolic, and mean blood pressure are displayed. If an interesting event is noted, a 1-hr display can give a better evaluation of data (as shown in Fig. 4).

gas results can be displayed only on this screen (as trend curves) along with the ventilation settings.

RESULTS

During a 12-month period 53 sick newborns (Table I) were monitored with this computer based system (birth weight: 2001 ± 753 g (mean ± SD); gestational age: 34 ± 2.9 weeks), eight being very low birth weight infants (less than 1200 g). Forty-four had respiratory disorders, and 35 of these had to be ventilated. Six out of the 53 infants died. Although no statistical and no definite results can be given from such a small group, evaluation of the system as to simplicity, efficiency, and usefulness is possible.

a. Simplicity is evident since, except for the blood gases which have to be entered into the VT 55 keyboard, parameters are automatically acquired from bedside monitoring system, so that no additional work is required from the medical staff. Furthermore, this system would appear to be a time saving device. In critically ill newborn care, parameters have to be checked very often; the medical staff spends time recording parameter values and trying to compare them in order to evaluate the precise clinical course of the illness. In the system described, since the monitored parameters are automatically recorded, the staff and nurses are freed of this routine chore and can devote their time to other important tasks. Trend curves are displayed continuously and comparisons between them are easily visualized, so that monitoring failure is quickly seen. Consequently, hourly survey of newborn (by checking heart rate,

TABLE I

Clinical Data

	CASES	B.W.[*] (g)	G.A.[*] (w)	ASSISTED VENTILATION	DEATH
RESPIRATORY DISTRESS	45	2186 ±665	34.7 ±2.2	36	4
Asphyxia	10			8	0
IRDS	30			26	3
Transient Tachyp.	3			1	0
Pneumonia	1			0	0
Hydrops Foetalis	1			1	1
VLBW[**] (≤ 1 200 g)	8	985 ±165	30 ±3.5	0	2
TOTAL	53	2001 ±753	34 ±2.9		6

   *   mean (± SD)

  **   Very Low Birth Weight

respiratory rate, ventilator setting) can be replaced by a glance at the screen. These result in a lower level of newborn disturbance which is not a negligible point, as these babies are usually in an unstable clinical condition. Blood gas results have to be entered into the VT 55 keyboard, and one might imagine this to be somewhat complicated. In fact, Reynolds et al.[1] demonstrated that type writing blood gas results into a keyboard was no more time-consuming than handwriting them. Furthermore, there is the advantage of having immediate tabulations and trend curves of the results (Fig. 3) plus copy which can be kept in the infant's chart, thereby facilitating case presentation for teaching or discussion purposes.

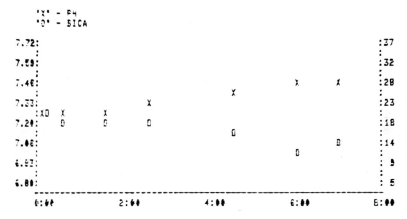

Fig. 3. An 8-hr shift hard copy of the VT 55 screen shows blood gas evolution along with ventilator settings. Either pH and bicarbonate (as shown here) or P_aO_2 and P_aCO_2 can be displayed as trend curves (pH 731 stands for 7.31; bicarbonates are in mEq/liter; P_aCO_2 and P_aO_2 in mmHg; p peak (ventilation peak pressures), PEEP (positive end expiratory pressures) are expressed in cm H_2O; FiO_2 100 stands for 1, FiO_2 90 stands for 0.9; I/E ratio: 1/2 = 0.50; 1/1.5 = 0.75; 1/1 = 100; 1.5/1 = 150; 2/1 = 200).

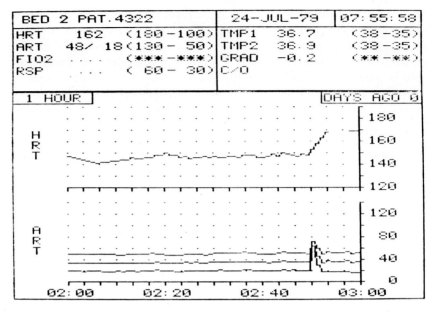

Fig. 4. A 1-hr extended display of heart rate (beats/min) and arterial pressure (mmHg) trend curves of a ventilated patient.

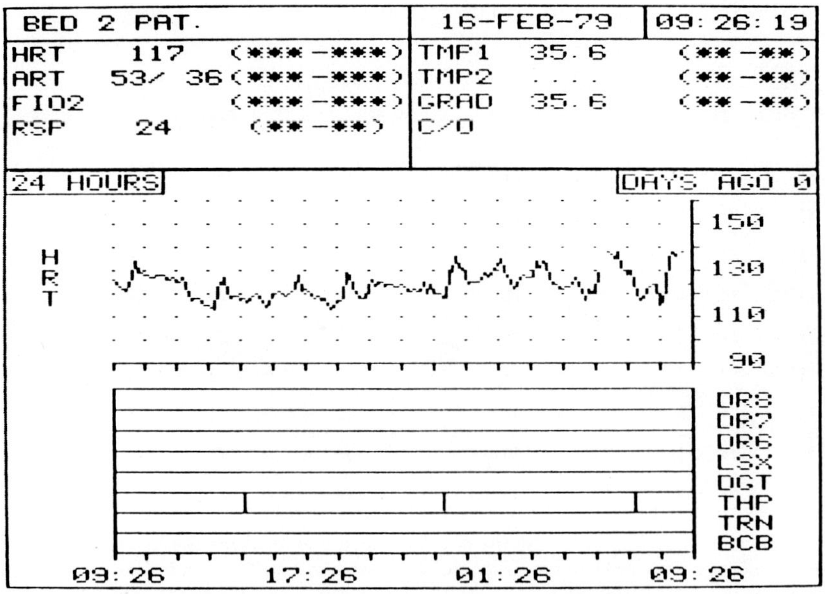

```
BED 2 PAT.          16-FEB-79   09:26:19
HRT     117  (*** -***) TMP1   35.6    (** -**)
ART     53/ 36 (*** -***) TMP2   ....    (** -**)
FIO2         (*** -***) GRAD   35.6    (** -**)
RSP     24   (** -**)   C/O
24 HOURS              DAYS AGO 0
                                        150
 H
 R                                      130
 T
                                        110

                                        90

                                        DR8
                                        DR7
                                        DR6
                                        LSX
                                        DGT
                                        THP
                                        TRN
                                        BCB
   09:26      17:26      01:26      09:26
```

Fig. 5. A 24-hr display showing comparison between heart rate and theophylline (THP) administration.

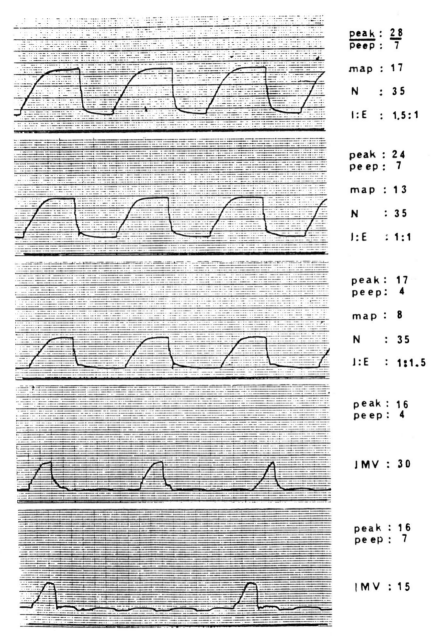

Fig. 6. Pressure waves evolution during ventilation of an infant with respiratory distress syndrome. (1) Waveforms generated by ventilation settings (written on the right) and (2) the exact effect of ventilation setting modifications are clearly seen (peak, PEEP, and MAP are in cm H_2O; N = rate/min; I:E = inspiratory/expiratory ratio).

b. Efficiency results of several areas. Continuously recorded parameters and trend curves visualisation give more precise information than the usual hourly recorded data. Figure 2 gives an example of a 24-hr shift display for heart rate and blood pressure; ventilation pressures, FiO_2, respiratory rate, and temperature, for which monitoring importance has been recently underlined,[5] can be displayed as well. Furthermore, if precisions of a specific event are required on a 24-hr shift, a 1-hr extended curve (Fig. 4) gives an immediate and almost minute by minute record of the memorized parameters. This information could not be otherwise collected by nurses without automated monitoring.

Comparison between the evolution of parameters is an important point in clinical evaluation: Nurse's notes are not always indicative of this evolution and the actual drawing of trend curves can not be replaced. As shown in Figures 2 and 4; with the video system this information is constantly available as well as a comparison between parameters and treatment (Fig. 5), making clinical evaluation easier and more rapid.

Better control of administered ventilation is part of the management of distressed neonates. In our system, airway pressures are measured at the endotracheal tube connector using a standard pressure transducer and a standard pressure display module. As seen in Figure 6 any ventilation setting modification is clearly visualized and recorded. Our experience with mean airway pressure (MAP) monitoring is in agreement with Boro's data[2,3] showing a good correlation between MAP and PaO_2. But as seen in Figure 6 the same MAP may result in different pressure waveforms, so that visualisation of them appears to be important in order to evaluate accurately mechanical ventilation risks and thereby reduce them. Furthermore, ventilation pressure monitoring has shown that ventilation pressure is a very important point for assay and for teaching new medical residents ventilation management.

c. The usefulness of such a system seems obvious in that it gives precise and continuous recording of all monitored parameters; data are clearly displayed and information is quickly available. The *cost* of this system for two beds was 100,000 U.S. dollars in 1978. It seems expensive but if we consider the burden of newborn care which is removed from the shoulders of the staff and nurses plus the maximal observation efficiency, plus a 3-day recall of recorded data and a reduction in the risk factor of human error, we feel that the system has proven its worth.

We have concluded that this computer based monitoring system has shown itself to be an efficient tool in a newborn intensive care unit because of a marked improvement in data handling and display. Simple to use by medical staff, it permits better evaluation of clinical problems and better monitoring of administered therapeutic agents.

ACKNOWLEDGMENTS

The authors are grateful to Hospices Civils de Lyon for their financial support, to Service Informatique des Hospices Civils de Lyon for their help, and to Mennen-Greatbach Company for their technical advice.

REFERENCES

1. Allen, L. P., Clifton, J. S., Ingram, D., Le Souef, P. N., Reynolds, E. O. R., and Wimberley, P. D., Computer system for recording and display of data from newborn infants with respiratory distress. *Arch. Dis. Child.* **53,** 169 (1978).
2. Boros, S. O., Matalon, S. V., Ewald, R., Leonard, A. S., and Hunt, C. F., The effect of independent variations in inspiratory-expiratory ratio and end expiratory pressure during mechanical ventilation in hyaline membrane disease: the significance of mean airway pressure. *J. Pediatr.* **91**(5)**,** 794 (1977).
3. Boros, S. J., Variations in inspiratory:expiratory ratio and airway pressure wave form during mechanical ventilation: the significance of mean airway pressure. *J. Pediatr.* **94**(1)**,** 114 (1979).
4. Gersony, W. M., Duc, G. V., Dell, R. B., and Sinclair, J. C., Oxygen method for calculation of right to left shunt: new application in presence of right to left shunting through the ductus arteriosus. *Cardiovasc. Res.* **6,** 423 (1972).
5. Perlstein, P. H., Edwards, N. K., Atherton, H. D., and Sutherland, J. M., Computer-assisted newborn intensive care. *Pediatrics* **57,** 494 (1976).
6. Sanik, D. S., Swarner, O. W., Henriksen, K. M., and Wyman, H. L., A computerized simple entry system for recording and reporting data on high risk newborn infants. *J. Pediatr.* **93,** 519 (1978).

41

Transcutaneous Oxygen Tension and Behavioural State in the Neonate

A. OKKEN and N. HANSON

INTRODUCTION

In the past few years several reports on continuous monitoring of arterial oxygen tension (PaO_2) and transcutaneous oxygen tension ($tcPO_2$) have demonstrated that in sick newborn infants large fluctuations in PaO_2 and in $tcPO_2$ may occur.[1, 4-6, 11, 15, 16] In contrast little is known about the fluctuations in PaO_2 or in $tcPO_2$ in healthy, newborn infants.[12] We therefore recorded $tcPO_2$ continuously in normal preterm and in normal term infants.

PATIENTS AND METHODS

Transcutaneous oxygen tension ($tcPO_2$) was continuously monitored and behavioural state evaluated in a group of 10 normal preterm infants and 10 normal term infants. In the preterm infant group birth weight was 1505 ± 154 g, gestational age was 32.2 ± 2.3 weeks, and postnatal age was 8.4 ± 5.1 days (mean ± SD). In the term infant group birth weight was 3245 ± 247 g, gestational age was 39.9 ± 0.3 weeks, and postnatal age was 6.3 ± 3.4 days (mean ± SD). All infants were studied at their neutral environmental temperature appropriate for their birth weight and postnatal age.[8] Term infants were bottle-fed at the commencement of the study. Preterm infants were fed by nasogastric drip.

A Dräger electrode heated at 44°C was used to monitor $tcPO_2$. In all infants the electrode was placed in the upper right thoracic region and a "warm-up" time of 30 min was allowed before commencing the study. Respiration was monitored using an impedance pneumogram. A continuous tracing was made throughout the study. Body temperature was measured with thermistor probes

Department of Pediatrics, Division of Neonatology, University of Groningen, The Netherlands

at two sites (footsole and rectal) at the beginning and end of the study. Room and incubator temperature were monitored continuously throughout the study. The infant's behavioral state was continuously observed and recorded. Assessment was based on the clinical criteria of Prechtl.[17] The criteria are:

state 1: eyes closed, no movements, regular respiration
state 2: eyes closed, no gross movements, irregular respiration
state 3: eyes open, no gross movements
state 4: eyes open, gross movements, no crying
state 5: eyes open or closed, crying

The respiratory pneumogram was used as an aid in distinguishing states 1 and 2 as regular, and irregular breathing patterns could readily be distinguished using the tracing. The study terminated when all states had been observed or after 3 hr had elapsed. A mean $tcPO_2$ level for each behavioural state in each infant was calculated excluding the first 100 sec of each state period. No periods of state 3 longer than 100 sec were observed in our infants, thus excluding state 3 from further analyses. The total duration of states 1, 2, 4, and 5 analysed for $tcPO_2$ level were 142, 352, 73, and 68 min, respectively, in the preterm infant group and 185, 279, 98, and 63 min, respectively, in the term infant group.

RESULTS

Transcutaneous PO_2 levels expressed as mean and standard deviation in the preterm and in the term infant group in states 1, 2, 4, and 5 are summarised in Tables I and II. In one infant in the preterm infant group state 1 could not be recorded, in an other infant state 4 could not be recorded. A paired comparison of $tcPO_2$ levels between all states was made. In the preterm infants $tcPO_2$ levels in states 1, 4, and 5 were significantly increased ($p < 0.05$) when compared to state 2. There was no significant difference between $tcPO_2$ levels

TABLE I

Mean Transcutaneous PO_2 Levels ($tcPO_2$) in Preterm Infants in Different Behavioural States

Infant Code	$tcPO_2$ State 1 (mmHg)	$tcPO_2$ State 2 (mmHg)	$tcPO_2$ State 4 (mmHg)	$tcPO_2$ State 5 (mmHg)
1	58.1	49.4	58.5	60.7
2	85.6	84.4	87.6	91.0
3	70.5	61.3	—	69.0
4	48.0	48.9	50.7	54.0
5	99.1	93.9	99.8	99.5
6	49.7	47.1	57.0	66.0
7	—	61.6	71.1	71.0
8	74.7	66.3	67.0	72.7
9	82.2	74.4	75.0	85.0
10	45.6	42.0	62.2	59.5
Mean	68.2	62.9	69.9	72.8
SD	18.9	17.1	15.6	14.6

in states 1 and 4 and states 1 and 5; however, $tcPO_2$ levels in state 5 were significantly increased ($p < 0.05$) when compared to state 4.

In the preterm infant group mean $tcPO_2$ level in state 2 was 62.9 ± 17.1 mmHg (mean ± SD). Mean $\Delta tcPO_2$ in state 1 was +5.3 mmHg (range −0.9 to +9.2 mmHg), mean $\Delta tcPO_2$ in state 4 was +7.0 mmHg (range +0.6 to +20.0 mmHg), and in state 5 was +9.9 mmHg (range +5.1 to +19.9 mmHg). In the term infants $tcPO_2$ levels in states 1, 4, and 5 were significantly increased ($p < 0.05$) when compared to state 2. There was no significant difference between $tcPO_2$ levels in states 1 and 4, 1 and 5, and 4 and 5. In the term infant group mean $tcPO_2$ level in state 2 was 64.5 ± 9.6 mmHg (mean ± SD). Mean $\Delta tcPO_2$ in state 1 was +5.7 mmHg (range −1.2 to +11.0 mmHg), mean $\Delta tcPO_2$ in state 4 was +8.1 mmHg (range +2.2 to 32.3 mmHg), and in state 5 was +4.5 mmHg (range −1.6 to +26.5 mmHg). There were insufficient data to evaluate $tcPO_2$ levels during state 3 ("quiet awake state").

DISCUSSION

In our study we observed a mean 7.9% decrease in $tcPO_2$ in the preterm infant group and a mean 8.3% decrease in $tcPO_2$ in the term infant group in state 2 when compared to state 1. In both infant groups there was an increase in $tcPO_2$ in the awake states 4 and 5 to levels similar to those of state 1. Our data demonstrate that in normal infants $tcPO_2$ is maintained at a constant level throughout the different behavioural states except for state 2.

Several authors have tried to explain the fall in $tcPO_2$ occurring in the sleep state 2. Kairam, et al.[9] suggested that the transition from NREM (state 1) to REM sleep (state 2) is accompanied by widespread alterations in autonomic functions, which could reflect instability and/or vulnerability of control mechanisms during this period. Martin, et al.[12] suggested that as a result of motor neuron inhibition during "active sleep" (state 2)[7] accompanied by asynchro-

TABLE II

Mean Transcutaneous PO_2 Levels ($tcPO_2$) in Term Infants in Different Behavioural States

Infant Code	tcPO_2 State 1 (mmHg)	tcPO_2 State 2 (mmHg)	tcPO_2 State 4 (mmHg)	tcPO_2 State 5 (mmHg)
1	63.3	54.5	86.8	81.0
2	82.9	76.1	78.3	72.9
3	81.4	70.4	76.8	81.6
4	70.9	72.1	74.7	74.5
5	65.5	57.4	63.8	60.7
6	82.8	79.6	83.2	78.0
7	62.1	55.3	66.2	59.2
8	63.7	59.8	67.3	50.7
9	69.1	65.7	70.4	72.0
10	60.2	53.6	58.1	59.0
Mean	70.2	64.5	72.6	69.0
SD	8.9	9.6	9.0	10.7

nous ribcage movements, local areas of atelectasis might develop, leading to a decrease in ventilation/perfusion ratios. Increased oxygen consumption in state 2 might be a factor contributing to the fall in $tcPO_2$ if there is a greater venous admixture within the lung. Assuming that in our infants oxygen consumption and minute ventilation were increased in state 2 with a further increase in states 4 and 5,[9, 13, 20, 21] this did not affect $tcPO_2$ levels in states 4 and 5. In spite of cardiorespiratory changes in the different states, the infants were able to maintain $tcPO_2$ at a constant level throughout states 1, 4, and 5 but not in state 2. Although it seems likely that the fall in $tcPO_2$ in state 2 is the result of an increased ventilation/perfusion imbalance, our data indicate that a limited response to arterial oxygen tension in regulation of breathing in state 2 cannot be excluded.

When $tcPO_2$ levels during states 4 and 5 are compared, levels were significantly higher ($p < 0.05$) in state 5 in the preterm infant group; there was no significant change in the term infant group. In all preterm infants crying resulted in an increase in $tcPO_2$. Of the term infants, four had an increase in $tcPO_2$, and six had a decrease in $tcPO_2$ during crying. Apparently circulatory and respiratory changes that occur during crying[2, 10] may result in either an increase or a decrease in $tcPO_2$. The mechanisms responsible for the direction of the change in $tcPO_2$ during crying are not yet fully understood. Presumably crying affects ventilation/perfusion ratios as increases in intrathoracic pressure of 40 cm H_2O or more in crying newborn infants have been measured.[10] It is therefore possible that in the infants with an increase in $tcPO_2$ during crying, local areas of atelectasis have disappeared, leading to increased ventilation/perfusion ratios. From this point of view crying may be an important physiological mechanism, compensating for atelectasis that may have developed during state 2. Assuming that in the infants with a decrease in $tcPO_2$ during crying ventilatory changes were similar to those in the other infants, the fall in $tcPO_2$ can only be explained by circulatory changes resulting in an increased right-to-left shunt. In these infants increased pulmonary vascular resistance and right-to-left shunting through the foramen ovale during crying may play a role. Pulmonary vascular resistance drops markedly immediately after birth with a further gradual decline in the first weeks of life.[18, 19] There are, however, marked individual differences;[18] and pulmonary vascular resistance may have been increased in some of our infants. Our finding that there is no fall in $tcPO_2$ levels in the majority of our infants when active or crying, is contrary to the observation in sick infants, where restlessness or crying usually results in a fall in $tcPO_2$ levels.[3, 14] It is evident that the response of sick infants to these situations is different from that of normal infants. Measuring $tcPO_2$ levels during activity and crying may be of particular clinical value in monitoring infants with cardiorespiratory disease.

REFERENCES

1. Boyle, R. L., and Oh, W., Transcutaneous PO_2 monitoring in infants with persistent fetal circulation who are receiving tolazoline therapy. *Pediatrics* **62**, 605 (1978).

2. Buda, A. J., Pinsky, M. R., Ingels, N. B., Daughters, G. T., Stinson, E. B., and Alderman, E. L., Effect of intrathoracic pressure on left ventricular performance. *N. Engl. J. Med.* **301,** 452 (1979).

3. Dangman, B. C., Hegyi, T., Hiatt, M., Indyk, L., and James, L. S. The variability of PO$_2$ in normal infants in response to routine care (Abstract). *Pediatr. Res.* **10,** 422 (1976).

4. Ekert, W. D., Apitz, J., König, C., and Schenk, H. W., Apnoen, Herz-frequenz-Änderungen und transkutane PO$_2$ Änderung bei atemgestörten Früh- und Neugeborenen. *Monatsschr. Kinderheilkd.* **125,** 425 (1977).

5. Fenner, A., Müller, R., Busse, H. G., Junge, M., and Wolsdorf, J., Transcutaneous determination of arterial oxygen tension. *Pediatrics* **55,** 244 (1975).

6. Fox, W. W., Schwartz, J. G., and Schaffer, T. H., Pulmonary physiotherapy in neonates: physiologic changes and respiratory management. *J. Pediatr.* **92,** 977 (1978).

7. Gabriel, M., Albani, M., and Schulte, F. J., Apneic spells and sleep states in preterm infants. *Pediatrics* **57,** 142 (1976).

8. Hey, E. N., and Katz, G., The optimum thermal environment for naked babies. *Arch. Dis. Child.* **45,** 328 (1970).

9. Kairam, R., Schulze, K., Koeningsberger, M., and James, L. S., The effects of changing sleep states on autonomic functions in the newborn (Abstract). *Pediatr. Res.* **13,** 498 (1979).

10. Kraus, A. N., Klain, D. B., Dahms, B. B., and Auld, P. A. M., Vital capacity in premature infants. *Am. Rev. Respir. Dis.* **108,** 1361 (1973).

11. Le Souëf, P. N., Morgan, A. K., Soutter, L. P., Reynolds, E. O. R., and Parker, D., Comparison of transcutaneous oxygen tension with arterial oxygen tension in newborn infants with severe respiratory illness. *Pediatrics* **62,** 692 (1978).

12. Martin, R. J., Okken, A., and Rubin, D., Arterial oxygen tension during active and quiet sleep in the normal neonate. *J. Pediatr.* **94,** 271 (1979).

13. Mestyán, J., Jarai, I., and Fekete, M., The total energy expenditure and its components in premature infants maintained under different nursing and environmental conditions. *Pediatr. Res.* **2,** 161 (1968).

14. Okken, A., Rubin, I. L., and Martin, R. J., Intermittent bag ventilation of preterm infants on positive airway pressure. *J. Pediatr.* **93,** 279 (1978).

15. Peabody, J. L., Gregory, G. A., Willis, M. M., and Tooley, W. H., Huch transcutaneous PO$_2$ electrode in sick infants (Abstract). *Pediatr. Res.* **10,** 430 (1976).

16. Peabody, J. L., Neese, A. L., Philip, A. G. S., Lucey, J. F., and Soyka, L. F. Transcutaneous oxygen monitoring in aminophylline-treated apneic infants. *Pediatrics* **62,** 698 (1978).

17. Prechtl, H. F. R., The behavioural states of the newborn infant (a review). *Brain Res.* **76,** 185 (1974).

18. Riggs, T., Hirschfeld, S., Bormuth, C., Fanaroff, A., and Liebman, J., Neonatal circulatory changes: An echocardiographic study. *Pediatrics* **59,** 338 (1977).

19. Rudolph, A. M., The changes in the circulation after birth: their importance in congenital heart disease. *Circulation* **41,** 343 (1970).

20. Scopes, J. W., and Iqbal Ahmed, Minimal rates of oxygen consumption in sick and premature newborn infants. *Arch. Dis. Child.* **41,** 407 (1966).

21. Stothers, J. K., and Warner, R. M., Oxygen consumption and neonatal sleep states. *J. Physiol.* **278,** 435 (1978).

42

Stimulation Characteristics of Nursery Environments for Critically Ill Preterm Infants and Infant Behavior

JUARLYN L. GAITER, Ph.D.,[1] GORDON B. AVERY, M.D., Ph.D.,[2]
CASSANDRA J. TEMPLE, B.S.,[3] ALIX A. S. JOHNSON, M. PHIL.,[4]
and NATHANIEL B. WHITE, M. PHIL.[5]

INTRODUCTION

Currently there is controversy concerning the nature of preterm nursery environments. Little is known about the effects of prolonged special care on infant behavior or the psychological needs of infants who require such care. Recent findings strongly suggest that the long-term developmental prognosis of preterm infants is highly dependent upon the nature of the environment in which they grow.[26] A special item in this long-term prognosis is the presence or absence of sensitive and supportive caregiving by parenting figures. Consequently, a number of research investigations have examined the nature of interactions which occur between parents and their preterm new-

[1] Departments of Neonatology and Pediatric Psychology, Children's Hospital National Medical Center, Department of Child Health and Development, School of Medicine and Health Sciences, George Washington University, Washington, D.C.

[2] Department of Neonatology, Children's Hospital National Medical Center, Department of Child Health and Development, School of Medicine and Health Sciences, George Washington University, Washington, D.C.

[3] Department of Neonatology, Children's Hospital National Medical Center, Washington, D.C.

[4] Department of Neonatology, Children's Hospital National Medical Center, Department of Psychology, George Washington University, Washington, D.C.

[5] Epidemiology and Biometry Research Program, National Institute of Child Health and Human Development, Bethesda, Maryland

borns.[2, 10, 11, 15, 19] Such explorations assume that parent-infant interactions are facilitated by predictable opportunities for parents and infants to learn each other's signals and thereby establish a successful relationship.[4, 14, 22] The specialized nursery care required for the preterm infant interferes with the establishment and progression of this partnership. There is a growing data base which describes the interaction difficulties peculiar to early and prolonged parent-infant separation.[3, 11, 12, 16, 30]

We decided to study special instances of nursery staff and newborn interactions as they may be regarded as antecedents to the negotiation of parent-infant relationships. Thus, these patterns of interactions may serve as a model for understanding the social interactive consequences of preterm birth and prolonged therapeutic confinement.

The healthy newborn possesses social interaction behaviors described as preadapted to elicit from caregivers the behavioral organization which the newborn is yet to develop.[1] In contrast, the preterm infant is relatively incompetent behaviorally but must function in an environment for which it is not fully prepared. The therapeutic environment of the special care nursery makes extraordinary demands on the organization and adaptability of the preterm newborn. In order to facilitate optimal developmental and successful early interactive outcomes for such infants, it is imperative that we understand the nature of their therapeutic environment and how they behave there.

A number of studies have concluded that special care nursery environments are monotonous and understimulating compared with the range of kinesthetic, social, auditory, and vestibular stimulation typically experienced by term infants.[17, 27-29] Consequently, a number of investigators have labelled the special care nursery a "depriving" environment for preterm infants. In contrast to this argument, Cornell and Gottfried[7] and Korones[20] have suggested that the presence of nursery personnel, monitoring equipment, and work shift activity probably provide preterm infants with large amounts of differentiated stimulation. At the present time we lack functional criteria for normative environmental stimulation for children. Therefore, in the absence of specific behavioral criteria, characterizations of preterm nursery environments as depriving or overstimulating have limited value.

There has not been a clear delineation of the stimulation present in the preterm nursery in the context of interactions which occur there. Although some aspects of infant-nursery staff interactions have been examined by others,[5, 9] previous studies have not related their findings to parent-infant relationships.

Objectives of the Study

A major objective of the observational study was to describe the stimulation experiences of a relatively homogeneous sample of sick preterm infants. Other objectives were to (1) differentiate the nursery environment into major categories of stimulation, (2) obtain patterns of change across time in the content and frequency of stimulation infants received during intensive, intermediate, and predischarge care, and (3) suggest appropriate interventions to facilitate the behavioral development of preterm infants and their adaptation to parenting during prolonged hospital care.

Hypotheses

Our hypotheses were: (1) that caregiver-infant interactions would be strongly influenced by the degree of infant illness (intensive vs. intermediate vs. predischarge care), (2) that caregiver social stimulation would be less when the infants were relatively inaccessible (isolette vs. open crib), and (3) that the morning shifts, when medical rounds occur, would be more stimulating than late night shifts.

Subjects and Procedures

Ten preterm infants, five males and five females with clinically diagnosed hyaline membrane disease (HMD) evidenced by respiratory distress within 4 hr of birth, tachypnea, retractions and an x-ray indicating reticulogranular diffuse densities, and air bronchograms, constituted the study sample. All subjects received some form of ventilatory assistance via a respirator or CPAP during intensive care therapy. The mean gestational age of the sample was 30.5 weeks with a range of 28–33 weeks. The mean birth weight of the newborns was 1362 g with a range of 1078–1469 g. Of the ten newborns, six were first borns and the remaining four were later borns. The mean age of the infants' mothers was 24 years.

A time-sampling observation system was designed to record data at the infants' bedside. Two trained observers having attained high inter-observer reliability (0.86) recorded data on precoded observation forms. The observers coded the frequency of occurrence of 33 behavioral variables in the following four categories of stimulation experienced by the infants: (1) caregiving, (2) social, (3) animate auditory, and (4) medical. A fifth behavioral category consisted of 10 frequently occurring infant behaviors: looks, sounds, smiles, suck, vocalization, fuss-cry, limb movements, and body movements. A tenth category was labeled "absence of activity."

The observation procedure allowed recording of the behavioral data for each variable in the five behavioral categories every 5 sec. Each hour of observation utilized 60 precoded forms consisting of twelve 5-sec rows with frequency columns, which represented 1 min of recording time per form. A tape delivered an auditory signal to the observer via earphones at 5-sec intervals for 60 min. At the sound of the auditory signal the observer recorded which precoded behaviors were observed to occur during the previous 5-sec interval. Thus, the continuous recording generated 720 frequency counts for each of 33 behavioral events during each 60-min observation. The 10 subjects were each observed on six different occasions for 60 min, thereby generating 4320 frequency counts of behavioral data per infant. Each of the two observers independently recorded data on one half of the 10 infants and on subsequent sessions observed the same infant.

Each infant was observed for two 1-hr periods at three separate sessions during nursery care: intensive, intermediate, and predischarge. One observation period occurred between 8 and 10 AM and the other occurred between 2 and 4 AM. The first pair of observations were done on the second day following the infant's admission to the intensive care nursery. The mean age of infants at the time of the first two intensive care observations was 2 days with a range of 2–3 days.

A second pair of observations occurred during intermediate care therapy. The criteria for these observations were that the infants had been extubated, were in isolettes, and gavage- or bottle-fed. The mean age of infants during the intermediate care observations was 20.7 days with a range of 11–55 days.

The third pair of observations were completed during the week prior to the expected date of the infant's discharge to their home environments. At this time infants received growing premature care in open cribs. At predischarge the mean age of infants was 44.1 days with a range of 25–70 days of age.

Other stimulation data were recorded during each observation to provide information concerning the inanimate environment in the nursery. A Bruel and Kjaer type 2213 sound level meter (A-weighted scale) was used at the infant's bedside to record noise levels in decibel units. In addition, a General Electric light meter measured illumination near the infant's bedside in foot candles.

Study Analysis

The study used a 3×2 (intensive, intermediate, and predischarge care periods by morning and night observations) repeated measures analysis of variance design. The repeated measures were on both factors (care periods and early and late observations). Thus, each infant appeared in all six cells of the design. The data base consisted of five groups of dependent variables (caregiving, social, animate auditory, medical, and infant behaviors) represented by 33 behavioral events which were observed across morning and nighttime periods.

The actual data were the frequency counts of behavioral events coded in 5-sec intervals for six 1-hr observations. Frequency data for each of the behavioral events within the five groups of dependent variables were analyzed separately using the repeated measures analysis of variance procedure. Duncan's multiple range tests were used to determine whether the intensive, intermediate, and predischarge care periods differed significantly from each other.

A stepwise linear regression analysis was used to determine which specific infant behavioral variables were most highly associated with the caregiver behavioral variables. The regression model assumed that the infant and caregiver behavioral variables were linearly related. Thus, the model entered in a sequential fashion the infant behavioral variable which explained the most variability in the caregiver behavioral variable. The criterion for the number of infant variables which entered the final regression equation was the minimum number of infant behavioral variables required to explain at least 75% of the variability in the caregiver variable. Particularly significant were those caregiver variables which were explained by only a few infant variables.

RESULTS

Our data indicated that for most variables there was no significant difference between the morning and night observations. Therefore, for the final analysis, the mean (per hr) of the pooled morning and night frequencies were used as the best estimates of the events for the three periods of care. Table I (at bottom) shows that the overall frequency of handling the infants during 5-sec intervals was not different during intensive, intermediate, and predischarge care. Also, Figures 1a, 1b, and 1c show that the overall frequency of caregiving during 5-sec intervals was not different across care periods. Most of the social stimulation, as predicted, occurred during the intermediate and predischarge care periods, as shown in Figures 1a, 1b, and 1c. These figures also include the medical events data, which shows an expected decrease from intensive care to intermediate and predischarge care. (Table I contains the means and standard deviation data for all the stimulation variables in the study.)

Morning and Night Shift Differences

Animate auditory stimulation in the form of staff conversations were significantly more likely to occur during the late night observations ($F = 7.9$, $df = 1, 18, p < 0.01$). Figures 1a, 1b, and 1c show the mean frequency of the total 5-sec interval and standard deviation data for the variable "vocalizations to others." In contrast to staff conversations, which occurred more often at night, the infants were talked to at almost equal rates during day and night shifts across the three periods of care.

Infant Behaviors

Infant looking behavior significantly increased from intensive care to predischarge care ($F = 9.4$, $df = 2, 18, p < 0.001$) as shown in Figures 2a, 2b, and 2c. Looking behavior during intermediate and predischarge care did not differ. In contrast to the data on looking behavior, infants tended to move their limbs at about equally high rates during all levels of care. However, limb activity was significantly more evident during the late night observations ($F = 6.3$, $df = 1$, $18, p < 0.02$). Figure 3 shows the mean frequency of 5-sec intervals and standard deviation data for this variable. Infant body movements were relatively less frequent than limb movements (Figures 2a, 2b, and 2c) and showed similar rates of occurrence across care periods. Fuss-cry behavior occurred more frequently while infants were in the acute phase of illness (intensive care) and during predischarge care. Significantly less irritable activity was observed during intermediate care therapy ($F = 2.84$, $df = 2, 18, p < 0.08$). Refer to Figures 2a, 2b, and 2c.

TABLE I

Summary Table of Means and Standard Deviations for All Caregiver Stimulation Data (Medical, Animate Auditory, Social, and Caregiving)

CAREGIVER BEHAVIORS	INTENSIVE CARE		INTERMEDIATE CARE		PREDISCHARGE CARE	
MEDICAL STIMULATION	MEAN	S.D.	MEAN	S.D.	MEAN	S.D.
Suctioning	3.60**	4.71	1.30**	2.75	0.00**	0.00
Heelstick, Injections	4.55**	6.56	0.65**	1.88	0.00**	0.00
Wrapping/Taping	6.55***	7.37	0.00***	0.00	0.00***	0.00
Blood Gas	10.30**	15.87	0.30**	0.95	0.00**	0.00
Special Procedures	13.50**	18.42	2.15**	4.61	0.00**	0.00
Stimulate Breathing	9.10	15.41	0.50	1.41	0.60	1.15
Overall Medical Stimulation	71.85****	61.46	11.40****	10.02	7.30****	7.14
ANIMATE AUDITORY	MEAN	S.D.	MEAN	S.D.	MEAN	S.D.
Vocalizations to Baby	24.65	13.86	16.20	12.39	33.90	46.68
Vocalizations to Staff	145.50	99.08	116.10	102.07	69.90	77.72
SOCIAL STIMULATION	MEAN	S.D.	MEAN	S.D.	MEAN	S.D.
Cuddling	6.90	9.00	16.85	38.87	12.50	23.94
Rocking	.20	.35	11.10	19.05	11.00	18.96
Smiling	0.00	0.00	0.05	0.16	0.30	0.53
Kissing	0.50	0.16	1.00	1.91	1.65	2.93
Overall Social Stimulation	7.15	8.96	29.00	43.33	25.45	41.89
CAREGIVING	MEAN	S.D.	MEAN	S.D.	MEAN	S.D.
Feeding	3.30*	9.92	53.55*	83.90	20.45*	26.41
Handling	33.80	17.67	29.05	18.48	34.60	40.98
Burping	.40**	1.26	4.70**	8.68	10.85**	19.57
Provide Pacifier	.20**	.42	1.00**	1.47	3.25**	3.93
Incidental Touching	20.35	17.05	4.80	4.98	25.20	71.36
Abdominal Measuring	24.25**	15.14	6.50**	6.96	6.70**	6.96
Overall Caregiving Stimulation	58.05	35.05	93.10	100.23	94.35	111.02

*p < .10

**p < .05

***p < .01

****p < .001

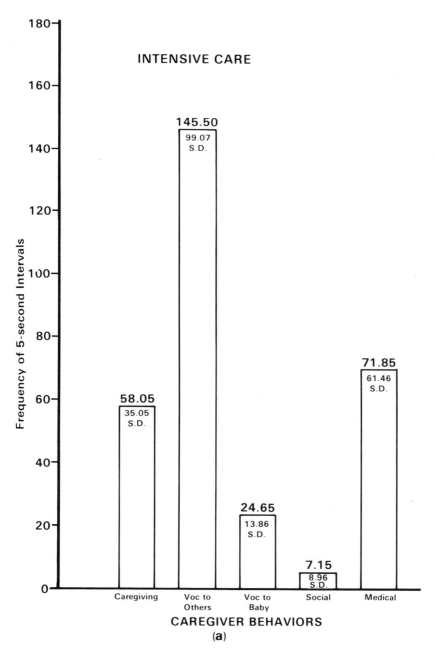

Fig. 1a. Total mean frequencies of 5-sec intervals for caregiving behaviors during intensive care.

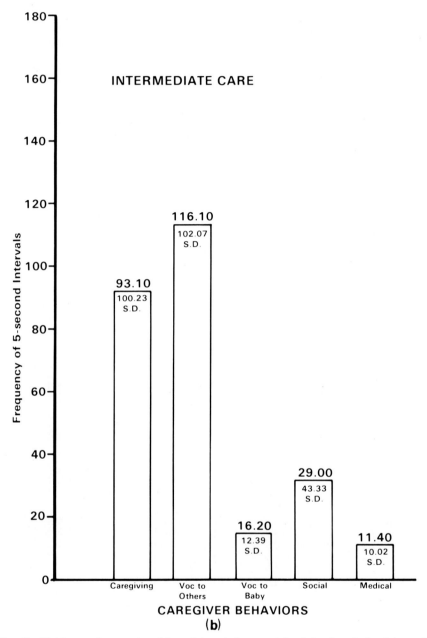

Fig. 1b. Total mean frequencies of 5-sec intervals for caregiving behaviors during intermediate care.

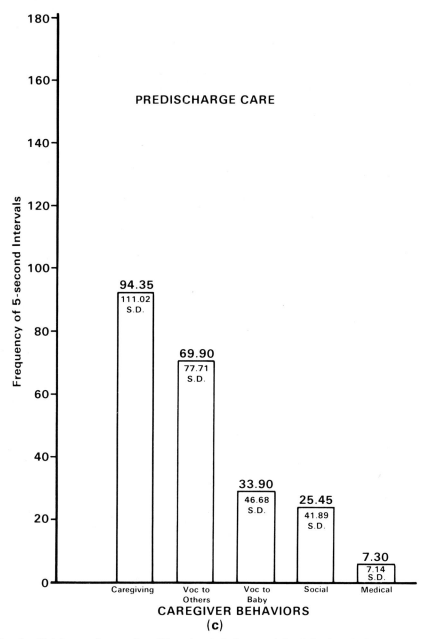

Fig. 1c. Total mean frequencies of 5-sec intervals for caregiving behaviors during predischarge care.

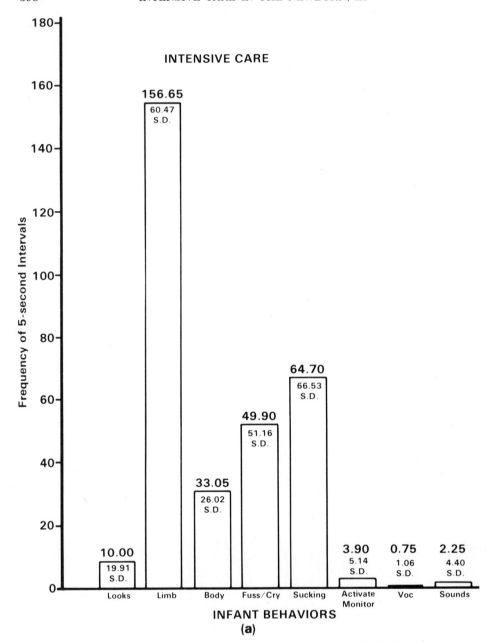

Fig. 2a. Total mean frequencies of 5-sec intervals for infant behavior during intensive care.

STEPWISE REGRESSION ANALYSIS

An attempt was made to determine how infant behaviors were related to the variability in caregiver behavior. From the variables which were included in the regression equation, those which were significantly correlated with caregiver variables will be discussed. Refer to Tables II, III, and IV for regression analysis relationships.

Physical Contact Interactions

Infant looking behavior accounted for 31% of the variance in caregiver handling of the prematures during the intensive care period (Table II). This

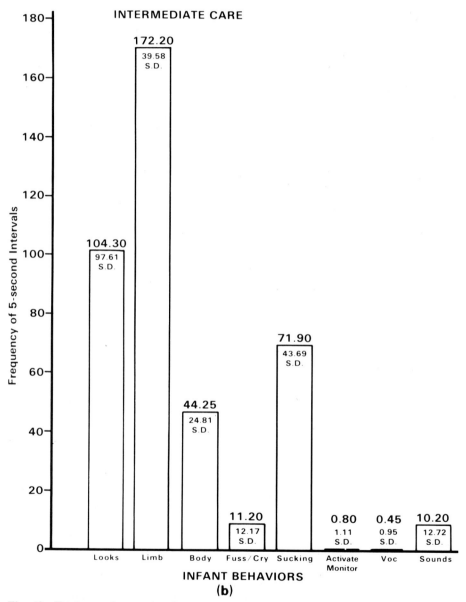

Fig. 2b. Total mean frequencies of 5-sec intervals for infant behavior during intermediate care.

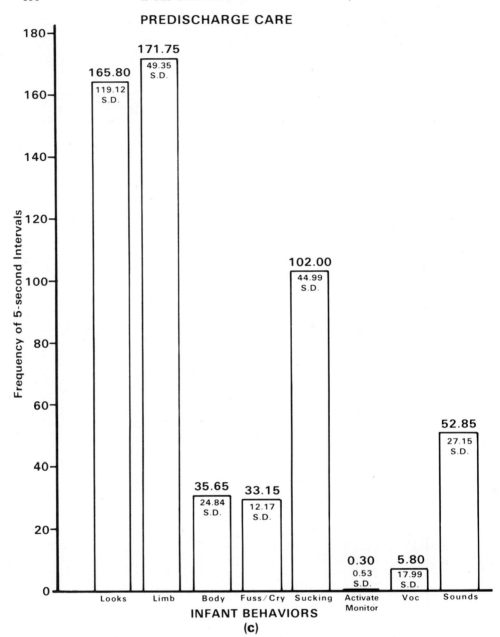

Fig. 2c. Total mean frequencies of 5-sec intervals for infant behavior during predischarge care.

relationship grew stronger across care periods and was significant at predischarge care ($r = 0.73, p < 0.01$). Infant looking was also closely associated with caregiver behavior such as feeding, accounting for 60% of the variance in feeding behavior during predischarge care ($r = 0.77, p < 0.01$) (see Table II).

Social-physical Contact Stimulation

Infant fuss-cry behavior was closely associated with caregiver rocking behavior and explained 70% of the variance in this caregiver variable ($r = 0.83$, $p < 0.002$) during predischarge care. Refer to Table III (Rocking) for these relationships. Activation of monitoring alarms by infants was related to caregiver kissing behavior during intensive care and accounted for 86% of the variance ($r = 0.92$, $p < 0.0001$). During predischarge care it accounted for 43% of the variance ($r = 0.65$, $p < 0.03$) (see Table III, Kissing).

Animate Auditory Stimulation

The infant irritability variable "fuss-cry" was significantly associated with the occurrence of nursery staff vocalizations to infants during intensive care treatment (56% of variance), ($r = 0.74$, $p < 0.01$) and again during predischarge care (38% of the variance) ($r = 0.61$, $p < 0.05$). (Refer to Table III, Vocalize to Baby). Staff conversations in close proximity to the infants showed a negative

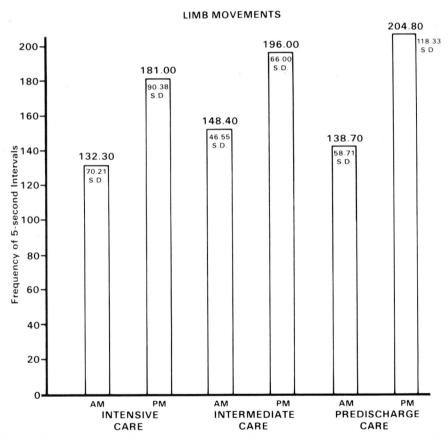

Fig. 3. Mean frequencies of 5-sec intervals for infant limb movements during morning and night observations across three periods of care ($N = 10$).

TABLE II

Figures in Parentheses Are *r*-Values for Correlation between Caregiving Stimulation Variables
and Infant Behavioral Variables

CAREGIVING STIMULATION

CAREGIVER BEHAVIORS	INFANT BEHAVIORS		
	INTENSIVE CARE	INTERMEDIATE CARE	PREDISCHARGE CARE
Handling	Looks (.55) Activate Monitor (.48)	Looks (.52) Limb movements (-.14) Smiles (-.21)	Looks (.73)** Suck, mouth (-.43)
Incidental Handling	Activate monitor (.82)* Looks (.03)	Smiles (-.48) Suck, mouth (.18) Looks (.17) Fuss, cry (-.02) Activate monitor (-.02) Sounds (.03)	Smiles (.44) Looks (.17) Vocalize (-.12) Limb movements (.41) Activate monitor (-.19)
Abdominal Measuring	Activate monitor (.65)* Suck, mouth (.42) Limb movements (-.04)	Activate monitor (-.46) Looks (-.22) Vocalize (-.25)	Vocalize (.58) Limb movements (.56) Suck, mouth (.004)

CAREGIVING STIMULATION

CAREGIVER BEHAVIORS	INFANT BEHAVIORS		
	INTENSIVE CARE	INTERMEDIATE CARE	PREDISCHARGE CARE
Feeding	Sounds (.93)***	Looks (.40) Limb movements (-.23) Activate monitor (.12) Sounds (-.08)	Looks (.77)* Suck, mouth (-.34)
Burping	Fuss, cry (.84)* Smiles (-.15)	Sounds (.63)* Smiles (-.26) Body movements (.21)	Looks (.70)* Suck, mouth (-.38) Vocalize (-19)
Provide Pacifier	Suck, mouth (.61)* Fuss, cry (.44)	Fuss, cry (.64)* Looks (.22) Sounds (-.22) Body movements (-.12)	Fuss, cry (.64)* Smiles (.19) Vocalize (-.29)

· p < .05
·· p < .01
··· p < .001
···· p < .0001

association with infant fuss-cry behaviors explaining 41% of the variance ($r = -0.64$, $p < 0.04$). During predischarge care staff conversations were positively associated with the infant alertness variable "looking" by explaining 41% of variance in staff vocalization behaviors ($r = 0.64$, $p < 0.04$) (Table III, Vocalize to Others).

Medical Stimulation Relationships

Most of the medical procedures was concentrated in the intensive care period. However, the only significant relationship was between caregiver stimulation of infants to encourage breathing and infant activation of monitoring alarm equipment, which explained 79% of caregiver stimulation at predischarge care ($r = 0.88$, $p < 0.001$) (refer to Table IV, Stimulate to Breathe).

TABLE III

Figures in Parentheses Are r-Values for Correlation between Social Stimulation Variables and Infant Behavioral Variables and between Animate Auditory Stimulation Variables and Infant Behavioral Variables

SOCIAL-STIMULATION

CAREGIVER BEHAVIORS	INFANT BEHAVIORS		
	INTENSIVE CARE	INTERMEDIATE CARE	PREDISCHARGE CARE
Cuddling	Sounds (.68)* Activate monitor (.57)	Looks (.38) Sounds (-.07) Body movement (.01) Fuss, cry (-.20)	Fuss, cry (.50) Smiles (.23) Vocalize (-.18) Looks (.40)
Rocking	Suck, mouth (.81)* Looks (.06) Limb movement (.06)	Fuss, cry (.54) Sounds (.46) Limb movements (.32) Body movements (.09)	Fuss, cry (.83)* Smiles (-.02) Suck, mouth (.17)
Smiling			Looks (.76) Smiles (-.66) Sounds (-.22)
Kissing	Activate monitor (.92)****	Looks (-.60) Sounds (.09) Body movements (.16)	Activate monitor (.65)* Sounds (.52) Limb movements (.51) Smiles (.03) Suck, mouth (-.19)

ANIMATE AUDITORY STIMULATION

CAREGIVER BEHAVIORS	INFANT BEHAVIORS		
	INTENSIVE CARE	INTERMEDIATE CARE	PREDISCHARGE CARE
Vocalize to Baby	Fuss, cry (.74)** Limb movements (.19) Suck, mouth (-.07)	Looks (.42) Smiles (-.30) Suck, mouth (.37) Limb movements (.14)	Fuss, cry (.61)* Suck, mouth (-.07) Smiles (-.01) Looks (.60) Body movement (.34)
Vocalize to Others	Looks (.37) Fuss, cry (-.22) Vocalize (-.15) Sounds (-.11) Body movements (-.14)	Fuss, cry (-.64)* Body movements (.63) Smiles (.22)	Looks (.64)* Fuss, cry (.37) Suck, mouth (-.39) Limb movements (.15)

*	$p < .05$
**	$p < .01$
***	$p < .001$
****	$p < .0001$

TABLE IV

Figures in Parentheses Are *r*-Values for Correlation between Medical Stimulation Variables and Infant Behavioral Variables

MEDICAL STIMULATION

CAREGIVER BEHAVIORS	INFANT BEHAVIORS		
	INTENSIVE CARE	INTERMEDIATE CARE	PREDISCHARGE CARE
Suctioning	Vocalize (.54) Suck, mouth (.42) Looks (-.15)	Smiles (-.46) Suck, mouth (.06) Fuss, cry (.23) Activate monitor (.37)	
Heelstick Injection	Activate monitor (.71) Suck, mouth (.48)	Smiles (-.42) Activate monitor (-.26) Looks (-.36)	
Bloodgas (central line)	Activate monitor (.90)	Looks (.41) Sounds (-.08) Body movements (.05) Fuss, cry (-.18)	

MEDICAL STIMULATION

CAREGIVER BEHAVIORS	INFANT BEHAVIORS		
	INTENSIVE CARE	INTERMEDIATE CARE	PREDISCHARGE CARE
Special Procedures	Activate monitor (.90)	Fuss, cry (-.36) Activate monitor (.50)	
Wrap/tape	Activate monitor (.78) Looks (.08) Suck, mouth (.18)		
Stimulate To Breathe	Limb movements (-.54) Sounds (.07) Body movements (-.43) Vocalize (-.38) Activate monitor (.24) Fuss, cry (-.24)	Suck, mouth (-.45) Activate monitor (-.19) Sounds (-.24)	Activate monitor (.88)*

    ·   p < .05
    ··   p < .01
    ···   p < .001
    ····   p < .0001

Inanimate Stimulation

The mean noise levels in the nurseries were remarkably similar throughout care periods. The mean noise level during intensive care therapy was 61.1 dB (A), SPL (sound pressure level) SD = 8.1, 63.09 dB (A), SPL SD = 1.45 during intermediate care, and 59.1 dB (A), SPL SD = 6.7 at predischarge care, respectively. Noise levels ranged from a low of 46 dB (A), SPL to a high of 75.7

dB (A), SPL. These average noise levels are not unlike those found in a large business office environment.[24] There were no significant differences between morning and night observation measurements.

In contrast to the finding of similarity in noise levels in the nursery environments, we found that because of bilirubin light therapy (for nine of the 10 infants) illumination levels were significantly higher during intensive care observations than during any of the subsequent observations, ($F = 12.61$, $df = 2, 13$, $p < 0.01$). The mean illumination level during intensive care was 350.7 footcandles (fc), SD = 153.5, compared to means of 64.8 fc (SD = 34.3) and 72.5 fc (SD = 54.6) during intermediate and predischarge care periods, respectively. The illumination levels during intermediate and predischarge care were not different.

DISCUSSION

This study sought to document the stimulation experienced by sick, preterm infants by describing the nature of interactions caregivers have with infants during hospital confinement.

Caregiving Stiulation

Throughout the course of hospitalization the most salient characteristic of caregiving involved handling the infants. These data agree with that of Marton, et al.,[23] who reported that their intensive and intermediate care babies received relatively even rates of caregiver handling. In general, these results tend to support our finding that the diapering, positioning, holding, and bathing of infants are such routine procedures that they are not closely related to the degree of infant illness. This aspect of care is in contrast to the minimal contact procedures typical of early traditional medical management of preterm infants.[8]

The regression analyses revealed a pattern of initial infant vulnerability and behavioral disorganization. For example, during intensive care, handling was associated with negative changes in infant medical status. Other physical contact variables such as incidental handling and abdominal measuring all showed relationships to the infant monitor alarm variable. Since the data did not indicate directional effects, it is possible that some aspects of caregiver handling may have elicited negative changes in infant condition. Support for this interpretation was shown by the number of intensive care physical contact variables of a nonmedical nature which were related to negative changes in newborn medical status. It is also possible, however, that sicker infants required more handling for adequate management. Minimal handling of vulnerable preterm infants during management of the acute phase of illness may decrease the frequency of negative changes in their condition. Klaus (personal communication[18]) has indicated that minimal caregiver contact for some of his intensive care newborns has shown evidence of improvement in their medical status.

Social Stimulation

Relatively little social-physical contact between infants and nursery staff was observed in comparison to caregiving and medical contact. Most social interactions involved cuddling and occurred more frequently during periods of partial recovery (intermediate and predischarge care). Although an increase in social stimulation was noted during intermediate care, it was not statistically significant because of the large amount of variability between infants. This increase in social stimulation occurred despite the physical barrier effect of the isolette, which was assumed to have an inhibiting influence on social interactions between infants and nursery staff. At predischarge care when infants were relatively more accessible in open cribs, rates of social contact were similar to rates at intermediate care. Overall, these modest rates of social interaction suggest that, in comparison to other caregiver behavior, social interactions occur infrequently and that these babies lack capabilities to evoke social responsivity in caregivers.

Medical Stimulation

As expected, medical events were highly characteristic of intensive care and were infrequently observed during subsequent care periods.

Animate Auditory Stimulation

Staff conversations occurred at rates two to six times more frequent than instances when staff spoke directly to babies. The finding that staff tended to engage in more conversational behavior in the evenings and that at these times infants evidenced significantly high rates of limb activity raises the possibility that caregiver conversations may be stimulating infant activity during late night hours. However, Phillips, et al.[25] found that limb activity was more frequent in the evenings in a study of the spontaneous activity of normal newborns. Condon and Sanders[6] reportedly have demonstrated a synchrony between infant limb movements and some aspects of adult speech.

Illumination and Inanimate Auditory Stimulation

Infants were exposed to extraordinary levels of illumination under phototherapy for the treatment of elevated bilirubin levels during intensive care. These high illumination levels dropped significantly at later recovery periods to levels more typical of well lighted environments. However, fluorescent overhead lighting was constant despite one complete wall of window in each of the intermediate and predischarge nursery rooms. Regarding phototherapy effects on infants, Telzrow, et al.[31] reported that phototherapy contributes to lethargy and reduced responsivity in infants. Presently, it is difficult to determine the consequences for infants of phototherapy and abrupt changes in high intensity light exposure during confinement. Consideration should be given to gradually reducing illumination intensity as the infant recovers to approximate changes in the natural diurnal cycle. It is not unusual for parents of preterm infants to comment that their baby sometimes shows aversive reactions to overhead illumination in the home environment. In the nursery phototherapy and high intensity fluorescent illumination may have an additive effect such that both conditions may interfere with infant state regulation. Therefore, parents should be made aware of the likelihood of this effect on infant responsivity. Infants in their home environment may show increased alertness when illumination levels are low.

Noise measurements were made using a sound level meter with an A-weighting filter which simulates the frequency response of the human ear. The noise levels in the nurseries were moderately above those found in office settings where adult conversational speech is around 52–54 dB. However, noise levels did not approach the high levels reportedly measured in some other nurseries. Lawson, et al.[21] recorded highs of 98 dB in their growing nursery rooms using a linear scale which measures frequencies within ranges which are less sensitive to the human ear. Therefore, the actual auditory effects resulting from the high levels reported by these investigators may be somewhat less than what one would anticipate. Gadeke, et al.[13] reported that noise levels in most intensive care environments exceed the high threshold of infant tolerance for noise. Unfortunately, Gadeke, et al.[13] also used a linear weighting scale when taking their nursery measures. As in the Lawson, et al.[21] study, we found that noise levels in the intensive care nurseries were somewhat lower, though not statistically so, than levels in either intermediate or predischarge nurseries. Typically, in these latter rooms there was a constant clicking sound of infant monitoring equipment. The acoustic energy of this equipment was of low frequency sound, which probably facilitated the ability of nursery staff to habituate to these sounds. It is also possible that infants are able to habituate to these sounds as well.

Infant Behavior

Limb movements and visual and sucking responses were the major infant activities which were frequently evident during confinement. Of all infant behaviors, limb movements were observed to occur most frequently. It seemed that infants tended to activate those systems most readily available to them. The typical "froglike" posture of the premature probably restricts activation of the trunk while limb restraints (for medical purposes) may further limit infant motor responses. Subsequent delays seen in the preterm infant's ability to raise the head and trunk or to sit with and without support may be partially due to the inability of infants to exercise the motor components of these developmental milestones during confinement.

Greater organization of physiological and behavioral functions was a significant accomplishment of the intermediate care infant. During this period of care there was a discernible increase in the number of infant variables which showed slight to moderate relationships with caregiver variables. Whitelaw, et al.[32] found similar results with infant data which indicated increased responsivity in infants who had partially recovered from critical illness. They cited more visual, limb, and mouthing behaviors as evidence of infant recovery, which are the same activities identified in this study which showed increases over their intensive care levels at predischarge care. One might assume that these increases may be attributed to greater maturation of the infants systems. However, we correlated infant gestational age at each period of care with infant behaviors at comparable care periods and found virtually no significant relationships. Similarly, Whitelaw, *et al.*[32] reobserved their infant sample approximately 2 weeks following their initial observations and found no significant differences for visual and limb responses, although there was a significant increase in mouthing behavior. Thus, they concluded that increased infant responsivity was probably attributed to recovery from illness.

Despite the increase in responsivity observed during intermediate care, it is not until one looks at the predischarge care relationships that there is a sense of some degree of mutuality or feedback between infants and caregivers. Of the 13 caregiver behaviors for which predischarge regression relationships were found, eight of them were associated with infant visual behavior. Caregiver behaviors such as feeding, cuddling, smiling, and talking to the babies either evoked infant visual interest or seemed to be responsive to infant signals. Evidence of infant ability to signal more effectively was shown at predischarge care by the infant irritability variable "fuss-cry" which was associated with five of 13 caregiver behaviors. Fuss-cry behavior appeared to elicit caregiver cuddling, rocking, vocalizations, provision of pacifiers, and staff vocalizations. Dramatic increases in infant receptiveness to stimulation was evident in the successive strengthening of relationships between caregiver handling and infant visual behavior over the three periods of care.

The preterm infant at recovery from serious respiratory illness, although not as robust or vocal as the healthy term infant, is visually active, and has best quiet alert periods in low illumination. The premature may be motorically active at night and may demonstrate increasing communication capabilities through irritable responses. Parents who take their infant home following prolonged special care need to learn the behavioral characteristics of their baby before he or she is discharged from the nursery. These study findings suggest that it may be wise to encourage early parent-newborn contact which involves more vocal and visual interactions than physical contact. Later during intermediate care more active handling of the infants in ways more typical of parent-newborn relationships may be appropriate. Particular attention should be given to encourage parents to be sensitive to individual differences in responsivity, behavior rhythms, and temperament of the baby so that parents may experience some early success in adapting to the infant's needs.

REFERENCES

1. Als, H., Lester, B. M., and Brazelton, T. B., Dynamics of the Behavioral Organization of the Premature Infant: A Theoretical Perspective, in *Infants Born at Risk*, Field, T., Sostek, A., Goldberg, S., and Shuman, H. H., Eds. Spectrum Publications, Jamaica, N. Y., 1979.
2. Barnett, C. R., Leiderman, P. H., Grobstein, R., and Klaus, M., Neonatal separation: The maternal side of interactional deprivation. *Pediatrics* **45**(2), (1970).

3. Brazelton, T. B., Koslowski, B., and Main, M. The Origins of Reciprocity: The Early Mother-Infant Interaction, in *The Effect of the Infant on Its Caregiver*, Lewis, M. and Rosenblum, L. A., Eds. John Wiley and Sons, New York, 1974.

4. Brown, J. V., and Bakeman, R., Behavioral dialogues between mothers and infants: The effect of prematurity. Unpublished paper, April 1977.

5. Chamorro, I. L., Davis, M. L., Green, D., and Kramer, M., Development of an instrument to measure premature infant behavior and caretaker activities. *Nurs. Res.* **22**(4), (1973).

6. Condon, W. S., and Sander, L., Synchrony demonstrated between movements of the neonate and adult speech. *Child Dev.* **45**, (1974).

7. Cornell, E. H., and Gottfried, A. W., Intervention with premature infants. *Child Dev.* **47**, (1976).

8. Crosse, M. V., *The Premature Baby*, 5th ed. Little, Brown Co., Boston, 1961.

9. David, M., and Appell, G., A Study of Nursing Care and Nurse-Infant Interaction, in *Determinants of Infant Behavior*, Foss, B. M., Ed. London, 1959.

10. DiVitto, B., and Goldberg, S., The effects of newborn medical status on early parent-infant interaction, in *Infants Born at Risk*, Field, T., Sostek, A., Goldberg, S., and Shuman, H. H., Eds. Spectrum Publications, Jamaica, N. Y., 1979.

11. Field, T. M., Effects of early separation, interactive deficits, and experimental manipulations on mother-infant interaction. *Child Dev.* **48**, (1977).

12. Field, T. M., The three Rs of infant-adult interactions: rhythms repertoires, and responsivity. *J. Pediatr. Psychol.* **3**(3), (1978).

13. Gadeke, R., Doring, B., Keller, F., and Vogel, A., The noise level in a children's hospital and the wake-up threshold in infants. *Acta Paediatr. Scand.* **58**, (1969).

14. Goldberg, S., Social competence in infancy: a model of parent-infant interaction. *Merrill Palmer Q.* **23**, (1977).

15. Goldberg, S., Brachfeld, S., and DiVitto, B., Feeding, Fussing and Play: Parent-Infant Interaction in the First Year as a Function of Newborn Medical Status, in *Interactions of High Risk Infants and Children*, Field, T., Goldberg, S., Stern, D., and Sostek, A., Eds. Academic Press, New York, in press.

16. Goldberg, S., Premature birth: Consequences for the parent-infant relationship. *Am. Sci.* **67**, (1979).

17. Katz, V., Auditory stimulation and developmental behavior of the premature infant. *Nurs. Res.* **20**, (1971).

18. Klaus, M. H., personal communication, 1979.

19. Klaus, M. H., Kennell, J. H., Plumb, N., and Zuehlke, S., Human maternal behavior at the first contact with her young. *Pediatrics* **46**, (1970).

20. Korones, S. B., Disturbance and infant's rest, in Iatrogenic Problems in Neonatal Intensive Care. Proceedings of the 69th Press Conference on Pediatric Research, Columbus, Ohio, 1976.

21. Lawson, K., Daum, C., and Turkewitz, G., Environmental characteristics of a neonatal intensive care unit. *Child Dev.* **48**(4), (1977).

22. Lozoff, B., Brittenham, G. M., Trause, M. A., Kennell, J. H., and Klaus, M. H., The mother-newborn relationship: limits of adaptability. *J. Pediatr.* **91**(1), (1977).

23. Marton, P., Dawson, H., and Minde, K., The interaction of ward personnel with infants in the premature nursery. *Pediatrics* **61**(3), (1977).

24. Peterson, A. P. G., and Gross, E. E., Eds., *Handbook of Noise Measurement*, 5th ed. General Radio Co., Boston, 1963.

25. Phillips, S., King, S., and DuBois, L., Spontaneous activities of female versus male newborns, *Child Dev.* **49**, (1978).

26. Sameroff, A., and Chandler, M., Reproductive Risk and the Continuum of Caretaking Casualty, in *Review of Child Development Research*, Vol. 4, Horowitz, F. D., Hetherington, M., Scarr-Salapatek, S., and Siegel, G., Eds. University of Chicago Press, Chicago, 1975.

27. Scarr-Salapatek, S., and Williams, M. L., The effects of early stimulation on low-birth weight infants. *Child Dev.* **44**, (1973).

28. Segal, M. E., Cardiac responsivity to auditory stimulation in premature infants. *Nurs. Res.* **21**, (1972).

29. Solkoff, N., Yaffe, S., Weintraub, D., and Blase, B., Effects of handling on the subsequent development of premature infants. *Dev. Psychol.* **1**, (1969).
30. Stern, D. N., Mother and Infant at Play, in *The Effect of the Infant on Its Caregiver*, Lewis, M. and Rosenblum, L., Eds. Wiley and Sons, New York, 1974.
31. Telzrow, R., Snyder, D., Tronick, E., Als, H., and Brazelton, T. B., The effects of phototherapy on neonatal behavior. Unpublished manuscript, March 1977.
32. Whitelaw, A., Minde, K., and Brown, J., The effects of severe physical illness on the behavior of very small premature infants. Unpublished manuscript, 1979.

Subject Index

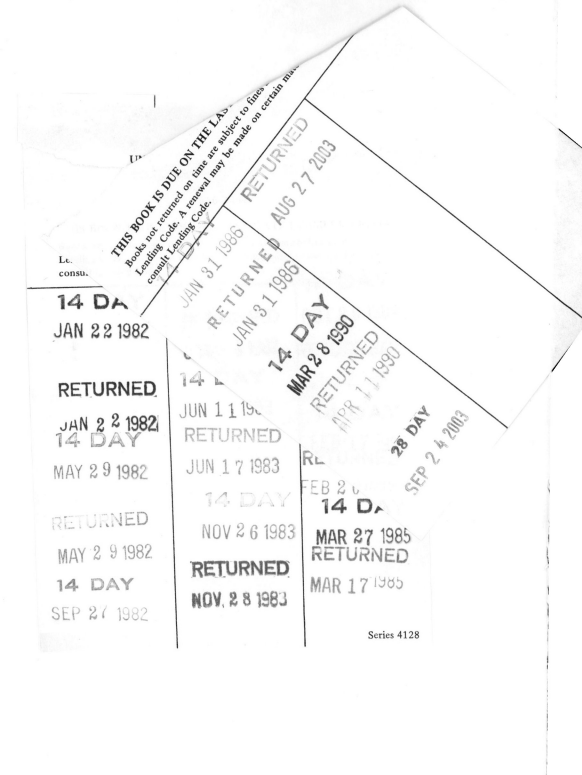

THIS BOOK IS DUE ON THE LAST
Books not returned on time are subject to fines
Lending Code. A renewal may be made on certain
consult Lending Code.

14 DAY

JAN 22 1982

RETURNED

JAN 22 1982
14 DAY

MAY 29 1982

RETURNED

MAY 29 1982

14 DAY

SEP 27 1982

JAN 31 1986

RETURNED
JAN 31 1986

14 D

JUN 11 19

RETURNED

JUN 17 1983

14 DAY

NOV 26 1983

RETURNED

NOV. 28 1983

RETURNED
AUG 27 2003

14 DAY

MAR 28 1990

RETURNED
APR 11 1990

28 DAY
SEP 24 2003

FEB 2

14 D

MAR 27 1985
RETURNED

MAR 17 1985

Series 4128